Viral Diseases

History and new developments in diagnostics and therapeutics

Online at: https://doi.org/10.1088/978-0-7503-4987-1

Viral Diseases

History and new developments in diagnostics and therapeutics

Edited by
Arvind K Singh Chandel
Department of Chemical System Engineering, The University of Tokyo, 7-3-1 Hongo Bunkyo-Ku, Tokyo 113-8655, Japan

Bhakti Tanna
Department of Medical Writing, Bosker Medico Services, Ahmedabad, Gujarat, India

Amisha Parmar
University of Veterinary Medicine, Vienna, Austria

Gopal Patel
Lakshmi Narain College of Pharmacy, Kalchuri Nagar, Raisen Road, Bhopal, Madhya Pradesh, India

Neeraj S Thakur
Department of Pharmaceutical Sciences, College of Pharmacy, University of Oklahoma Health Sciences (OUHS), Oklahoma City, OK, USA

IOP Publishing, Bristol, UK

ISBN 978-0-7503-4987-1 (ebook)
ISBN 978-0-7503-4985-7 (print)
ISBN 978-0-7503-4988-8 (myPrint)
ISBN 978-0-7503-4986-4 (mobi)

DOI 10.1088/978-0-7503-4987-1

Version: 20250401

IOP ebooks

British Library Cataloguing-in-Publication Data: A catalogue record for this book is available from the British Library.

Published by IOP Publishing, wholly owned by The Institute of Physics, London

IOP Publishing, No.2 The Distillery, Glassfields, Avon Street, Bristol, BS2 0GR, UK

US Office: IOP Publishing, Inc., 190 North Independence Mall West, Suite 601, Philadelphia, PA 19106, USA

Contents

Preface

The ongoing evolution of viral infections, coupled with the emergence of new pathogens, has posed significant challenges to global health. Despite remarkable advances in biomedical research, including the advent of proteogenomic and RNA-based vaccine technologies, the current landscape of viral diagnostics and therapeutics remains both promising and incomplete. The purpose of this book is to cast light on the advantages and limitations of existing diagnostic and therapeutic approaches, aiming to refine current techniques and foster the development of new, precise, and robust antiviral strategies. In light of past viral outbreaks, the first part of this book serves to acquaint readers with the historical context of viral infections. It delves into the biology of viruses, exploring their modes of infection and transmission, the consequences of human interference with ecological systems, and the resultant threats posed by viral pathogens. This foundational knowledge is crucial for understanding the complexities of viral diseases and the ongoing battle to combat them.

The second and third parts focus on the spectrum of diagnostic and therapeutic approaches available today. From traditional methods to cutting-edge technologies, these chapters provide a comprehensive overview of how viral diseases are identified and treated. The book then progresses to discuss the need for a deeper understanding of specific viral biology, which is essential for developing more accurate diagnostic techniques. Furthermore, this part highlights potential viral targets for the creation of novel therapeutic agents and vaccines, aiming to prevent and mitigate the impact of both emerging and established viruses. In the concluding parts, the book addresses the process of antiviral drug discovery and development, including the intricate regulatory requirements essential for bringing therapeutics from the research bench to the patient bedside. These insights are critical for understanding the path that new treatments must follow to reach the market and ultimately benefit public health.

The motivation for this book stems from the urgent need to bridge the gaps in our current understanding of viral diseases and their management. While numerous books on human viral diseases exist, many were published years ago and fail to address the full scope of modern diagnostic and therapeutic innovations. Recent publications have focused primarily on SARS-CoV-2, leaving a void in comprehensive resources that cover the history, diagnostic approaches, treatment strategies, and regulated development of therapeutics for a broader range of viral diseases.

This book aspires to fill that gap. It will serve as an all-encompassing guide for chemists, biologists, clinicians, biotechnologists, and pharmaceutical scientists. By compiling knowledge across multiple disciplines including chemistry, biology, nanotechnology, material science, pharmaceutical science, chemical engineering, biotechnology, and regulatory affairs this book provides a multidisciplinary perspective on the development of diagnostics and therapeutics for viral diseases.

In summary, this book is designed to equip its readers with the knowledge necessary to advance the fight against viral infections. It will enable scientists, researchers, and healthcare professionals to better understand viral diseases, identify new therapeutic targets, and contribute to the development of effective diagnostics and treatments, ultimately helping to prepare for and combat future outbreaks.

Editor biographies

Arvind K Singh Chandel

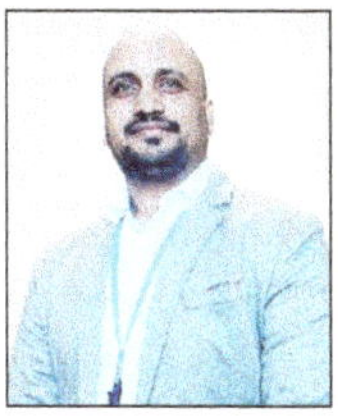

Dr Arvind K Singh Chandel is a researcher and educator specializing in pharmaceutical biotechnology, polymer chemistry, and tissue engineering. He completed his B. Pharmacy at Barkatullah University, Bhopal, in 2011 and his MS Pharm. at NIPER, Hajipur, in 2013. He earned his PhD in biological sciences from AcSIR-CSIR-CSMCRI, Bhavnagar, in 2018. Dr Chandel received the Japan Society for the Promotion of Science (JSPS) postdoctoral fellowship and has conducted research at the University of Tokyo. His work focuses on the design of polymeric materials for biomedical applications, advanced drug delivery systems, and water desalination. Currently an Assistant Professor at the University of Tokyo, Dr Chandel has published 35 peer-reviewed papers, holds eight patents, and has contributed to 20 book chapters. He has received awards like the Marie Skłodowska-Curie Individual Postdoctoral Fellowship and the M.K. Bhan Young Researcher Fellowship. His research is known for its interdisciplinary approach, advancing innovation in healthcare.

Bhakti Tanna

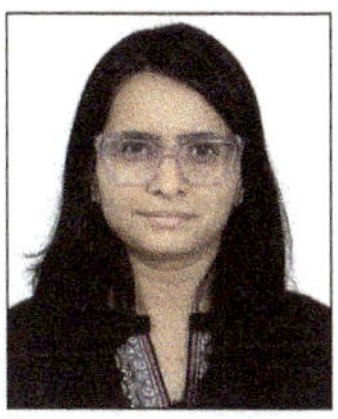

Dr Bhakti Tanna has a PhD from CSIR-CSMCRI (Council of Scientific And Industrial Research–Central Salt And Marine Chemicals Research Institute) with her own CSIR (Council of Scientific & Industrial Research) JRF fellowship awarded on June 2014. Currently, she is working at GBRC (Gujarat Biotechnology Research Centre), Gandhinagar, India as a Technical Assistant. Before this, she has also worked as guest lecturer at Harivandana college, Rajkot for a brief period in 2020 in which she has given a webinar on 'Vaccine will they sort things out?' for COVID-19 which is freely available on YouTube—https://www.youtube.com/watch?v=9k8dWx2G4Xo&t=3s. In her PhD work, she selected the topic 'Non-targeted metabolite profiling of selected seaweeds along the Gujarat coast'. She completed her PhD in February 2020. She completed her master MS Pharm. from NIPER (National Institute of Pharmaceutical Education and Research), Mohali in Traditional Medicine-Department of Natural Products in 2013. She completed her B.Pharm. from NIRMA University, Ahmedabad in 2011.

Amisha Parmar

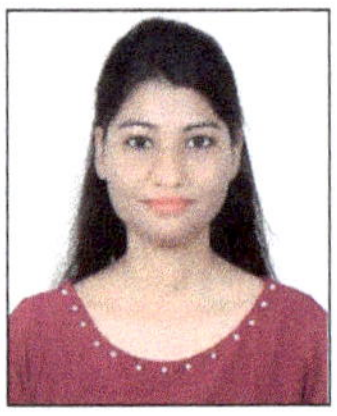

Ms Amisha Parmar has pursued her bachelor's in Pharmacy from Gujarat University and obtained her master's in pharmacology and toxicology from NIPER, Mohali where she studied the influence of local inflammation and oxidative stress on testicular toxicity in dextran sulphate sodium-induced ulcerative colitis in mice. Later, she embarked on an industrial research career where she gained around four years of experience in early discovery research companies in India. She began her professional career as a research trainee at Dabur Research Foundation, Ghaziabad, later joining the *in vivo* team in the Department of Neuroscience, Jubilant Biosys Ltd, Bangalore where she extensively contributed in *in vivo* preclinical studies in research areas such as neurodegenerative diseases and neuropathic pain. Moreover, she further gained experience in the triple negative breast cancer *in vivo* model development and efficacy studies at Sun Pharma Advanced Research Center, Vadodara. Later, due to a strong interest in neuroscience, she undertook a one-year research project at University of Central Lancashire. Her research project entailed investigating the role of RE-1 Silencing Transcription factor in adult mouse brain using molecular biology techniques and transcriptomics. Currently, she is involved in assessing gene therapy approach for motor neuron disease at Sheffield Institute for Translational Neuroscience, United Kingdom.

Gopal Patel

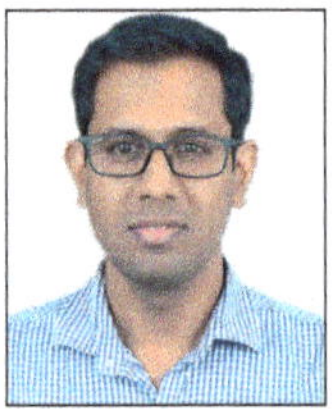

Dr Gopal Patel obtained MTech (2013) and PhD (2018) degrees from the department of Pharmaceutical Biotechnology, National Institute of Pharmaceutical Education and Research (NIPER), SAS Nagar, India; which is one of the well-known and premier institutes of pharmacy in India. He worked as Assistant Professor (Sep 2018–May 2019) School of Biotechnology, Rajiv Gandhi Proudyogiki Vishwavidyalaya (State Government University), Bhopal Madhya Pradesh. He is currently working as a post-doctoral research scholar in the College of Pharmacy, Zhejiang Chinese Medical University, Hangzhou, China (from May 2019 to till now). He has 10 years of working experience in the field of pharmaceutical biotechnology, plant biotechnology, fermentation and nanobiotechnology. He has a brilliant academic record and qualified with various national level highly competitive examinations (DBT JRF—2013–14 and CSIR-National Eligibility Test (JRF), June 2014) which provided funding during his PhD. Apart from this, he also received various national and international travel grants to attend international conferences.

Neeraj S Thakur

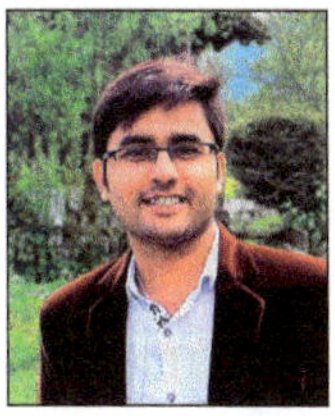

Dr Neeraj S Thakur leads advanced research in theranostics, biomaterials, drug delivery systems and nanomaterials. With a PhD and MTech in pharmaceutical technology (biotechnology) from the National Institute of Pharmaceutical Education and Research (NIPER), Mohali, India, Dr Thakur has extensive expertise in nanoformulation, theranostics, and advanced drug delivery platforms. His research spans international laboratories in the USA, Europe, and Asia, including appointments at the University of Oklahoma Health Sciences (OUHS, USA), the University of Geneva (Switzerland) and the Center of Innovative and Applied Bioprocessing (India). A recipient of prestigious scholarship awards including the John B. Bruce Award, the Swiss Government Excellence Scholarship and DST-INSPIRE Fellowship, Dr Thakur has published >29 peer-reviewed papers, secured five patents, authored one book and six book chapters, and mentored numerous graduate students and continues to push boundaries in pharmaceutical and biomedical innovations.

List of contributors

Vibhuti Agrahari
Department of Pharmaceutical Sciences, College of Pharmacy, University of Oklahoma Health Sciences (OUHS), Oklahoma City, OK, USA

Bhavya Bhargava
Floriculture Laboratory, Agrotechnology Division, CSIR–Institute of Himalayan Bioresource Technology, Palampur, Himachal Pradesh, India

Meha Bhatt
Gujarat Biotechnology Research Centre (GBRC), Gandhinagar, Gujarat, India

Nutan Bhingaradiya
Department of Biomaterials, Graduate School of Medicine, Dentistry and Pharmaceutical Science, Okayama University, Okayama, Japan

Urvi Budhbhatti
Gujarat Biotechnology Research Centre (GBRC), Gandhinagar, Gujarat, India

Kanak Chahar
Department of Pharmaceutical Quality Assurance, ISF College of Pharmacy, Moga, Punjab, India

Arvind K Singh Chandel
Department of Chemical System Engineering, The University of Tokyo, Tokyo, Japan

Rupal Dubey
Vidhyapeeth Institute of Pharmacy, Vidhyapeeth Group of Institutions, Bhopal, Madhya Pradesh, India

Luca Ghigliotti
Brain and Cognitive Sciences, University of Amsterdam, Amsterdam, The Netherlands

Niyati Gupta
Dr Hari Singh Gour Central University, Sagar, Madhya Pradesh, India

Pratyusha Janaswamy
PRADO Preclinical Research Organisation Pvt. Ltd, Pune, Maharashtra, India

Madhav Kumar
Gut Microbiome Division, SKAN Research Trust, Bengaluru, 560034, Karnataka, India

Raghawendra Kumar
Floriculture Laboratory, Agrotechnology Division, CSIR–Institute of Himalayan Bioresource Technology, Palampur, Himachal Pradesh, India

Lakshmi Kumari
Department of Pharmaceutics, ISF College of Pharmacy, Moga, Punjab, India

Balak Das Kurmi
Department of Pharmaceutics, ISF College of Pharmacy, Moga, Punjab, India

Ashwani Mishra
Assistant Professor, School of Pharmacy and Technology Management (NMIMS), Shirpur, Maharashtra, India

Lopamudra Mishra
Department of Pharmaceutics, ISF College of Pharmacy, Moga, Punjab, India

Dharm Pal
Department of Chemical Engineering, National Institute of Technology, Raipur, Chhattisgarh, India

Raikishore Pandey
Department of Surgery, School of Medicine, University of Missouri, Columbia, Missouri, USA

Amisha Parmar
University of Veterinary Medicine, Vienna, Austria

Gopal Patel
Lakshmi Narain College of Pharmacy, Kalchuri Nagar, Raisen Road, Bhopal, Madhya Pradesh, India

Neha P Patel
Bioinformatics Department, Transdisciplinary Biology, RGCB Bio Innovation Center-Rajiv Gandhi Centre for Biotechnology, Thiruvananthapuram, Kerala, India

Preeti Patel
Department of Pharmaceutical Chemistry, ISF College of Pharmacy, Moga, Punjab, India

Anil Kumar Poonia
Department of Chemical Engineering, National Institute of Technology, Raipur, Chhattisgarh, India

M V S Sandhya
PRADO Preclinical Research Organisation Pvt. Ltd, Pune, Maharashtra, India

Muniappan Sankar
Department of Chemistry, Indian Institute of Technology Roorkee, Roorkee, Uttarakhand, India

Simran Sharma
Department of Veterinary Pathobiology, Bond Life Science Center, University of Missouri, Missouri, USA

Sonal Sharma
Gujarat Biotechnology Research Centre, Gandhinagar, Gujarat, India

Yash Sharma
Department of Pharmaceutical Quality Assurance, ISF College of Pharmacy, Moga, Punjab, India

Dilpreet Singh
Department of Pharmaceutics, ISF College of Pharmacy, Moga, Punjab, India

Priyambada Singh
Department of Microbiology, Kalinga University, Raipur, Chhattisgarh, India

Bhakti Tanna
Department of Medical Writing, Bosker Medico Services, Gujarat, India

Neeraj S Thakur
Department of Pharmaceutical Sciences, College of Pharmacy, University of Oklahoma Health Sciences (OUHS), Oklahoma City, OK, USA

Pradeep Singh Thakur
Centre for Nanotechnology, Indian Institute of Technology Roorkee, Roorkee, Uttarakhand, India

Yesha Upadhyaya
Gujarat Biotechnology Research Centre, Gandhinagar, Gujarat, India

Aditi Wangikar
PRADO Preclinical Research Organisation Pvt. Ltd, Pune, Maharashtra, India

Prahlad Wangikar
PRADO Preclinical Research Organisation Pvt. Ltd, Pune, Maharashtra, India

Venkteshwar Yadav
Department of Chemical Engineering, National Institute of Technology, Raipur, Chhattisgarh, India

Chapter 1

The effect of human interference on ecology and infectious diseases

Neha P Patel, Vibhuti Agrahari and Neeraj S Thakur

Human-centric activities have negatively impacted the Earth's ecosystem, leading to the emergence and re-emergence of infectious diseases threatening the survival of animals, plants, and humans. These activities include industrialization, agriculture, urbanization, landscape change, deforestation, wildlife poaching, global trade, and tourism. These activities have led to biodiversity loss, global climate change, and increased antimicrobial resistance (AMR). This chapter discusses the impact of these activities on ecology and infectious diseases, as well as the efforts to combat and mitigate the impact of these diseases on human, animal, and plant life.

1.1 Humans, ecology, and infectious disease

An ecosystem consists of abiotic and biotic components that interact for nutrient and energy flow. Humans are part of the ecosystem, but their actions have significantly impacted its functioning. Anthropogenic activities like industrialization, agriculture, urbanization, landscape change, deforestation, wildlife poaching, global trade, and tourism are transforming the Earth's ecosystem, leading to increased infectious diseases in humans, plants, and animals. Some key definitions related to infectious diseases are mentioned in table 1.1.

Emerging infectious diseases (EIDs) are contagious agents that are newly identified or newly evolved in a population, or a known infectious agent that is rapidly increasing in incidence or expanding geographical range [1]. In 2022, 60% of EIDs were of zoonotic origin, accounting for approximately 54.3% (bacteria), 25.4% (virus or prions), 10.7% (protozoa), 6.3% (fungi), and 3.3% (helminths) [2]. EIDs have increased in incidence in humans and have typically been given temporal boundaries over the past two decades. Examples include the COVID-19 pandemic, which is caused by the SARS-CoV-2 (Severe Acute Respiratory Syndrome Coronavirus-2) virus, which may have come in contact with humans due to wild

doi:10.1088/978-0-7503-4987-1ch1

Table 1.1. Some key definitions related to infectious disease.

Term	Definition	References
Infectious disease	An illness due to a pathogen or its toxic product, which arises through transmission from an infected person, an infected animal, or a contaminated inanimate object to a susceptible host.	[6]
Host and pathogen	The infected organism (e.g., human being) is called the host, and the infecting microorganisms are called pathogens (bacteria, viruses, protozoa, etc).	[6]
Vector-borne disease	An intermediary agent (usually a biting insect or arthropod) that spreads a pathogen to humans is known as a vector, and an infection so transmitted is a vector-borne disease.	[6]
Anthroponotic infections	Infections spreading between humans without another animal reservoir host being involved (whether an intermediate host or vector is involved) are termed as anthroponotic infections.	[7]
Zoonotic infection	An infection that can be maintained in vertebrate animal populations, and is transmissible between animals or from animals to humans, is known as a zoonotic infection.	[7]
Spillover' events	Refers to the pathogen transmission from a reservoir host population to a novel host population.	[2]
Species barrier	The natural mechanisms that prevent a virus or disease from spreading from one species to another.	[2]

animal food consumption or avoidable interaction between humans and wild animals. Global connectivity for trade and tourism has amplified the spread of the virus, negatively affecting humans and animals. Re-emerging diseases, such as malaria and tuberculosis disease, have declined dramatically and become health problems for a significant proportion of the population again [3, 4]. Other examples of EIDs in 2022 include the monkeypox disease, which has caused a multi-country outbreak in over 35 countries across Europe, North America, Asia, Latin America, the Middle East, and the Pacific regions [3]. The transmission of the virus from animals to humans is believed to be due to the proximity of humans to infected wild animals and eating undercooked meat and other animal products [5]. Table 1.2 lists the infectious diseases reported in 2022–23, which have resulted in significant human deaths. On the other hand, human pathogens like respiratory syncytial virus (HRSV), human metapneumovirus (HMPV), and human coronavirus subtype OC43 are being transferred to wild animals, including apes and chimpanzees, posing genetic threats to wildlife [3].

Infectious diseases arise from human interference with ecosystems and infectious disease-causing agents. Understanding these interferences is crucial for predicting future impacts and developing effective measures to mitigate the effects of emerging and re-emerging diseases on humans, animals, and plants. This chapter details

Table 1.2. Some examples of infectious diseases that occurred in 2022–23 and their direct or indirect link with human activities.

Infectious disease	Threat	Human activities
Nipah virus infection	Since 4 January 2023 and as of 13 February 2023, 11 cases (10 confirmed and one probable) including eight deaths (Case Fatality Rate (CFR) 73%) have been reported across two divisions in Bangladesh.	Consumption of raw date palm sap during harvesting season.
Measles	In 2022, a cumulative of 3509 suspected measles cases were reported from 18 regions in Somalia and ~35 319 suspected measles cases from Afghanistan.	Complex humanitarian crisis due to conflict and droughts, and related displacements.
Japanese encephalitis	From Dec 2021-April 2022, a cumulative of 37 human cases of Japanese encephalitis (25 laboratory-confirmed cases and 12 probable cases) were reported in four states in Australia.	International travel, consuming contaminated meat from an infected animal, climate change, biodiversity change.
Lassa fever	Lassa fever is endemic in the West African countries of Benin, Ghana, Guinea, Liberia, Mali, Sierra Leone, and Nigeria and is likely present in other West African countries. In 2022, a Lassa fever outbreak was reported from the Guéckédou prefecture in the southeast of Guinea, Togo, United Kingdom of Great Britain, and Northern Ireland.	Direct contact with infected Mastomys rodents or through food or household. Items contaminated with the urine or feces of infected rodents.
Middle East respiratory syndrome coronavirus (MERS-CoV)	Till 15 May 2022, the total number of laboratory-confirmed MERS-CoV infection cases reported globally to WHO is 2591, which includes 894 associated deaths.	International travel and trade. Direct or indirect contact with dromedary camels is the natural host and zoonotic source of the MERS-CoV infection.
Influenza A(H1N1)	Between 2003 and 31 March 2022, a total of 864 cases and 456 deaths of influenza A (H5N1) human infection were reported worldwide from 18 countries.	Contact with swine farm workers, poultry facility, global travel, contact with birds

(Continued)

Table 1.2. (*Continued*)

Infectious disease	Threat	Human activities
Avian Influenza A (H3N8)	In April 2022, one confirmed case was reported from Henan Province in China.	Poultry industry.
Crimean-Congo Hemorrhagic Fever (CCHF)	Between 1 January and 22 May 2022, 212 cases of CCHF have been reported to the WHO by the Iraqi health authorities.	Direct contact with animals, and were livestock breeders or butchers.
Monkeypox	From January 2022 to June 2022, a multi-country outbreak of monkeypox (approx. 3413 lab-confirmed cases and one death) were reported from 50 countries/territories in five WHO Regions.	International travel, Increased contact between wildlife and humans, and human to human.
Severe acute hepatitis	Severe acute hepatitis of unknown etiology in children was reported (~1010 cases) from 35 countries in five WHO Regions, which include 22 deaths as of 8 July 2022.	Climate change impact—heavy rains causing flooding and sanitation problems.
Marburg virus	On June 2022, two Marburg virus diseases (MVD) were reported from the Ashanti region, Ghana.	Dense population, Travel, Forest encroachment.
Dengue	In Rohingya refugee/Forcibly Displaced Myanmar Nationals (FDMN) camps in Cox's Bazar—Bangladesh, a total of 7687 confirmed cases and six deaths were reported in July, with 93% (7178) of the cumulative number of cases being reported since the end of May 2022. Also, on 13 May 2022, the first reported dengue outbreak was in São Tomé and Príncipe.	Forced population displacement, climate change, Increase in vector density.
Ebola virus disease	In 2022, the third Ebola virus outbreak (EVD) was reported in Equateur province and the sixth in the Democratic Republic of the Congo since 2018. Previously from this country, 13 EVD outbreaks have been reported since 1976.	It may be linked with deforestation, wildlife trade, etc.

Yellow fever	Yellow fever is endemic to East, West, and Central Africa. Twelve countries have reported 184 confirmed and 274 probable cases, including 21 deaths from Jan 2021–Aug 2022.	Low population immunity, population movements, viral transmission dynamics, and climate and ecological factors have contributed to the spread of *Aedes* and *Haemagogus* mosquitoes.
Poliomyelitis	A re-emerging infectious disease caused by Sabin-like type 2 poliovirus or Wild poliovirus type 1 (WPV1) or Vaccine-derived poliovirus 2 (cVDPV2), or vaccine-derived poliovirus type 3 (cVDPV3). From February to May 2022, wild poliovirus type 1 (WPV1) cases were reported in Mozambique and Malawai. From April–July, cases of cVDPV2 were reported from Tamanrasset province, southern Algeria, and Rockland County. cVDPV2 was detected in wastewater from Algeria, the United Kingdom of Great Britain and Northern Ireland, and the USA in 2022. cVDPV3 was detected in an unvaccinated child from Jerusalem city, Israel.	Contaminated water or food. Mutated from the strain originally contained in the oral polio vaccine (OPV).

Source: https://www.who.int/emergencies/disease-outbreak-news/1 [3].

human activities and their impact on ecology and infectious disease-causing agents, highlighting efforts like One Health at global and national levels.

1.2 Human activities interfering with the ecosystem functioning

The ecosystem provides essential resources and services for survival, but humans extract and modify it for greed. Major human activities disrupt the natural balance and increase the risk of infectious diseases, affecting the ecosystem's overall health. Here the major human activities disturbing the natural balance of the ecosystem and increasing the risk of infectious disease are discussed in brief (figure 1.1).

1.2.1 Human population dynamics

The increasing human population, estimated at 10 billion by 2057, is a major contributor to the rise in infectious diseases [9]. This growth in population demands

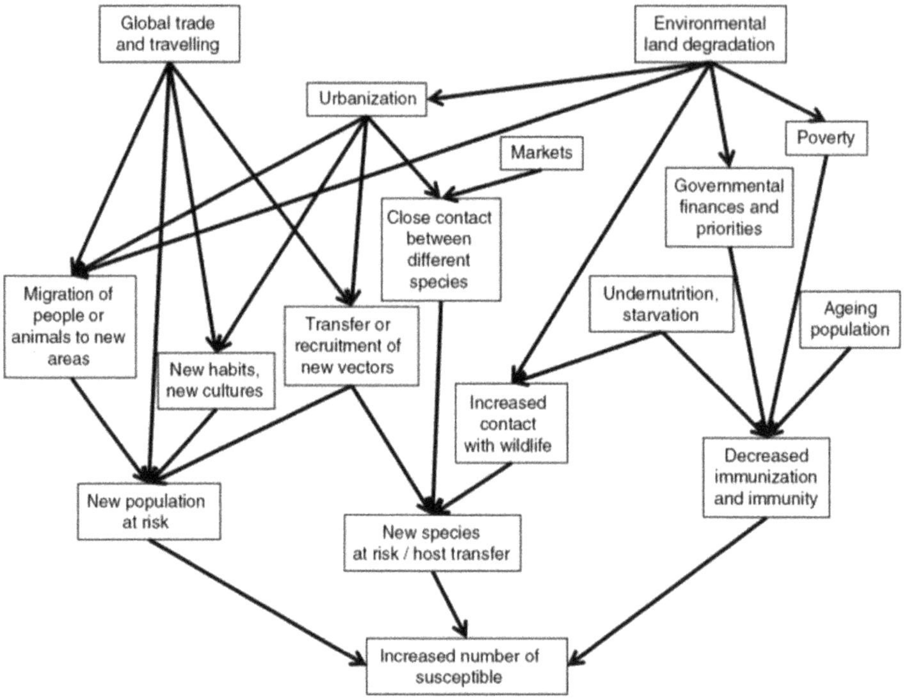

Figure 1.1. Factors leading to increases in the number of susceptible individuals [8], Adapted from reference [8], copyright (2015) with permission from Taylor & Francis Ltd.

more living resources, burdening the natural ecosystem. Human activities like agriculture, urbanization, and pollution contribute to the emergence and spread of infectious agents, disrupting the ecosystem's natural balance and increasing the risk of contagious diseases.

1.2.2 Deforestation/landscape modification

Deforestation is the conversion of forests to other lands, often driven by human-induced factors. Since 1990, the world has lost 178 million hectares of forest, driven by the need for agricultural, settlement, and commercial activities [10]. Deforestation is also driven by the need to boost economies by building roads and infrastructure. With global connectedness and liberalization in trade policies, land clearance and deforestation become financially attractive for developing national economies, especially in countries with vast forest reserves and under debt [10]. Deforestation has numerous negative consequences for the health of living beings, including destroying the natural habitat of wild animals, birds, and insects, leading to biodiversity loss, forcing them to intrude into human settlements, allowing pathogens to cross species barriers, causing extreme climate change, and causing large, economically driven migration to meagerly inhabited areas. Additionally, forest loss reduces the chances of discovering drugs to treat existing or emerging infections, increasing the chances of diseases and their spread [11]. To conserve forest ecosystems, initiatives have been taken at regional, national, and global levels, including forest plantation. The GFRA (Global Forest Resources Assessment) reports that the planted forest area has increased by 123 million hectares since 1990, covering around 3% of the global forest area and 45% of the total area of planted forests [10]. However, forest plantation also introduces foreign species to native land, creating opportunities for infectious diseases and contributing to the decrease in naturally regenerating forests. Anthropogenic forest plantations may decrease naturally regenerating forests and reduce biodiversity, increasing the risk of infectious diseases in plants, animals, and humans [12]. Landscape modification, such as dam construction, disrupts local ecology and influences the spread of infections. This can lead to gastroenteritis outbreaks, toxic cyanobacterial growth, and schistosomiasis [13]. Therefore, deforestation and landscape change could significantly contribute to global climate change and pollution, which essentially drives infectious disease emergence and spread.

1.2.3 Agriculture, animal husbandry, and aquaculture activities

Food is essential for human survival, and increasing crop and animal production will be necessary to meet the growing population by 2100. However, this demand will come at the cost of the natural ecosystem, as the agriculture sector uses over two-thirds of the worlds freshwater, promoting a two-fold increase in irrigation projects. Additionally, the use of pesticides, fertilizers, and antibiotics will increase the risk of diseases in humans, animals, and plants [14]. Excessive use of fertilizers can alter host/parasite densities and behavior, modify the micro–macro community composition, affecting the populations of intermediate hosts and parasites. Moreover, nutrient enrichment due to excess fertilizers can benefit vectors carrying parasites, such as mosquitoes transmitting malaria and West Nile Virus [15]. Furthermore, the excessive use of chemicals will lead to the development of resistance in human, animal, or plant pathogens, making controlling vector-borne infectious diseases more challenging [16]. The unregulated use of antibiotics in aquaculture and animal production will also develop resistance in disease-causing pathogens, increasing the risk of spreading infectious agents to other animals [17].

Agriculture and animal activities increase contact rates between host and parasite/pathogens, promoting 'spillover' events [18]. Over half of all recognized human and animal pathogens have zoonotic origin, responsible for 60%–76% of recent infectious disease events. Agriculture also contributes to over 25% of all and 50% of zoonotic infectious human diseases [14]. Many chemicals used in agriculture or animal production are immunomodulators, modifying host immune susceptibility to pathogens or disrupting immunity downstream. These chemicals cost immense energy for detoxification by the host system, reducing the available energy resource required for resisting the infectious agent [14]. Additionally, the use of chemicals disturbs the structure and function of the native micro/macro-biota, contaminates natural land/animals, and causes malnutrition, impacting the host's immune system to defend against pathogen attacks. This promotes the emergence of infectious diseases in humans and livestock [14, 19].

1.2.4 Urbanization

Urbanization is the shift from rural areas to urban areas, with high population density and well-developed infrastructures. By 2030, two-thirds of the world's population will live in urban areas [7]. Rapid urbanization is driven by factors such as population explosions, industrialization, and advanced technology development. For example, Latin America's urban growth is primarily due to increased migration and industrialization. Macroeconomic policies like SAPs (Structural Adjustments Programs) and trade liberalization threaten rural communities' livelihoods, forcing them to relocate to urban and peri-urban areas for better employment in the manufacturing or tourism sectors [7].

Urban populations face higher risks of infectious diseases compared to rural populations due to rapid population growth, unplanned emigration, and poor sanitation facilities [20]. Most of the urban areas are overcrowded, concentrated, and lack access to safe drinking water, making them more susceptible to water- and vector-borne infections. Additionally, at least 30%–50% of waste generated in urban areas is left unmanaged, accumulating in public or private places. This solid waste can breed pathogens and vectors causing infectious diseases, such as cysticercosis. Emigrants to urban areas may bring new infectious diseases or put them at higher risk of developing infections. Urban areas are associated with greater mobility and inter-mixing, which promotes the transmission of infectious diseases. Urban activities are also responsible for global climate change, impacting the ecology of infectious agents and hosts. Extreme weather events, such as hurricanes and floods, can overwhelm or damage basic urban public health infrastructures, leading to epidemics of waterborne infections. New biological areas have encroached to accommodate the increasing population in urban areas, increasing the risk of non-urban infections. For instance, urban areas developed by replacing rural environments facilitate exposure to insect or arthropod vectors like malaria, filariasis, dengue, and schistosomiasis in parts of South America, Africa, and Asia. Overcrowding, air, water, and soil pollution, and lack of healthy food and safe drinking water intensify the susceptibility of urban inhabitants to new or existing infectious diseases, especially those related to the respiratory and digestive systems [20, 21].

1.2.5 Population mobility, tour, and travel

Humans often migrate for survival reasons, such as food, water, and security. The United Nations High Commissioner for Refugees (UNHCR) estimates that over 70 million people are forcibly displaced, with 25.9 being refugees. This migration increases the risk of infectious diseases, such as acute respiratory infections, tuberculosis, endemic diarrhea, measles, malaria, cholera, cutaneous leishmaniasis, dengue, hepatitis E, poliomyelitis, meningitis, skin infections, intestinal helminth infections, SARS, MERS (Middle East Respiratory Syndrome), and Zika disease [22]. Over 840 000 confirmed or suspected cases of infectious diseases were reported in 48 destination countries/territories due to forcible displacement. Several reasons contribute to the high frequency of infectious disease outbreaks in displaced populations. These include socio-economic and political limitations in surveillance of infectious diseases, extreme events like natural disasters or war, overcrowded refugee camps or temporary shelters, amplified person-to-person contact, and the potential for non-endemic regions where refugees may not be immune to local infectious pathogens. For example, in 2022, WHO reported the Rohingya refugee/ Forcibly Displaced Myanmar Nationals (FDMN) camp in Bangladesh experienced an acute surge in dengue cases in 2022, highlighting the need for better health and protection for displaced populations [23]. Voluntary migration within or across countries due to wage differences encourages workers' movement, leading to contact between populations with different susceptibility to infectious agents from diverse geographic and environmental regions. This interaction accelerates and amplifies the spread of infectious diseases to new communities. For example, the re-emergence of TB in urban areas of many high-income countries has been linked to migrant populations from South Asia who stayed in such living conditions that enabled the infection to spread [22]. Tourism is another major voluntary reason for travel, with enhanced global connectivity through communication and transport systems. The United Nations World Tourism Organization (UNWTO) in 2022 reported tripled international tourist arrivals from January to May 2022 compared to the previous year, despite the COVID-19 pandemic and Monkeypox diseases. Travelers tend to explore new niches, particularly tropical regions and unexplored destinations, which may pose significant health risks to people in their homes and destination countries. Traveling is considered the foremost reason for the reckless spread of infectious diseases in the mass population living in widely dispersed areas and communities worldwide. Global connectivity through network and transport systems enhances the potential of rapid geographical spread, as most infectious diseases have an incubation period of approximately 36 h [24]. The globalization of financial services, trade, and industry has increased the need for travel for business, increasing the risk of spreading infection in diverse and distant populations [22, 25].

1.2.6 Global trade of goods, services, and wildlife

Global trading of capital, goods, and services has increased significantly due to rapid development in the transportation and communication sectors. This has led to increased cargo movement, including flowers and food from Africa and Asia to Europe and North America [7]. However, this transportation poses risks of emerging infectious diseases through vector or pathogen transport. Animals, such as rodents and cockroaches, often carry pathogens, such as the Hantavirus, which causes HPS (Hantavirus Pulmonary Syndrome) and HFRS (Hemorrhagic Fever Renal Syndrome) in humans [7]. Transporting vehicles can also spread pathogens to new areas, as shipping introduced non-indigenous species to new regions through ballast water [7]. Transporting non-human goods also exposes handlers to new or existing pathogens, like blood trade, which can spread viral and other infections between countries. For example, the Marburg virus was discovered after handling blood and tissues from African green monkeys in Uganda. Additionally, transport of materials can indirectly increase the risk of infection if ecosystems are altered to facilitate breeding pathogens or vectors that spread disease. For example, plant species introduced to environments can provide new protective habitats for vectors like mosquitoes, leading to malaria outbreaks. Arthropod-borne viruses, such as chikungunya, dengue, and Zika, are a global concern due to their rapid spread across continents [13]. The processing, storage, and transport of food materials, particularly meat food products from animal origin, require extra precautions and care due to high chances of contamination with infectious agents. For example, Salmonellosis outbreaks in the US were linked to imported melons from Mexico contaminated with *Salmonella Poona* during production and packaging at source farms. Low-income countries often cultivate non-indigenous crops to boost their economy, which may be susceptible to local pathogens. Mass production of food products from animal and plant origin uses centralized processing and distribution infrastructures, which may lead to the widespread dissemination of contaminated foods [26]. Wildlife trade involves trading wild animals, their parts, and their derivatives for consumption as food, decoration, or pharmaceutical or healthcare industries [27]. Globalization has led to legal or illegal wildlife trade, increasing the risk of infectious disease emergence and spread. Examples include the H5NI type A influenza virus outbreak in 2005 and the Ebola outbreak in central Africa among hunters harvesting and handling infected gorillas and chimpanzee cadavers for meat consumption. Factors contributing to the high risk of infectious diseases due to wildlife trade include increased contact between wild animals and people living in diverse geographical ranges, trading mixed animal populations, and contaminated vehicles and cages used for transporting animals [28].

1.2.7 Other activities

- **Translocation of animals for conservation and non-trade purposes:** Other than trading, the two main reasons for the translocation of animals are increasing interest in owning pets and others for wildlife conservation. Even though both reasons have a good motive, they risk spreading infectious diseases. In captive wildlife, animals are more prone to pathogens/parasites, either prevalent or newly brought, in the new habitat [28].
- **The use of vaccines derived from animal sources** may transfer unknown infections from animals to humans. For example, WHO, in 2022, reported re-emergence of Poliomyelitis reported from multiple countries like southern Algeria, the United Kingdom of Great Britain, Northern Ireland, and the USA, which was attributed to the Vaccine-derived poliovirus 2 or 3 (cVDPV2 or cVDPV3). These strains were mutated from the strain originally contained in the oral polio vaccine (OPV).
- **War:** The infectious agents used in war as weapons pose a serious threat to living on earth. For instance, anthrax spores were intentionally distributed in the US in 2001 for terrorist purposes [29].

1.3 Overall impact of human activities interfering with the ecology and infectious disease

Human activities cause global problems like climate change, biodiversity loss, pollution, and antimicrobial resistance. These consequences contribute to the emergence and re-emergence of infectious diseases in humans, animals, and plants (figure 1.2).

1.3.1 Global climate change

Climate change due to human interventions is becoming a threat to both humans and the environment. Physical threats include flooding from melting glaciers, drought from deforestation, and increased temperature due to environmental

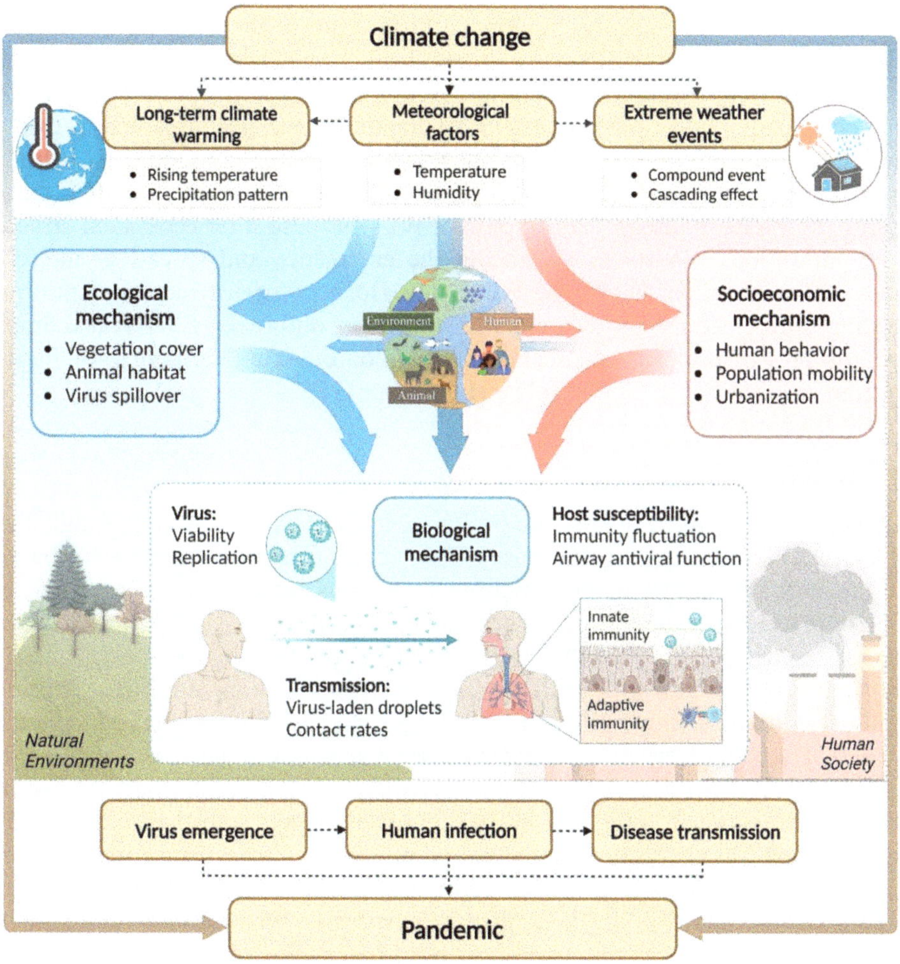

Figure 1.2. Mechanistic pathways through which climate change influences viral respiratory infections (VRIs). Adapted from reference [30], copyright (2023), with permission from Elsevier.

pollutants. These threats eventually lead to biological threats, including infectious disease-causing pathogens like bacteria, viruses, and parasites. Climate change affects infectious diseases' prevalence, incidence, burden, and distribution by modifying pathogens' abundance, competence, transmission, and survival, as well as their vectors and intermediate hosts [31]. For example, stagnant water accumulated after rain promotes malaria mosquito populations [32]. Climate change also impacts the ecology of parasites and their host snails, causing schistosomiasis in humans [33]. The Intergovernmental Panel on Climate Change (IPCC) predicts that climate change will expand the geographical distribution of vector-borne diseases like malaria, dengue, and leishmaniasis from tropical to higher altitudes and latitudes [34]. Warmer sea temperatures and ocean acidification (OA) are critical factors affecting marine flora and fauna in ocean worlds [35]. OA promotes the proliferation of algal blooms, which can be toxic to marine life and humans. Fluctuation in local oceanic climates supports the proliferation of planktonic populations that may harbor human pathogens, such as *Vibrio cholera*. Ocean warming is also linked to alteration in regular oceanic climatic norms, such as El Niño and La Niña Southern Oscillation events, leading to changes in the distribution and spread of infectious diseases [31]. Climate change, accompanied by extreme weather events (EWEs), results in severe public health consequences. Disaster situations, such as floods in Mozambique, often lead to epidemics like gastroenteritis, respiratory disease, and typhus. EWEs can also alter ecosystem structure and composition, potentially advancing the emergence and spread of infectious diseases. For example, heavy rainfall in the Horn of Africa increased mosquito breeding sites, leading to the rift valley disease outbreak. EWEs also impact predator–prey relationships, as seen in the 1993 outbreak of Hantavirus pulmonary syndrome caused by the Sin Nombre Hantavirus [36].

1.3.2 Biodiversity loss

Biodiversity refers to the diverse life on Earth, including plant, animal, fungi, algae, protists, archaea, bacteria, and viruses. These organisms work together to balance and support life on Earth, participating in various ecological processes such as primary production, respiration, energy flow, carbon, water, and nutrient cycling. Human dominance has led to the loss of approximately one million species out of an estimated eight million, with anthropogenic activities such as hunting, overfishing, alien species introduction, pollution, and climate change contributing to biodiversity loss [37]. The loss of one species can have a far-reaching impact on the ecological process, such as the food web and infectious diseases [38]. Studies have shown that high host diversity can dilute the impact of Lyme disease, and the 'dilution effect' suggests that biodiversity losses may promote disease transmission [12]. Additionally, human-caused global change alters the natural forest ecosystem, challenging the survival of threatened tree species [39]. The loss in flora will ultimately impact fauna and microbes, resulting in the emergence of infectious diseases in animals and humans.

1.3.3 Pollution

Pollution is the introduction of substances by humans into the environment, causing health hazards including the emergence and spread of infectious diseases. Pollutants alter the structural and functional composition of native microbes, leading to the proliferation of pathogenic microbes [40]. Plastics, such as macro/microplastics, can spread harmful bacteria by providing support and protection for microbial biofilm formation [41]. They are also prone to antibiotics and chemical pollutants, modifying the exposure of pathogens or vectors to these substances. Microplastics are the physical vector for the spread of antibiotic-resistant bacteria, leading to the global problem of antimicrobial resistance. Studies have shown that microplastics selectively enrich antibiotic-resistant bacteria and genes, and can alter vector-borne infectious disease transmission by altering the population dynamics of interacting species [41, 42].

1.3.4 Antimicrobial resistance (AMR)

Antimicrobials, including antibiotics, antivirals, antifungals, and antiparasitic drugs, are essential for preventing and treating infections in humans, animals, and plants. However, their widespread unregulated use has made them major pollutants in the environment, particularly in soil and water systems [40]. Human activities, such as overcrowding, inadequate water and sanitation, and food facilities in shelters and refugee camps, contribute to the increased use of antibiotics. Additionally, excessive use of antibiotics in animal and aquaculture farms can lead to the selection of antibiotic-resistant microbes, which may interact with pathogens in the environment [17]. This can lead to the development of antibiotic resistance in clinical pathogens. Increased microbial resistance poses challenges in preventing infectious diseases, such as the emergence of drug-resistant HIVDR (Human Immunodeficiency Virus Drug Resistance). HIV patients receiving antiretroviral drugs may acquire HIVDR or infect healthy people. The prevalence of HIVDR is high, with over 50% of infants newly diagnosed with HIV carrying a virus resistant to non-nucleoside reverse-transcriptase inhibitors (NNRTIs) in sub-Saharan Africa [43]. AMR also has economic implications, as it increases hospital stays and healthcare costs, affecting the accessibility of poor citizens to healthcare facilities. Extended hospital stays also affect the work of patients and healthcare givers, ultimately affecting the economy of their employers and the country. The World Bank estimates that AMR will cost around 3.4 trillion US dollars by 2050, further fueling the emergence and spread of infectious diseases in humans and animals [43].

1.4 Current initiatives to combat emerging infectious diseases

Emerging infectious diseases pose a significant threat to humans, animals, and plants, requiring collaboration across various disciplines. The One Health Initiative Task Force (OHITF) aims to address infectious hazards, epidemics, antimicrobial resistance, food security, and climate change. This interdisciplinary approach involves professionals from human, environmental, and animal health sectors, including law enforcement, policymakers, farmers, communities, and pet owners. The One Health approach benefits from increased information sharing among sectors, enabling the development of new eco-inspired technologies and therapies to control infectious diseases. Regular surveillance of pathogens improves early warning systems, allowing for the development of prevention strategies to control the spread of infectious diseases. The Quadripartite Collaboration for One Health (QCoU) aims to strengthen cooperation and optimize the health of humans, animals, plants, and the environment [44–46]. However, the One Health approach faces challenges such as lack of harmonized definitions, coordination difficulties, insufficient core competencies, and limitations in knowledge sharing due to regional, national, and international borders. To fully benefit human, animal, and environmental health, the One Health approach must overcome these challenges and find ways to harness the full benefits of these approaches (table 1.3) [47].

Table 1.3. Some success stories of the One Health initiatives.

Ecological countermeasures for Lyme disease	• Japanese barberry increases Lyme disease risk by supporting pathogen vectors (ticks) and hosts (mice). • The risk is mitigated by Japanese barberry eradication and native plant restoration.
Rabies disease control in India	• Elimination of human rabies in Goa and Tamil Nadu through One Health approach.
Crowdsourcing to report and respond to zoonotic diseases	• In Thailand, farmers, local health volunteers, and human and animal health officers use mobile technology to report zoonotic diseases that pose a severe threat to the health of people and animals.
Schistosomiasis control in the People's Republic of China	• A new mitigation program for schistosomiasis integrated case detection and morbidity control in humans, molluscicide treatment, health education, surveillance, and environmental management and livestock control initiatives. • The integrated program created a net benefit for the society of $6.20 per $1 invested.
Human and animal vaccination delivery to remote nomadic communities in Chad	• A joint human–livestock vaccination campaign resulted in a 15% cost reduction in operational costs compared with separate vaccination campaigns, in addition to benefits from increased vaccination of humans.
SARS-CoV2 pandemic management in India	• Significant efforts by healthcare, research, government, and private sectors, plus common people, come together to fight the COVID-19 pandemic.

	• CO-Win mobile app for tracking COVID-19 cases, surveillance, vaccination, and related updates by the government of India.
Sewage water surveillance	• Even though at a developmental stage, many countries like India, Italy, US are working to establish a wastewater framework for monitoring diverse human and animal pathogens in the environment [48, 49].
Tackling AMR in people and animals	• Several countries like India, Canada, UK have initiated programs for surveillance and management of AMR, like The Canadian Integrated Program for Antimicrobial Resistance Surveillance, The UK's Five-year national action plan for tackling AMR-2019–24, National Policy for containment of AMR, India 2011 [50].

Source: CDC, Publications and News (https://www.cdc.gov/onehealth/in-action/index.html) [51].

Eco-Health, Planetary health, One Medicine, and One Welfare are frameworks that aim for an integrated perspective on health and the environment [52]. These frameworks focus on novel pathogen surveillance in hotspot countries, strategic funding for transdisciplinary research, and funding for One Health projects. The Emerging Pandemic Threats-2 program, Wellcome Trust's 'Our Planet, Our Health' initiative, and the Network for Evaluation of One Health (NEOH) are all initiatives aimed at reducing infectious disease risk in humans, animals, and plants.

1.5 Conclusion

Infectious diseases are crucial for ecosystem functioning and balance species. However, they cannot be completely eradicated. To reduce their impact, humans can slow down or minimize activities that disturb the ecosystem's structure. The COVID-19 pandemic has demonstrated that reducing human activities can allow Nature to rejuvenate, but it will also impact human lives. To achieve a balance between humans and nature, approaches like One Health can be used. Preventing the emergence of infectious diseases is essential, and understanding the ecology of infectious diseases and human interference can strengthen the pathogen and disease surveillance system. Diagnostic technologies and treatment measures can be developed to address these issues.

Abbreviations

AMR	Antimicrobial resistance
COVID-19	Coronavirus disease of 2019
EIDs	Emerging infectious diseases

EWEs	Extreme weather events
FDMN	Forcibly displaced myanmar nationals
GFRA	Global forest resources assessment
HFRS	Hemorrhagic fever renal syndrome
HIVDR	Human immunodeficiency virus drug resistance
HMPV	Human metapneumovirus
HPS	Hantavirus pulmonary syndrome
HRSV	Human respiratory syncytial virus
IPCC	Intergovernmental panel on climate change
MERS	Middle East respiratory syndrome
NEOH	Network for evaluation of one health
NNRTIs	Non-nucleoside reverse-transcriptase inhibitors
OA	Ocean acidification
OHITF	One health initiative task force
QCoU	Quadripartite collaboration for one health
SAPs	Structural adjustments programs
SARS-CoV-2	Severe acute respiratory syndrome Coronavirus-2
UNHCR	United Nations High Commissioner for Refugees
UNWTO	United Nations World Tourism Organization
WHO	World Health Organization

References

[1] McArthur D B 2019 Emerging infectious diseases *Nurs. Clin. North Am.* **54** 297–311

[2] Kock R and Caceres-Escobar H 2022 Situation analysis on the roles and risks of wildlife in the emergence of human infectious diseasesGland, Switzerland: IUCN https://portals.iucn.org/library/node/49880

[3] Disease Outbreak News 2022 Multi-country monkeypox outbreak: situation update. https://www.who.int/emergencies/disease-outbreak-news/item/2022-DON396

[4] Sharma A, Tiwari S, Deb M K and Marty J L 2020 Severe acute respiratory syndrome coronavirus-2 (SARS-CoV-2): a global pandemic and treatment strategies *Int. J. Antimicrob. Agents* **56** 106054

[5] Di Giulio D B and Eckburg P B 2004 Human monkeypox: an emerging zoonosis *Lancet Infect. Dis.* **4** 15–25

[6] Barreto M L, Teixeira M G and Carmo E H 2006 Infectious diseases epidemiology *J. Epidemiol. Community Health* **60** 192–5

[7] Saker L, Lee K, Cannito B, Gilmore A and Campbell-Lendrum D 2002 Globalization and infectious diseases: a review of linkages (WHO) *Special Topics in Social, Economic and Behavioural (SEB) Research* TDR/STR/SEB/ST/04.2 https://iris.who.int/bitstream/handle/10665/68726/TDR_STR_SEB_ST_04.2.pdf

[8] Lindahl J F, Grace D and Strand T 2015 The consequences of human actions on risks for infectious diseases: a review *Infect. Ecol. Epidemiol.* **5** 30048

[9] Worldometer 2023 Worldometer—Real Time World Statistics https://www.worldometers.info/

[10] FAO 2020 Global forest resources assessment 2020Food and Agriculture Organization of the United Nations https://www.fao.org/interactive/forest-resources-assessment/2020/en/

[11] Guégan J F, Ayouba A, Cappelle J and De Thoisy B 2020 Forests and emerging infectious diseases: unleashing the beast within *Environ. Res. Lett.* **15** 083007

[12] Keesing F and Ostfeld R S 2021 Impacts of biodiversity and biodiversity loss on zoonotic diseases *Proc. Natl. Acad. Sci. USA* **118** e2023540118

[13] Crowl T A, Crist T O, Parmenter R R, Belovsky G and Lugo A E 2008 The spread of invasive species and infectious disease as drivers of ecosystem change *Front. Ecol. Environ.* **6** 238–46

[14] Rohr J R *et al* 2019 Emerging human infectious diseases and the links to global food production *Nat. Sustain.* **2** 445–56

[15] Johnson P T J, Townsend A R, Cleveland c c, Glibert P M, Howarth R W, Mckenzie V J, Rejmankova E and Ward M H 2010 Linking environmental nutrient enrichment and disease emergence in humans and wildlife *Ecol. Appl.* **20** 16–29

[16] Hemingway J, Hawkes N J, McCarroll L and Ranson H 2004 The molecular basis of insecticide resistance in mosquitoes *Insect Biochem. Mol. Biol.* **34** 653–65

[17] Sundberg L R, Ketola T, Laanto E, Kinnula H, Bamford J K H, Penttinen R and Mappes J 2016 Intensive aquaculture selects for increased virulence and interference competition in bacteria *Proc. R. Soc. B Biol. Sci.* **283** 20153069

[18] Borremans B, Faust C, Manlove K R, Sokolow S H and Lloyd-Smith J O 2019 Cross-species pathogen spillover across ecosystem boundaries: mechanisms and theory *Philos. Trans. R. Soc. B Biol. Sci.* **374** 20180344

[19] Trivellone V, Hoberg E P, Boeger W A and Brooks D R 2022 Food security and emerging infectious disease: risk assessment and risk management *R. Soc. Open Sci.* **9** 211687

[20] Combs M A, Kache P A, VanAcker M C, Gregory N, Plimpton L D, Tufts D M, Fernandez M P and Diuk-Wasser M A 2022 Socio-ecological drivers of multiple zoonotic hazards in highly urbanized cities *Glob. Chang. Biol.* **28** 1705–24

[21] Bradley C A and Altizer S 2007 Urbanization and the ecology of wildlife diseases *Trends Ecol. Evol.* **22** 95–102

[22] Findlater A and Bogoch I I 2018 Human mobility and the global spread of infectious diseases: a focus on air travel *Trends Parasitol* **34** 772–83

[23] Coyne C J, Duncan T K and Hall A R 2021 The political economy of state responses to infectious disease *South. Econ. J.* **87** 1119–37

[24] Muley D, Shahin M, Dias C and Abdullah M 2020 Role of transport during outbreak of infectious diseases: evidence from the past *Sustain* **12** 7367

[25] Montiel I, Park J, Husted B W and Velez-Calle A 2022 Tracing the connections between international business and communicable diseases *J. Int. Bus. Stud.* **53** 1785–804

[26] Matos R A, Adams M and Sabaté J 2021 Review: The consumption of ultra-processed foods and non-communicable diseases in Latin America *Front. Nutr.* **8** 622714

[27] Nawtaisong P *et al* 2022 Zoonotic pathogens in wildlife traded in markets for human consumption, Laos *Emerg. Infect. Dis.* **28** 860

[28] Price S J, Garner T W J, Cunningham A A, Langton T E S and Nichols R A 2016 Reconstructing the emergence of a lethal infectious disease of wildlife supports a key role for spread through translocations by humans *Proc. R. Soc. B Biol. Sci.* **283** 20160952

[29] Rathish B, Pillay R, Wilson A and Pillay V V 2021 *Comprehensive Review of Bioterrorism* (St. Petersburg, FL: StatPearls)

[30] He Y, Liu W J, Jia N, Richardson S and Huang C 2023 Viral respiratory infections in a rapidly changing climate: the need to prepare for the next pandemic *eBioMedicine* **93** 104593

[31] El-Sayed A and Kamel M 2020 Climatic changes and their role in emergence and re-emergence of diseases *Environ. Sci. Pollut. Res.* **27** 22336–52

[32] Ludwig A, Zheng H, Vrbova L, Drebot M, Iranpour M and Lindsay L 2019 Increased risk of endemic mosquito-borne diseases in Canada due to climate change *Can. Commun. Dis. Rep.* **45** 91–7
[33] Stensgaard A S, Vounatsou P, Sengupta M E and Utzinger J 2019 Schistosomes, snails and climate change: current trends and future expectations *Acta Trop.* **190** 257–68
[34] Matthew R, Chiotha S, Orbinski J and Talukder B 2022 Research note: Climate change, peri-urban space and emerging infectious disease *Landsc. Urban Plan.* **218** 104298
[35] Flahault A, de Castaneda R R and Bolon I 2016 Climate change and infectious diseases *Public Health Rev.* **37** 269–76
[36] McMichael A J 2015 Extreme weather events and infectious disease outbreaks *Virulence* **6** 543–7
[37] Schmeller D S, Courchamp F and Killeen G 2020 Biodiversity loss, emerging pathogens and human health risks *Biodivers. Conserv.* **29** 3095–102
[38] Selakovic S, De Ruiter P C and Heesterbeek H 2014 Infectious disease agents mediate interaction in food webs and ecosystems *Proc. R. Soc. B Biol. Sci.* **281** 20132709
[39] Burgess T I, Oliva J, Sapsford S J, Sakalidis M L, Balocchi F and Paap T 2022 Anthropogenic disturbances and the emergence of native diseases: a threat to forest health *Curr. For. Reports* **8** 111–23
[40] Khan A H *et al* 2022 Impact, disease outbreak and the eco-hazards associated with pharmaceutical residues: a critical review *Int. J. Environ. Sci. Technol.* **19** 677–88
[41] Loiseau C and Sorci G 2022 Can microplastics facilitate the emergence of infectious diseases? *Sci. Total Environ.* **823** 153694
[42] Bank M S, Ok Y S and Swarzenski P W 2020 Microplastic's role in antibiotic resistance *Science* **369** 1315
[43] Tenover F C and McGowan J E 2008 Antimicrobial resistance *Int. Encycl. Public Heal.* 211–9
[44] Barrett M and Osofsky S 2013 One Health: interdependence of people, other species, and the planet *Jekel's epidemiology, biostatistics, preventive medicine, and public health* (Cornell University) pp 364–77
[45] Adisasmito W B *et al* 2022 One health: a new definition for a sustainable and healthy future *PLoS Pathog.* **18** e1010537
[46] Sinclair J R 2019 Importance of a one health approach in advancing global health security and the sustainable development goals *Rev. Sci. Tech.* **38** 145–54
[47] van Herten J, Bovenkerk B and Verweij M 2019 One health as a moral dilemma: towards a socially responsible zoonotic disease control *Zoonoses Public Health* **66** 26–34
[48] Sarkate P P, Bera P, Kaundal N, Lovekesh , Sood S, Singh S K and Prakash C 2021 Sewage analysis as a tool for environmental surveillance of Sars-Cov-2: experience from Delhi, India *J. Commun. Dis.* **53** 1–13
[49] Deng Y, Xu X, Zheng X, Ding J, Li S, Chui H k, Wong T k, Poon L L M and Zhang T 2022 Use of sewage surveillance for COVID-19 to guide public health response: a case study in Hong Kong *Sci. Total Environ.* **821** 153250
[50] United Nations Environment Programme 2023 Antimicrobial resistance: a global threat *UNEP—UN Environment Programme* (UNEP)
[51] BVA 2019 *One health in action* British Veterinary Association https://www.bva.co.uk/media/3145/bva_one_health_in_action_report_nov_2019.pdf
[52] Khan M S, Rothman-Ostrow P, Spencer J, Hasan N, Sabirovic M, Rahman-Shepherd A, Shaikh N, Heymann D L and Dar O 2018 The growth and strategic functioning of one health networks: a systematic analysis *Lancet Planet. Heal.* **2** e264–73

IOP Publishing

Viral Diseases

History and new developments in diagnostics and therapeutics

Arvind K Singh Chandel, Bhakti Tanna, Amisha Parmar, Gopal Patel and Neeraj S Thakur

Chapter 2

History of viral disease

Rupal Dubey and Gopal Patel

This chapter provides a comprehensive overview of viral diseases, their origins, and the significance of studying their history and transmission modes. It explores the evidence of viral diseases in ancient civilizations, major pandemics throughout history, and emerging viral threats in the 21st century. The chapter delves into the classification of viruses, their structures, and the types of transmission, including airborne, direct contact, indirect contact, vector-borne, and foodborne. Specific viral diseases, such as influenza, HIV/AIDS, hepatitis, Ebola, and COVID-19, are examined in detail, including their transmission, symptoms, and treatments. The importance of continued research, education, and public health strategies to combat viral diseases is emphasized throughout.

2.1 Introduction

2.1.1 Overview of viral diseases

Diseases are caused by virus transmittable agents known as viral disease. These minute, non-living particles can only replicate inside a living cell, and once they contaminate a host, they can cause an extensive range of disease from mild to severe. Viral diseases can affect humans, animals, and plants, and they have been responsible for some of the deadliest pandemics in human history. Some examples of viral diseases that have an effect on humans include influenza, HIV/AIDS, hepatitis, measles, mumps, rubella, chickenpox, shingles, herpes, Ebola virus, Zika virus, and COVID-19. These viruses can cause a variety of symptoms, ranging from respiratory problems and fever to skin rashes, diarrhea, and neurological disorders [1].

Viral diseases can be classified based on their modes of transmission, such as airborne transmission (e.g., influenza), direct contact transmission (e.g., HIV), indirect contact transmission (e.g., norovirus), vector-borne transmission (e.g., West Nile virus), and foodborne transmission (e.g., hepatitis A). Virus prevention and control can involve a combination of strategies, such as vaccination, hand hygiene, quarantine, antiviral drugs, and public health policy. Despite advances in medical technology, viral

doi:10.1088/978-0-7503-4987-1ch2

diseases continue to pose a significant threat to global health, and there is a continued need for research, education, and public health measures to combat them [1].

2.1.2 The origin of viruses

The genesis and consequent progression of viruses are shrouded in mystery, thanks in part to the lack of a fossil record. On the other hand, recent advancements in the study of virus structure and reproduction have allowed for more knowledgeable assumptions on virus origins. Virologists are currently taking into consideration two major hypotheses. It has been claimed that some of the morc sophisticated enveloped viruses, such as proviruses and herpesviruses, evolved from small cells, most likely prokaryotic, that parasitized larger, more complicated cells. In a process known as retrograde evolution, these parasitic cells would grow increasingly basic and dependent on their hosts, much like multicellular parasites have. This hypothesis is damaged in various ways. Viruses are quite distinct from prokaryotes, and it is difficult to imagine the methods by which such an evolution might have occurred, as well as the selection pressures that led to it. Furthermore, one would anticipate finding transitional forms between prokaryotes, and at least the more intricate enclosed viruses, yet such forms have not been found [1].

The subsequent theory is that viruses are cellular nucleic acids that are moderately unconnected from the cell. A single mutation could transform nucleic acids that are only generated at particular periods into infectious nucleic acids whose replication is unmanageable. This hypothesis is reinforced by the fact that the nucleic acid of retroviruses and a few other viruses contain sequences that are quite similar to those of normal cells, plasmids, and transposons. Viroids are short, infectious RNAs with base sequences that complement transposons, the region around the boundary of mRNA introns, and a part of host DNA. This has given rise to skepticism that they result from introns or transposons [1].

2.1.3 Importance of studying the history of viral diseases and their mode of transmission

Understanding the history of viral diseases helps us identify patterns and trends in how these diseases have emerged and spread throughout history (figure 2.1). This knowledge can provide insight into the factors that contribute to the emergence and re-emergence of viral diseases and help us develop strategies to prevent and control future outbreaks. Secondly, knowing the history of viral diseases can inform the development of new treatments and vaccines. Many of the vaccines and antiviral drugs we use today were developed due to research into the history of viral diseases, and understanding the characteristics of specific viruses can help scientists develop new and more effective treatments [2].

Thirdly, understanding the history of viral diseases can help us prepare for future outbreaks. By learning from past experiences, we can develop more effective public health policies and emergency response plans and ensure that we are better equipped to contain and control viral disease outbreaks when they occur. Finally, studying the history of viral diseases can help us appreciate their impact on human societies

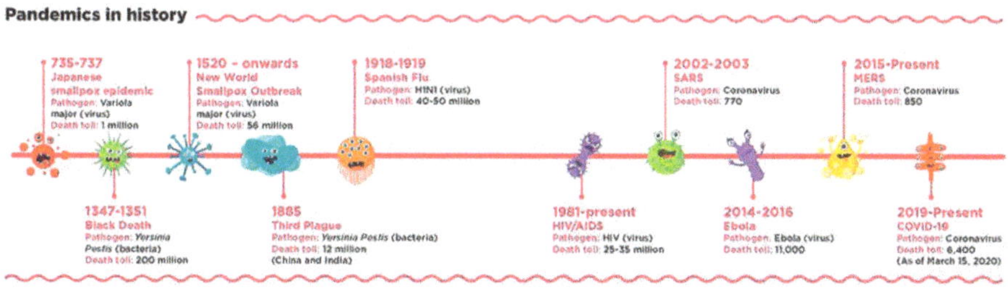

Figure 2.1. History of pandemics. Reprinted with permission from [2], copyright Down To Earth 2024. All rights reserved.

throughout history. By understanding their social and economic impacts, we can gain a greater appreciation for the significance of ongoing research and public health measures to prevent and control these diseases.

2.2 Early history of viral diseases

2.2.1 Evidence of viral diseases in ancient civilizations

Evidence suggests that viral diseases have been present in human populations for thousands of years. While it is difficult to identify specific viruses in ancient populations, researchers have identified various indicators of viral infections by studying historical records, archeological findings, and genetic analysis of ancient human remains. One of the earliest recorded viral epidemics was the outbreak of smallpox in ancient Egypt, which is thought to have occurred around 1500 BCE. Similarly, researchers have found evidence of viral infections in the skeletal remains of ancient populations. For example, studies of the remains of the Aztecs in Mexico have revealed evidence of infection with the variola virus, which causes smallpox. Genetic analysis of ancient human remains has also identified evidence of other viral diseases, including hepatitis B and C, HIV/AIDS, and influenza. Archeological findings have also provided evidence of viral infections in ancient civilizations. For example, the discovery of the remains of the Hittite civilization in Turkey revealed evidence of a viral epidemic that is believed to have occurred around 1650 BCE. The virus, which is thought to have been a strain of the influenza virus, caused a widespread epidemic that resulted in the deaths of many people [3].

Overall, while the specific viruses responsible for these ancient epidemics may not be known, there is ample evidence to suggest that viral diseases have existed in human populations throughout history. Understanding the impact of these ancient epidemics can offer essential insights into the emergence and spread of viral diseases and help inform efforts to prevent and control future outbreaks.

2.2.2 Bubonic plague, smallpox, and influenza in the Middle Ages

During the Middle Ages, several viral diseases had a noteworthy impact on the health and well-being of people in Europe and other areas of the world. Three of this period's most notable viral diseases were the bubonic plague, smallpox, and influenza.

2.2.2.1 The bubonic plague

The bubonic plague, also known as the Black Death, swept across Europe in the mid-14th century and was responsible for the deaths of an estimated 25 million people, or one-third of the European population at the time [2]. The disease was caused by the bacterium *Yersinia pestis*, carried by fleas that infested rats. The disease was highly contagious and spread rapidly, primarily through the movement of people and goods along trade routes.

Symptoms of the bubonic plague included high fever, chills, and the appearance of painful, swollen lymph nodes, or buboes, which gave the disease its name. The disease was often fatal, with death occurring within a few days of the onset of symptoms. The bubonic plague had a profound impact European society, causing widespread panic, economic disruption, and social upheaval.

2.2.2.2 Smallpox

Smallpox was another viral disease that significantly impacted the Middle Ages. It was caused by the variola virus and was highly contagious. Smallpox was spread through contact with infected individuals or contaminated objects, such as clothing or bedding. The disease had a mortality rate of around 30%, and survivors were often left with permanent scarring and other long-term health problems.

Smallpox had a significant impact on the Indigenous populations of the Americas, where it was introduced by European explorers and traders. The disease decimated entire communities and played a significant role in the European colonization of the Americas [3].

2.2.2.3 Influenza

Influenza, or the flu, was also present during the Middle Ages, although the exact strains and their impact are difficult to identify. Like the bubonic plague and smallpox, influenza was highly contagious and could spread rapidly through populations. Symptoms of the flu included high fever, cough, and respiratory problems. In severe cases, the disease could be fatal, especially among young children, the elderly, and those with weakened immune systems [4].

Influenza outbreaks were common during the Middle Ages, and the disease often significantly impacted local populations. However, because the virus was not well understood then, there were few effective treatments, and prevention efforts were limited to quarantine measures and herbal remedies.

Overall, these viral diseases had a profound impact on people's health and well-being during the Middle Ages. While modern medicine has made significant advances in preventing and treating these diseases, they continue to pose a significant threat to global health today.

2.2.3 Discovery of viruses and the beginning of modern virology

The discovery of viruses and the beginning of modern virology can be traced back to the late 19th and early 20th centuries. During this time, researchers began investigating the causes of infectious diseases and the role of microscopic agents in their transmission.

In 1892, a Russian scientist named Dmitry Ivanovsky conducted experiments on the tobacco plant, which was affected by a disease that any known bacteria or fungi could not explain. Ivanovsky discovered that the disease was caused by an infectious agent that was too small to be seen under a microscope. This agent was later identified as a virus, and Ivanovsky's work is now recognized as the beginning of modern virology.

In the years that followed, other scientists made important contributions to studying viruses and their impact on human health. In 1901, the German researcher Paul Ehrlich developed a technique for staining viruses, which allowed them to be visualized under a microscope. In 1905, the American scientist Walter Reed led the discovery of the virus responsible for yellow fever, a disease that devastated populations in the Americas and Africa.

Another breakthrough in the study of viruses came in 1935 when the American scientist Wendell Stanley crystallized the tobacco mosaic virus, the first virus to be purified and studied in detail. This work paved the way for further research into the structure and function of viruses and the development of vaccines and antiviral medications.

Today, virology is a complex and multidisciplinary field that encompasses the study of viruses' structure, function, and evolution, as well as their communications with the host and the immune system. This knowledge has enabled researchers to develop effective treatments and preventive measures for many viral diseases, including vaccines for polio, measles, and smallpox and antiviral medications for HIV/AIDS and hepatitis C.

2.3 Modern history of viral diseases

2.3.1 Major pandemics of the 20th century, including the Spanish flu, polio, and HIV/AIDS

In the 20th century, several viral diseases emerged and became widespread, causing pandemics affecting millions worldwide. The 1918 influenza pandemic, also known as the Spanish flu, was one of the most dangerous pandemics in history, killing around 50 million people at that time in the whole world. The polio epidemic in the 1950s and 1960s led to the development of the polio vaccine, which has appreciably abridged the incidence of the disease.

In the 1980s, the emergence of HIV/AIDS led to a global health crisis that continues to this day. In the early 2000s, the SARS outbreak in China and the H1N1 influenza pandemic brought global attention to the threat of emerging viral diseases [5].

2.3.2 Emerging viral diseases of the 21st century, including SARS, H1N1 influenza, and COVID-19 [4]

The 21st century has seen the emergence of several new viral diseases that have had a noteworthy role in global health. Some of this century's most notable emerging viral diseases include H1N1 influenza (swine flu), SARS (severe acute respiratory syndrome), and coronavirus disease 2019.

2.3.2.1 SARS

SARS was first identified in 2002 in the Guangdong province of China and quickly spread to other parts of the world. The disease was caused by a novel coronavirus similar to the virus that causes COVID-19. SARS primarily affects the respiratory system, causing severe acute respiratory distress syndrome (ARDS) and pneumonia. The disease had a high mortality rate, with around 10% of cases resulting in death.

The spread of SARS was primarily attributed to international travel and the movement of infected individuals across borders. The global response to SARS was swift and practical, with containment measures and public health interventions leading to the eventual eradication of the disease in 2004 [6].

2.3.2.2 H1N1 influenza

H1N1 influenza, also known as swine flu, emerged in 2009 and quickly spread to become a global pandemic. The disease was caused by a novel strain of the influenza virus, a combination of human, avian, and swine influenza viruses. H1N1 influenza primarily affects the respiratory system, causing symptoms such as fever, cough, and sore throat. The disease had a relatively low mortality rate, with most cases resulting in mild to moderate symptoms [7].

International travel and the movement of infected individuals across borders facilitated the spread of H1N1 influenza. The global response to H1N1 influenza was also swift, with containment measures and public health interventions leading to a decline in cases over time.

2.3.2.3 COVID-19

COVID-19 is the most recent emerging viral disease of the 21st century and has profoundly impacted global health and society. The disease was first identified in Wuhan, China, in December 2019 and has since spread to become a global pandemic. COVID-19 is caused by a novel coronavirus known as SARS-CoV-2, which primarily affects the respiratory system, causing symptoms such as fever, cough, and shortness of breath. COVID-19 is highly contagious and spreads primarily through respiratory droplets and contact with infected individuals. The disease has had a significant impact on global health, leading to millions of deaths and causing social and economic disruption on a worldwide scale.

The global response to COVID-19 has been extensive, with measures such as lockdowns, social distancing, and vaccination campaigns being implemented to contain the spread of the disease. Despite these efforts, the pandemic continues to impact global health and society, highlighting the ongoing threat of emerging viral diseases [7, 8].

2.4 Classification and characteristics of viruses

2.4.1 Overview of viral structure and replication

Viruses are infectious agents with a simple structure consisting of genetic material and a protein coat. They can infect living cells and cause various diseases in humans and animals. Understanding the structure and replication of viruses is essential in developing treatments and vaccines for viral diseases.

2.4.1.1 Structure

The structure of a virus consists of two main components: the genetic material and the protein coat. The genetic material can be either DNA or RNA, depending on the virus type. The protein coat, called a capsid, surrounds and protects the genetic material. Some viruses also have an outer envelope composed of lipids and proteins.

The capsid is made up of subunits called **capsomeres**, which can be arranged in different shapes, such as helical, icosahedral, or complex. The arrangement of the capsomeres determines the shape of the capsid and can influence the virus's ability to infect and replicate in host cells (figure 2.2) [8].

2.4.1.2 Replication

The replication of viruses is a complex process that involves several steps. The first step is attachment, where the virus attaches to specific receptors on the surface of host cells. Once attached, the virus enters the host cell and releases its genetic material.

The viral genetic material then takes over the host cell's machinery and begins to replicate itself. This process involves the synthesis of new viral proteins and the assembly of new virus particles. The new virus particles are then released from the infected host cell can infect new cells, continuing the cycle of infection and replication [8].

The replication of DNA viruses involves the viral DNA integrating into the host cell's genome or using the host cell's machinery to replicate its DNA. RNA viruses, on the other hand, use RNA-dependent RNA polymerase to replicate their RNA. Retroviruses, a special type of RNA virus, use reverse transcriptase to convert their RNA into DNA, which then integrates into the host cell's genome.

Viruses can also undergo genetic mutations during replication, which can result in the emergence of new virus strains with different properties. This can pose challenges in developing treatments and vaccines for viral diseases.

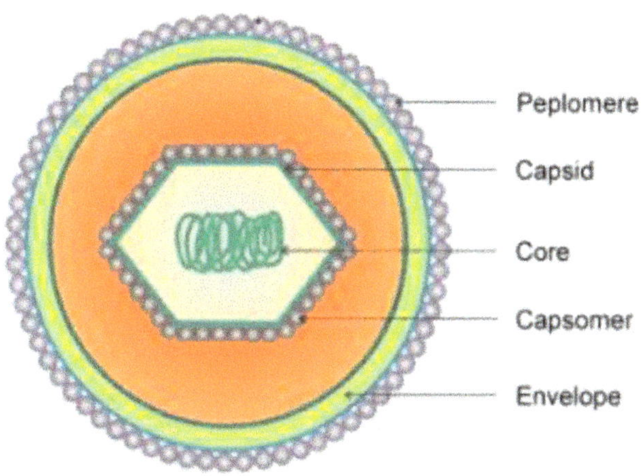

Figure 2.2. Basic structure of a virus. Reprinted from [9], copyright (2015), with permission from Elsevier.

Therefore, a virus's structure consists of genetic material and a protein coat, and the replication process involves several steps, including attachment, entry, replication, assembly, and release. Understanding the structure and replication of viruses is crucial in developing treatments and vaccines for viral diseases.

2.4.2 Types of viruses

There are two main types of viruses: DNA viruses and RNA viruses (table 2.1). These viruses differ in their genetic material and replication methods.

2.4.2.1 DNA viruses

DNA viruses have double-stranded DNA as their genetic material. DNA viruses include herpes simplex virus, varicella-zoster virus (the virus that causes chickenpox), and human papillomavirus (HPV). These viruses replicate by integrating their DNA into the host cell's genome or using the host cell's machinery to replicate their DNA.

2.4.2.2 RNA viruses

RNA viruses have single-stranded RNA as their genetic material. Examples of RNA viruses include influenza, measles, and human immunodeficiency (HIV). These viruses replicate by using RNA-dependent RNA polymerase to replicate their RNA. Retroviruses, a special type of RNA virus, use reverse transcriptase to convert their RNA into DNA, which then integrates into the host cell's genome.

2.4.2.3 RNA viruses can be further classified into four categories

(i) **Positive-sense RNA viruses:** These viruses have RNA that can be directly translated into proteins by the host cell's machinery. Examples include the common cold virus (rhinovirus) and the hepatitis C virus.

Table 2.1. Classification of virus based on nucleic acid, RNA viruses and DNA viruses. Data from [10].

RNA viruses	(−) RNA	Enveloped	Arenaviruses, Bunyaviruses Filoviruses, Orthomyxoviruses Paramyxoviruses, Rhabdoviruses
	(+) RNA	Non enveloped	Caliciviruses, Picornaviruses
		Enveloped	Coronaviruses, Flaviviruses, Togaviruses
	(−/+) RNA	Double capsid	Reoviruses
	(+) RNA via DNA	Enveloped	Retroviruses
DNA viruses	Double strand	Enveloped	Hepadnaviruses, Herpesviruses, Poxviruses
		Non enveloped	Adenoviruses, Papillomaviruses, Polyomaviruses
	Single strand	Non enveloped	Parvoviruses

(ii) **Negative-sense RNA viruses:** These viruses have RNA that needs to be converted into positive-sense RNA before it can be translated into proteins. Examples include the Ebola virus and the rabies virus.
(iii) **Double-stranded RNA viruses**: These viruses have two strands of RNA that can be directly translated into proteins by the host cell's machinery. Examples include rotaviruses (a common cause of gastroenteritis) and reoviruses (a cause of respiratory and gastrointestinal illnesses).
(iv) **Retroviruses:** As mentioned earlier, these viruses use reverse transcriptase to convert their RNA into DNA, which then integrates into the host cell's genome. Examples include HIV and the human T-cell leukemia virus.

Thus, viruses are classified based on their genetic material and how they replicate.

2.4.2.4 Characteristics of viruses

(i) Viruses are not considered living organisms because they cannot reproduce or carry out metabolic processes on their own. They require host cells to replicate and multiply.
(ii) Viruses are tiny and can only be seen under a microscope. They range in size from 20–300 nanometers in diameter.
(iii) Viruses have a simple structure consisting of a genetic material (DNA or RNA) surrounded by a protein coat called a capsid. Some viruses also have an outer envelope made of lipids.
(iv) Viruses are obligate intracellular parasites, which means they can only replicate inside a host cell. They enter host cells through attachment, where they bind to specific receptors on the cell surface. Once inside the cell, they use the host's cellular machinery to replicate and produce new viRus particles.
(v) Viruses have different replication modes depending on their genetic material. DNA viruses replicate using the host cell's DNA replication machinery, while RNA viruses use a unique enzyme called RNA-dependent RNA polymerase to replicate their genetic material.
(vi) Viruses can cause various diseases in humans and animals, from mild illnesses like the common cold to more severe illnesses like Ebola and COVID-19.
(vii) Viruses can undergo genetic mutations and evolve, which can lead to the emergence of new strains and the development of drug-resistant viruses.

In short, viruses are unique infectious agents that are classified based on their genetic material and morphological characteristics.

2.4.3 Characteristics of specific viral families and their associated diseases

Many families of viruses are associated with specific diseases. Here are some examples of viral families and their associated diseases, along with their unique characteristics:

(a) **Herpesviridae**: This family of viruses includes herpes simplex virus (HSV), varicella-zoster virus (VZV), and Epstein–Barr virus (EBV). These viruses are characterized by their ability to establish lifelong infections in the host and remain dormant until reactivation. They also have a unique ability to infect both neuronal and lymphoid cells.

(b) **Papillomaviridae:** This family of viruses includes human papillomavirus (HPV), a common cause of genital warts and cervical cancer. These viruses have a small, circular DNA genome transmitted through skin-to-skin contact.

(c) **Orthomyxoviridae:** This family of viruses includes influenza, which causes seasonal flu outbreaks. These viruses have a segmented RNA genome characterized by their ability to undergo frequent mutations, resulting in antigenic drift and the need for annual flu vaccines.

(d) **Retroviridae:** This family of viruses includes human immunodeficiency virus (HIV), which causes acquired immunodeficiency syndrome (AIDS). These viruses have a unique replication process that involves reverse transcription of their RNA genome into DNA, which is then integrated into the host cell's genome.

(e) **Coronaviridae:** This family of viruses includes severe acute respiratory syndrome coronavirus 2 (SARS-CoV-2), which causes COVID-19. These viruses have a large, positive-sense RNA genome characterized by their spike proteins that bind to the host cell's receptor, allowing for viral entry.

(f) **Flaviviridae:** This family of viruses includes Zika, dengue, and West Nile viruses. These viruses have a positive-sense RNA genome and are transmitted through mosquitoes. They are characterized by their ability to cause neurological complications, such as microcephaly in infants infected with the Zika virus.

(g) **Picornaviridae:** This family of viruses includes rhinovirus, a common cause of the cold. These viruses have a small, positive-sense RNA genome characterized by their ability to rapidly mutate, resulting in a high degree of genetic diversity.

Understanding the unique characteristics of different viral families is important for developing effective treatments and vaccines for viral diseases. It also helps in developing strategies for preventing the spread of viral infections.

2.5 Modes of transmission of viral diseases

Viral diseases can be transmitted in several ways, including:

(i) **Airborne transmission:** Some viruses can be transmitted through the air when an infected person coughs or sneezes, releasing virus-containing droplets into the air. Examples of viruses transmitted via airborne route include measles, chickenpox, and influenza.

(ii) **Direct contact transmission:** Viruses can be transmitted through direct contact with infected bodily fluids, such as blood, semen, vaginal secretions, or saliva. Examples of viruses transmitted via direct contact include HIV, hepatitis B and C, and herpes simplex virus.

(iii) **Indirect contact transmission:** Viruses can be transmitted indirectly through contact with contaminated objects or surfaces, such as doorknobs, telephones, or shared utensils. Examples of viruses transmitted via indirect contact include norovirus, rotavirus, and rhinovirus.

(iv) **Vector-borne transmission:** Some viruses are transmitted by vectors, such as mosquitoes or ticks, which are intermediaries in transmitting the virus from an infected person or animal to a new host. Viruses transmitted via vector-borne route include dengue fever, Zika virus, and West Nile virus.

(v) **Foodborne transmission:** Viruses can be transmitted through contaminated food or water. Examples of viruses transmitted via food or water include hepatitis A, norovirus, and rotavirus.

(vi) **Sexual transmission:** Some viruses can be transmitted through sexual contact with an infected person, such as HIV, herpes simplex virus, and human papillomavirus.

Preventing the spread of viral diseases involves understanding the modes of transmission and taking appropriate precautions. For example, practicing good hand hygiene, avoiding close contact with people who are sick, and wearing protective gear (such as masks or gloves) can help reduce the risk of transmission. Additionally, vaccines are available for many viral diseasesases, which can help prevent infection and reduce the spread of the virus in the community.

2.6 Viral diseases and society

The social and economic impacts of viral diseases can be significant and wide-ranging. Some of the major effects are:

Healthcare costs: Treating viral diseases can be substantial, particularly for those without access to affordable healthcare. Treatment costs include hospitalization, medications, diagnostic tests, and follow-up care. The economic burden of healthcare costs associated with viral diseases can be particularly high for low-income households and countries with limited healthcare resources.

Workforce disruptions: Outbreaks of viral diseases can lead to significant disruptions in the workforce. Sick employees may need to take time off work, leading to decreased productivity and lost wages. In addition, measures such as quarantine, social distancing, and business closures can significantly impact businesses and industries.

Stigma and discrimination: Some viral diseases are associated with stigma and discrimination. This can lead to social ostracism, discrimination in employment and housing, and limited access to healthcare and other services. The stigma associated with viral diseases can also discourage individuals from seeking medical care, which can lead to increased transmission of the virus.

Mental health: The impact of viral diseases on mental health can be significant. Fear, anxiety, and uncertainty associated with viral diseases can lead to psychological distress and even contribute to the development of mental health conditions such as depression and anxiety disorders.

Social disruption: The social disruption associated with viral diseases can be significant. Outbreaks can lead to school and business closures, restrictions on travel and public gatherings, and changes to how people interact and socialize. These disruptions can have a profound impact on mental health and well-being, particularly for vulnerable populations such as children, older people, and individuals with pre-existing medical conditions. The social and economic effects of viral diseases can be significant and wide-ranging. Healthcare costs, workforce disruptions, stigma and discrimination, mental health impacts, and social disruption are just a few of how viral diseases can affect society. Addressing these impacts requires a multi-faceted approach that includes prevention, early detection, effective treatment, and public health interventions to mitigate the spread of viral diseases.

2.7 Conclusion

In conclusion, the history of viral diseases spans thousands of years and has significantly impacted human societies throughout history. From the devastating pandemics of the past to the emerging viral diseases of the 21st century, the study of viral diseases has led to important discoveries about the nature of viruses and their modes of transmission. Over the centuries, researchers and public health officials have developed a range of strategies to prevent, detect, and treat viral diseases. These strategies have included vaccines, antiviral drugs, and public health interventions such as quarantine and contact tracing. As we continue to face new viral threats, studying viral diseases and their impact on human health and society remains critical. Advances in technology and research offer hope for new ways to prevent and treat viral infections, but many challenges remain to be overcome.

Through continued research, investment, and collaboration, we can better understand the complex nature of viral diseases and develop more effective strategies to control and mitigate their impact on human health and society.

Abbreviations

AIDS	Acquired immunodeficiency syndrome
COVID-19	Coronavirus disease 2019
DNA	Deoxyribonucleic ACID
EBV	Epstein–Barr virus
H1N1	Hemagglutinin Type 1 and Neuraminidase Type 1 (a subtype of the influenza virus)
HPV	Human papillomavirus
HSV	Herpes simplex virus
MRNA	Messenger ribonucleic acid
SARS	Severe acute respiratory syndrome
SARS-CoV-1	Severe acute respiratory syndrome Coronavirus 1

References

[1] Hendrix R W, Lawrence J G, Hatfull G F and Casjens S 2000 The origins and ongoing evolution of viruses *Trends Microbiol.* **8** 504–8

[2] https://downtoearth.org.in/news/young/secret-diary-of-a-virus-70564

[3] Hays J N 2006 *Epidemics and Pandemics: Their Impacts on Human History* (Oxford: ABC-CLIO)

[4] Wu X, Xiao L and Li L 2020 Research progress on human infection with avian influenza H7N9 *Front. Med.* **14** 8–20

[5] Worobey M, Han G Z and Rambaut A 2014 Genesis and pathogenesis of the 1918 pandemic H1N1 influenza A virus *Proc. Natl Acad. Sci. USA* **111** 8107–12

[6] Weinstein R A 2004 Planning for epidemics–the lessons of SARS *N. Engl. J. Med.* **350** 2332–4

[7] Viboud C, Miller M, Olson D, Osterholm M and Simonsen L 2010 Preliminary estimates of mortality and years of life lost associated with the 2009 A/H1N1 pandemic in the US and comparison with past influenza seasons *PLoS Curr* **2** RRN1153

[8] Teixeira R and Doetsch J 2020 The multifaceted role of mobile technologies as a strategy to combat COVID-19 pandemic *Epidemiol. Infect.* **148** e244

[9] Zhou X and Li Y 2015 Basic biology of oral microbes *Atlas of Oral Microbiology* (New York: Academic)

[10] https://onlinebiologynotes.com/classification-of-virus/

IOP Publishing

Viral Diseases
History and new developments in diagnostics and therapeutics
Arvind K Singh Chandel, Bhakti Tanna, Amisha Parmar, Gopal Patel and Neeraj S Thakur

Chapter 3

Contagiousness and threats of most prevalent viral diseases worldwide

Venkteshwar Yadav, Dharm Pal and Anil Kumar Poonia

As human populations move towards modernization, various health issues have emerged due to advancements in technology and substance use. In this context, medical emergencies caused by viral diseases have become a major concern. Over time, several newly mutated viruses have been identified, resulting in highly detrimental effects on both infected and healthy individuals. Furthermore, certain viral diseases such as coronavirus disease 2019 (COVID-19), human immunodeficiency virus/acquired immune deficiency syndrome (HIV/AIDS), and influenza-have become the most prominent diseases of our time. Due to the viral nature of these infecting agents, common disease transmission systems include direct contact or transmission through blood. This chapter discusses the contagiousness and threats posed by COVID-19, HIV/AIDS, and influenza. Additionally, protocols for precautions and currently available potential cures are also discussed.

3.1 Introduction

The health issue in living beings encompasses not only physical and mental well-being but also the economic burden posed by diseases [1–3]. Improvements in various aspects, such as proper garbage disposal, adequate hygiene and sanitation practices, access to clean water, optimal nutrition, and adherence to good medical practices, including antibiotics and vaccinations, can promote healthy human lives and contribute to income growth [4–7]. However, this improvement is also a major factor contributing to increasing several other issues because this process produces byproducts and waste [8]. These advancements, while making life easier for humans, ultimately lead to heightened pollution levels in the environment. This increase in pollution can facilitate the mutation and rapid proliferation of pathogenic substances [9, 10]. The polluted environment can create suitable conditions for the

doi:10.1088/978-0-7503-4987-1ch3

survival and resistance of pathogens to antibiotic drugs, rendering them ineffective against specific viral diseases [11, 12].

Currently, several factors contribute to the emergence of contagious diseases, including bacteria, viruses, parasites, and fungi [13–16]. However, viruses, in particular, have been responsible for numerous diseases, with their impact being particularly severe compared to other disease-causing agents. Human respiratory viruses constitute a diverse group of viruses that primarily spread through the respiratory secretions of infected individuals. These viruses target respiratory tract cells, leading to respiratory symptoms and various other manifestations. Clinical differentiation among respiratory viral infections is often challenging. Respiratory viruses belong to a broad family of viruses characterized by their viral and genomic architecture, susceptibility of certain populations, disease severity, seasonal circulation patterns, transmissibility, and routes of transmission [1]. Despite a decrease in the mortality rate associated with infectious diseases, they still present a significant threat to global health. In the ongoing battle against 21st century diseases such as coronavirus disease 2019 (COVID-19) and the human immunodeficiency virus (HIV)/acquired immune deficiency syndrome (AIDS), which has mutated or transferred from animal reservoirs [17]. Some infectious diseases, such as malaria and tuberculosis, are widespread and endemic, imposing significant and enduring burdens. Others, like influenza, exhibit fluctuations in intensity and prevalence, wreaking havoc in both developed and developing nations during epidemics (sharp rises in prevalence over larger areas or populations), pandemics (epidemics spanning multiple countries or continents), or outbreaks (sharp increases in prevalence in relatively small areas or populations) [4]. The first part of the book covered the widely and currently most concerning viral decease include covid-19, HIV/Aids, and influenza. The threat, precautions, and curing are covered in this part.

3.2 Current contagiousness viral decease

Currently, COVID-19, influenza, and HIV/AIDS are diseases caused by viruses, which will be discussed in subsequent sections, and table 3.1 contains the disease threats, precautions, and cures. Moreover, the symptoms of COVID-19, influenza, and HIV/AIDS are shown in figure 3.1.

3.2.1 COVID-19

The first pandemic situation in the 21st century was due to the COVID-19 viral disease. The origin of this viral disease was assumed to be in Wuhan city, where the seafood market was identified as the source of contagion. The initial case of COVID-19 was projected to be in March 2019, but the true origin of this worldwide virus remains uncertain [18]. Some intellectuals suggest that it was a genetically engineered virus produced in a Wuhan scientific laboratory. The first cases of this viral disease were reported worldwide in early 2020 by the National Health Commission of China. Subsequently, the World Health Organization (WHO) designated it with two terms: 'novel coronavirus 2019' (2019-nCoV) and 'severe acute respiratory syndrome coronavirus 2' (SARS-CoV-2), with international

Table 3.1. Various pharmaceutical companies from different countries have developed vaccines for viral diseases.

S. No.	Name of the disease	Name of the invented vaccine	Name of the company	Country	Period
1	COVID-19	Comirnaty	Pfizer-BioNTech	United States and Germany	Dec 2020
2	COVID-19	Moderna COVID-19	Moderna	United States	Dec 2020
3	COVID-19	Vaxzevria	Oxford-AstraZeneca	United Kingdom and Sweden	Dec 2020
4	COVID-19	Janssen	Johnson & Johnson	United States	Feb 2021
5	COVID-19	Novavax COVID-19	Novavax, Inc.	United States	Jan 2021
6	COVID-19	Sinopharm COVID-19	National Pharmaceutical Group (Sinopharm)	China	Feb 2021
7	COVID-19	CoronaVac	Sinovac Biotech	China	Jan 2021
8	COVID-19	Covaxin	Bharat Biotech	India	Jan 2021
9	COVID-19	Covishield	Oxford-AstraZeneca	India and United Kingdom	Dec 2020
10	Influenza A	Whole Inactivated Influenza Vaccine (IIV)	Various pharmaceutical companies	United States	1940
11	Influenza A	Live Attenuated Influenza Vaccine (LAIV)	Various pharmaceutical companies	United States	1960
12	Influenza A	Subunit Influenza A	Various pharmaceutical companies	United States, United Kingdom, and Australia	1970
13	Influenza A	Split-Virus Influenza A	Various pharmaceutical companies	Various contries	1970
14	Influenza A	Quadrivalent Influenza A	Sanofi, GlaxoSmithKline, Seqirus	United States, Europe, and Australia	2010
15	Influenza A	Recombinant Influenza A	Sanofi Pasteur	United States	2010
16	Influenza A	Cell-Based Influenza A	Seqirus, Sanofi Pasteur	United Kingdom and Germany	2010
17	HIV/AIDS	RV144 (ALVAC/AIDSVAX)	Sanofi Pasteur, Global Solutions	Thailand and USA	2009
18	HIV/AIDS	DNA vaccine[a]	GlaxoSmithKline, Merck, Johnson & Johnson	United States and Europe	1990
19	HIV/AIDS	Adenovirus-based vaccine[a]	Johnson & Johnson, National Institutes of Health	United States and Europe	2000
20	HIV/AIDS	Viral vector vaccine[a]	Johnson & Johnson, GeoVax, Inovio Pharmaceuticals	United States and Europe	2010
21	HIV/AIDS	mRNA vaccine[a]	Moderna, BioNTech	United States and Europe	2010
22	HIV/AIDS	Protein subunit vaccine[a]	Sanofi Pasteur, GlaxoSmithKline	United States and Europe	1990

[a] Represents the status of vaccines that are in the development stage.

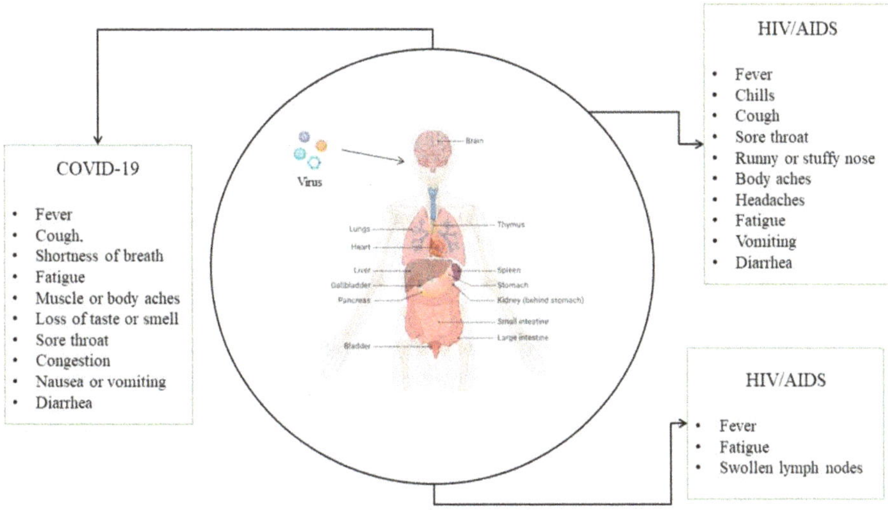

Figure 3.1. Symptoms of viral diseases.

committees playing a significant role [19]. Finally, the WHO designated the illness as 'coronavirus disease 2019' (COVID-19) [19, 20]. Despite this, China has denied any involvement, asserting that the viral outbreak originated from the Wuhan seafood market, where some consumers were infected after consuming contaminated food, though not all cases were linked to it. After some time, transmission pathways and media were identified, and it was widely accepted that the viral disease spread through human-to-human transmission via coughing and sneezing, with respiratory droplets or aerosols facilitating transmission. Furthermore, due to aerosol inhalation, which penetrates the upper respiratory tract and lungs, illness spread was reported in nearly every country on every continent, leading to a sharp increase in global case counts [21–23].

3.2.1.1 Threats, precautions and cures of COVID-19

The health sector has encountered significant new challenges during the pandemic period due to COVID-19. The presence of the virus has led to delays in the treatment of several other diseases because a COVID-19 test is mandatory for every patient before proceeding with any other treatment. It is crucial to highlight the occurrence of secondary bacterial pneumonias, which contributed to the fatal influenza outbreak of 1918 [24]. Both innate and adaptive antibacterial host defenses are compromised in respiratory viral illnesses such as influenza or COVID-19. During these infections, colonizing bacteria exploit this temporary breach in the physical and immunological barriers, leading to secondary bacterial pneumonias that worsen outcomes and can be fatal, particularly in patients with comorbidities and previously healthy individuals [25]. The rationale behind prescribing antibiotics to COVID-19 patients may be rooted in prior research indicating higher patient mortality rates from bacterial superinfection during influenza. Numerous studies have demonstrated secondary bacterial pneumonia or initial co-infection in hospitalized patients, as well as the challenge of ruling out bacterial co-infection based solely on the patient's presentation [26]. Furthermore, doctors are likely to err on the side of caution when administering broad-spectrum antibiotics to severely ill COVID-19 patients in whom the possibility of secondary bacterial infections remains uncertain. Consequently, a decrease in adherence to stewardship programs is observed among medical professionals as they strive to save COVID-19 patients [27].

Initially, the threat posed by COVID-2019 was that it was an unpredicted and incurable disease for which precautions had not been identified earlier. As the year 2020 progressed, some protocols were proposed to curb the widespread transmission of this viral disease. However, the identification of various aspects of the disease has posed a significant challenge for researchers, making inhibition efforts highly challenging. Major precautions for COVID-19 include measures such as social distancing, avoiding direct contact with infected individuals and unnecessary items, maintaining a healthy lifestyle, consuming nutritious food, practicing good hygiene, and frequent sanitization [23].

While human infections can be effectively treated with antibiotics and antivirals, infections caused by new pathogens typically respond less effectively to these treatments [28]. The discovery of vaccines serves as a reminder that our body's immune system is an intelligent weapon against invading pathogens. As a preventive approach, the effectiveness of vaccination has been demonstrated for numerous human pathogens, resulting in the saving of millions of lives through the use of subunit vaccines, non-replicating whole-virus or whole-bacteria vaccines, and attenuated live vaccines [29]. While candidate vaccines developed by Pfizer, Moderna, and AstraZeneca have shown promising results, detailed experimental data is yet to be published. Particularly, the efficacy of these vaccines in older individuals or those with underlying conditions, as well as their effectiveness in preventing severe disease in COVID-19 patients, remain unclear [30, 31]. However, in this race, Covishield and Covaxin have played significant roles in treating and reducing the rate of COVID-19-related deaths. These two vaccines are being used in several countries and have shown positive results in addressing the challenges posed by COVID-19 [32]. This is especially crucial given the challenges posed by microbial resistance to therapeutic drugs and the slow pace of vaccine development. In other words, microbial pathogens often demonstrate adaptability and resilience, highlighting the need for more sophisticated strategies to combat future pandemics [30].

3.2.2 Influenza

Public health experts began making preparations for a flu pandemic after the US centers for Disease Control and Prevention announced on April 21, 2009, that two people in California had contracted a novel influenza virus with swine origins [33]. Following recommendations from the World Health Organization, the current influenza outbreak was deemed to be pandemic-like. In response to the outbreak of the S-OIV infection, numerous schools were closed in Mexico, the US, Japan, and other nations, aiming to curb its spread. This highlights the danger posed by influenza viruses and the unpredictability of a novel influenza strain evolving into a deadly one. As of September 16, 2009, approximately 280 000 cases and 3200 deaths had been reported globally. During that same period, over 300 000 children worldwide succumbed to malaria, while over 600 000 children died from diarrheal illnesses [33, 34]. Because its segmented negative-sense RNA genome lacks systems for proofreading, mutations constantly accumulate in the influenza virus. Influenza viruses persist as a quasispecies due to ongoing processes known as antigenic drift and antigenic shift. Influenza A viruses undergo minimal evolution and typically cause inapparent disease in their natural reservoirs of aquatic birds and bats. However, once they spread to other species, influenza A viruses can undergo rapid evolution and trigger pandemics and epidemics of acute respiratory disease in humans, lower mammals, and domestic poultry [35, 36].

3.2.2.1 Threats, precautions and cures of influenza

With the introduction of frequent international air travel in the last few decades, the situation has drastically changed. Infected individuals can now be quickly transported into a vulnerable group and may even arrive before exhibiting symptoms. These days, pandemics like influenza might travel across continents and hemispheres in a matter of hours or days [37]. In addition to emerging during therapy, antiviral resistance in influenza can occasionally spread widely to supplant susceptible strains in situations where the medication was unavailable. The unpredictable nature of influenza viruses and the growing difficulties in treating influenza clinically, particularly in light of the limited number of available treatments [38]. Genetic drift and shift drive influenza risks, with point mutations in the virus's genes causing genetic drift due to RNA polymerase errors. This leads to recurrent influenza epidemics and necessitates annual vaccine updates as mutations affect antibody binding sites. Reassortment occurs when multiple influenza strains infect a single host cell, creating new combinations of the virus's surface glycoproteins, neuraminidase, and hemagglutinin [39].

Antiviral drugs are available for both treating and preventing influenza, serving as a valuable complement to vaccination. When used alongside other preventive measures such as immunization and isolation protocols, these drugs can significantly reduce influenza outbreaks in medical facilities. Published guidelines now exist for the use of antiviral drugs in healthcare facilities during influenza outbreaks. Various infection-control techniques are employed in healthcare institutions to reduce the risk of infectious agent transmission. Precautions based on transmission routes are tailored for diseases with multiple routes of transmission, focusing on the predominant route or routes of infection. With consistent adherence and efficient infection-control measures acting as barriers to the virus's transmission, isolation measures can play a significant role in combating the spread of respiratory viruses [40].

When it comes to inhibiting influenza, neuraminidase inhibitors like Oseltamivir and Relenza are typically the first choice. Additionally, amantadine and rimantadine, the other two authorized M2 ion-channel inhibitors, are also in use [41]. In 2009, phase 3 trials were conducted for peramivir (BioCryst Pharmaceuticals, Durham, NC, USA), another neuraminidase inhibitor, for both intravenous and intramuscular delivery methods [42]. In Japan, research was being conducted on the inhalation use of CS-8958, a different long-acting neuraminidase inhibitor [43]. In addition to being efficacious against the A, B, and C influenza viruses, the viral polymerase inhibitor T-705, also known as Favipiravir, has shown some efficacy against additional RNA viruses, such as certain hemorrhagic fever viruses [41]. Sialidase fusion protein inhibitor DAS181 (Fludase) is a fusion construct that can be mass-manufactured in *Escherichia coli* and contains the sialidase from Actinomyces viscosus, a common oral bacterium associated with a human-epithelium-manchoring domain [44]. The sialidase enzyme specifically targets the viral attachment process, which is a preliminary step in influenza virus reproduction. Cyanovirin-N and thiazolides, two viral hemagglutinin inhibitors, were also examined for H1N1 infection. Recently, several novel anti-influenza medications have been created, including Geldanamycin, an inhibitor of the viral polymerase assembly chaperone Hsp90, and mechanism-based covalent neuraminidase inhibitors. Furthermore, findings from a few clinical trials as well as animal models supported combination therapy with already available antivirals. According to Yuan, such combinations may reduce the likelihood of influenza virus strains becoming resistant [41].

3.2.3 HIV/AIDS

The report that coined the term AIDS was first published on June 5, 1981. It detailed the treatment of five young, previously healthy, homosexual men for *Pneumocystis carinii* pneumonia in three Los Angeles hospitals. Those who underwent testing showed signs of T-lymphocyte depletion, and two of them had died. Over the next few months, additional cases of *Pneumocystis carinii* pneumonia, other opportunistic infections, and Kaposi's sarcoma among males engaging in intimate activity with other males were reported from several US cities. Although the cause of the immunodeficiency remained unknown, cases in intercourse partners and findings from a national case-control study strongly suggested a sexually transmitted infection [45]. By January 1983, the primary routes of transmission for the as-yet-unidentified 'AIDS agent' had been identified. Reports of similar immunodeficiency in female intimate partners of males with AIDS in New York suggested heterosexual transmission [46]. Mother-to-child transmission was indicated by the unexplained immunodeficiency and opportunistic infections observed in infants born to women with AIDS-related diseases [45]. Multiple lines of evidence, including cases among injecting drug users and hemophiliacs, suggested transmission through blood and blood products. Additionally, it was reported that a baby in San Francisco developed the illness after receiving a platelet transfusion from a donor and subsequently developing *Pneumocystis carinii* pneumonia. Similarly, incidents where healthcare personnel were exposed to blood on the job were consistent with blood-borne transmission [47].

3.2.3.1 Threats, precautions and cures of HIV/AIDS

The resolution emphasized that 'if unchecked, this pandemic may pose a risk to stability and security,' in addition to expressing concern about the potential negative consequences of HIV/AIDS on UN peacekeeping forces. Since then, the idea that

HIV/AIDS poses a threat to national security has gained traction. Public health advocates who are concerned about HIV/AIDS may view the securitization of the disease positively. Indeed, governments in both wealthy and developing nations have started to take HIV/AIDS more seriously and have allocated more funds to its control. This includes improving the availability of life-prolonging drugs and implementing preventative efforts, all due to the perception that the disease constitutes a threat to national security [48]. The effectiveness of antiretroviral therapy as an HIV preventative measure is likely compromised for several reasons. However, some of the frequently highlighted reasons are: first, the perceived threat of AIDS diminishes as antiretroviral therapy transforms HIV infection into a chronic and manageable condition; second, individuals may become less inclined to use protection to prevent HIV transmission as physical intercourse gain a better understanding of how antiretroviral therapy impacts HIV transmission [49].

Based on current knowledge, some of the major precautions available to protect against HIV/AIDS include practicing safe intercourse, ensuring single usage of medical equipment for penetration, and avoiding transfusion of blood from an infected person to a healthy individual. Firstly, safe intercourse involves using protection during physical intimacy and limiting the number of sexual partners, as this is the primary mode of HIV transmission through direct contact. Additionally, ensuring the single use of medical equipment for penetration and preventing blood transfusions from infected individuals are essential medical precautions [50]. Even a small mistake in these practices can result in the transmission of the HIV virus to healthy individuals. Implementing these precautions diligently can have a significant impact on reducing the number of HIV/AIDS cases.

Thanks to effective antiretroviral treatment, new infection rates have slowed, saving millions of lives. Despite antiretroviral treatment's success in managing HIV as a chronic condition, challenges like cost, stigma, and toxicity persist. To address these, scientists aim to develop HIV cure strategies to eliminate the need for lifelong antiretroviral treatment, prevent transmission, and eradicate the virus from the body. Achieving a functional cure (sustained virus control without treatment) and a sterilizing cure (complete virus eradication) are ambitious goals in controlling the HIV pandemic. Progress has been made toward both, with cases like the 'Berlin patient' and 'London patient' showing promising results after complex procedures involving stem-cell transplants [51, 52]. However, these interventions carry high risks and are not scalable for all HIV-infected individuals. Despite this, ongoing studies aim to refine these strategies for broader application [53].

3.3 Summary

Most cases of viral diseases involve the transmission of viruses from contaminated surfaces or infected individuals to healthy individuals. In recent times, three major viral diseases have emerged as threats to humanity: COVID-19, HIV/AIDS, and influenza. Scientific advancements have enabled us to identify the reasons and origins of these threats. Furthermore, preventive measures for protection have been discovered, and awareness among the public has increased significantly, leading to their implementation based on this awareness and understanding. Currently, some antiviral vaccines and medications are available for treatment. However, viruses continue to mutate over time, posing unique challenges. In conclusion, the primary defense against these viral diseases is to adopt preventive measures and maintain a healthy lifestyle to strengthen immunity.

Acknowledgments

The authors greatly acknowledge the Department of Chemical Engineering of the National Institute of Technology Raipur for providing research opportunities.

Abbreviations

AIDS	Acquired immunodeficiency syndrome
COVID-19	Coronavirus disease 2019
H1N1	Hemagglutinin type 1 and Neuraminidase type 1 (a subtype of the influenza virus)
HIV	Human immunodeficiency virus
RNA	Ribonucleic acid
S-OIV	Swine-origin influenza virus

References

[1] Leung N H L 2021 Transmissibility and transmission of respiratory viruses *Nat. Rev. Microbiol.* **19** 528–45

[2] Upadhyay A, Pal D and Kumar A 2024 Interrogating *Salmonella typhi* biofilm formation and dynamics to understand antimicrobial resistance *Life Sci.* **339** 122418

[3] Upadhyay A, Pal D and Kumar A 2023 Deciphering target protein cascade in *Salmonella typhi* biofilm using genomic data mining, and protein–protein interaction *Curr. Genomics* **24** 1

[4] Bloom D E and Cadarette D 2019 Infectious disease threats in the twenty-first century: strengthening the global response *Front. Immunol.* **10** 1–12

[5] Upadhyay A, Pal D and Kumar A 2023 Combinatorial enzyme therapy: a promising neoteric approach for bacterial biofilm disruption *Process Biochem.* **129** 56–66

[6] Pattanayak D S, Pal D, Thakur C and Kumar A 2023 Techniques to stop spread and removal of resistance from wastewater *Antimicrobial Resistance in Wastewater and Human Health* (Elsevier) pp 101–30

[7] Pattanayak D S, Pal D, Mishra J and Thakur C 2023 Noble metal–free doped graphitic carbon nitride (g-C3N4) for efficient photodegradation of antibiotics: progress, limitations, and future directions *Environ. Sci. Pollut. Res.* **30** 25546–58

[8] Surana M, Pattanayak D S, Yadav V, Singh V K and Pal D 2024 An insight decipher on photocatalytic degradation of microplastics: mechanism, limitations, and future outlook *Environ. Res.* 118268

[9] Pattanayak D S, Pal D, Thakur C, Raut P and Wasewar K L 2022 Catalytic potential of phyto-synthesized silver nanoparticles for the degradation of pollutants *Sustainable Engineering, Energy, and the Environment* ed K L Wasewar and S N Rao (Apple Academic Press) pp 465–81

[10] Pattanayak D S, Behera A, Thakur C and Pal D 2023 Properties and adsorption mechanism of organic pollutants by carbon nanotubes *Water Treatment Using Engineered Carbon Nanotubes* (Elsevier) ch 9 pp 243–69

[11] Pattanayak D S, Pal D, Mishra J, Thakur C and Wasewar K L 2023 Doped graphitic carbon nitride (g-C3N4) catalysts for efficient photodegradation of tetracycline antibiotics in aquatic environments *Environ. Sci. Pollut. Res.* **30** 24919–26

[12] Pattanayak D S, Pal D and Thakur C 2024 The influence of various precursors on solar-light-driven g-C3N4 synthesis and its effect on photocatalytic tetracycline hydrochloride (TCH) degradation *Inorg. Chem. Commun.* **162** 112201

[13] Upadhayay A, Ling J, Pal D, Xie Y, Ping F F and Kumar A 2023 Resistance-proof antimicrobial drug discovery to combat global antimicrobial resistance threat *Drug Resist. Updat.* **66** 100890

[14] Upadhyay A, Pal D and Kumar A 2023 Substantial relation between the bacterial biofilm and oncogenesis progression in host *Microb. Pathog.* **175** 105966

[15] Upadhayay A, Pal D and Kumar A 2022 Salmonella typhi induced oncogenesis in gallbladder cancer: co-relation and progression *Adv. Cancer Biol.—Metastasis* **4** 2021–3

[16] Agrawal P, Upadhyay A and Kumar A 2024 microRNA as biomarkers in tuberculosis: a new emerging molecular diagnostic solution *Diagn. Microbiol. Infect. Dis.* **108** 116082

[17] Upadhayay A, Patel G, Pal D and Kumar A 2022 Frequently used allopathic and traditional medicine for COVID-19 treatment and feasibility of their integration *Chin. J. Integr. Med.* **28** 1040–7

[18] Fan Y, Zhao K, Shi Z L and Zhou P 2019 Bat coronaviruses in China *Viruses* **11** 27–32

[19] Wang C, Horby P W, Hayden F G and Gao G F 2020 A novel coronavirus outbreak of global health concern *Lancet* **395** 470–3

[20] Peretto G, Sala S and Caforio A L P 2020 Acute myocardial injury, MINOCA, or myocarditis? Improving characterization of coronavirus-associated myocardial involvement *Eur. Heart J.* **41** 2124–5

[21] Parry J 2020 China coronavirus: cases surge as official admits human to human transmission *Brit. Med. J.* **368** m236

[22] Riou J and Althaus C L 2020 Pattern of early human-to-human transmission of Wuhan 2019 novel coronavirus (2019-nCoV), December 2019 to January 2020 *Eurosurveillance* **25** 1–5

[23] Lotfi M, Hamblin M R and Rezaei N 2020 COVID-19: transmission, prevention, and potential therapeutic opportunities *Clin. Chim. Acta* **508** 254–66

[24] Chien Y-W, Klugman K P and Morens D M 2009 Bacterial pathogens and death during the 1918 influenza pandemic *N. Engl. J. Med.* **361** 2582–3

[25] Ginsburg A S and Klugman K P 2020 COVID-19 pneumonia and the appropriate use of antibiotics *Lancet Glob. Heal.* **8** e1453–4

[26] Klein E Y, Monteforte B, Gupta A, Jiang W, May L, Hsieh Y H and Dugas A 2016 The frequency of influenza and bacterial coinfection: a systematic review and meta-analysis *Influenza Other Respi. Viruses* **10** 394–403

[27] Ghosh S, Bornman C and Zafer M M 2021 Antimicrobial resistance threats in the emerging COVID-19 pandemic: where do we stand? *J. Infect. Public Health* **14** 555–60

[28] De Clercq E and Li G 2016 Approved antiviral drugs over the past 50 years *Clin. Microbiol. Rev.* **29** 695–747

[29] Ozawa S, Stack M L, Bishai D M, Mirelman A, Friberg I K, Niessen L, Walker D G and Levine O S 2011 During the 'decade of vaccines,' the lives of 6.4 million children valued at $231 billion could be saved *Health Aff.* **30** 1010–20

[30] Dai H, Han J and Lichtfouse E 2021 Smarter cures to combat COVID-19 and future pathogens: a review *Environ. Chem. Lett.* **19** 2759–71

[31] Christa L, Walker I, Rudan L and Liu H N 2020 Since January 2020 Elsevier has created a COVID-19 resource centre with free information in English and Mandarin on the novel coronavirus COVID-19 *Ann. Oncol.* **7** 19–21

[32] Machado B A S, Hodel K V S, Fonseca L M D S, Pires V C, Mascarenhas L A B, da Silva Andrade L P C, Moret M A and Badaró R 2022 The importance of vaccination in the context of the COVID-19 pandemic: a brief update regarding the use of vaccines *Vaccines* **10** 1–25

[33] Schnitzler S U and Schnitzler P 2009 An update on swine-origin influenza virus A/H1N1: a review *Virus Genes* **39** 279–92

[34] Wang T T and Palese P 2009 Unraveling the mystery of swine influenza virus *Cell* **137** 983–5

[35] Swayne D E 2016 Common aspects of animal influenza *Animal Influenza* (Wiley) p 656

[36] Webster R G and Govorkova E A 2014 Continuing challenges in influenza *Ann. N. Y. Acad. Sci.* **1323** 115–39

[37] Mathews J D, Chesson J M, Mccaw J M and Mcvernon J 2009 Understanding influenza transmission, immunity and pandemic threats *Influenza Other Respi. Viruses* **3** 143–9

[38] Hayden F G and De Jong M D 2011 Emerging influenza antiviral resistance threats *J. Infect. Dis.* **203** 6–10

[39] Asha K and Kumar B 2019 Emerging influenza D virus threat: what we know so far! *J. Clin. Med.* **8** 192

[40] Bridges C B, Kuehnert M J and Hall C B 2003 Transmission of influenza: implications for control in health care settings *Clin. Infect. Dis.* **37** 1094–101

[41] Yuan S 2013 Drugs to cure avian influenza infection multiple ways to prevent cell death *Cell Death Dis* **4** e835

[42] Yun N E *et al* 2008 Injectable peramivir mitigates disease and promotes survival in ferrets and mice infected with the highly virulent influenza virus, A/Vietnam/1203/04 (H5N1) *Virology* **374** 198–209

[43] Macdonald S J F *et al* 2004 Potent and long-acting dimeric inhibitors of influenza virus neuraminidase are effective at a once-weekly dosing regimen *Antimicrob. Agents Chemother.* **48** 4542–9

[44] Malakhov M P *et al* 2006 Sialidase fusion protein as a novel broad-spectrum inhibitor of influenza virus infection *Antimicrob. Agents Chemother.* **50** 1470–9

[45] De Cock K M, Jaffe H W and Curran J W 2012 The evolving epidemiology of HIV/AIDS *Aids* **26** 1205–13

[46] Anon 1983 Immunodeficiency among female sexual partners of males with Acquired Immune Deficiency Syndrome (AIDS)—New York *MMWR. Morb. Mortal. Wkly. Rep.* **31** 697–8

[47] Anonymous 1984 Needlestick transmission of HTLV-III from a patient infected in Africa *Lancet* **2** 1376–7

[48] Selgelid M J and Enemark C 2008 Infectious diseases, security and ethics: the case of HIV/AIDS *Bioethics* **22** 457–65

[49] Kalichman S C, Price D, Eaton L A, Burnham K, Sullivan M, Finneran S, Cornelius T and Allen A 2017 Diminishing perceived threat of AIDS and increasing sexual risks of HIV among men who have sex with men, 1997–2015 *Arch. Sex. Behav.* **46** 895–902

[50] Relevance C, Homeostasis L T, Patients I and Antiretroviral R 2014 *Patricia Ndumbi* **1** 245

[51] Gupta R K *et al* 2020 Evidence for HIV-1 cure after CCR5Δ32/Δ32 allogeneic haemopoietic stem-cell transplantation 30 months post analytical treatment interruption: a case report *Lancet HIV* **7** e340–7

[52] Hütter G *et al* 2009 Long-term control of HIV by CCR5 Delta32/Delta32 stem-cell transplantation *New Engl. J. Med.* **360** 692–8

[53] Bailon L, Mothe B, Berman L and Brander C 2020 Novel approaches towards a functional cure of HIV/AIDS *Drugs* **80** 859–68

IOP Publishing

Viral Diseases
History and new developments in diagnostics and therapeutics
Arvind K Singh Chandel, Bhakti Tanna, Amisha Parmar, Gopal Patel and Neeraj S Thakur

Chapter 4

Drug development process: clinical trials and regulations

Bhingaradiya Nutan, Arvind K Singh Chandel and Ashwani Mishra

This chapter provides a comprehensive overview of the drug development process, focusing on the pivotal roles of clinical trials and regulatory oversight. It delves into the phases of preclinical research, drug discovery, and the transition to clinical trials while outlining the legal frameworks of significant organizations such as the FDA and EMA. The chapter examines the various stages of clinical trials, including post-marketing surveillance, large-scale efficacy research, and early safety testing. It highlights advancements like personalized medicine, adaptive trial designs, and digital health technology while addressing current issues such as high prices, regulatory barriers, and patient recruitment. The chapter also discusses potential future paths, including emerging trends, prospective regulatory changes, and the ongoing need to enhance the drug development process to improve patient care and medical science.

4.1 Introduction

4.1.1 Overview of drug development

The drug development process, a complex yet crucial endeavor, is the cornerstone of improving patient outcomes and advancing medical science. Its goal is to discover, evaluate, and introduce novel pharmaceuticals to the market [1]. This process, from original medication discovery to market approval, involves several crucial steps, including discovery, preclinical research, clinical trials, and regulatory approval [2]. The whole process is summarised in figure 4.1.

Usually, the discovery phase of the drug development process is where scientists find and evaluate possible therapeutic targets. The main goals of this study phase are identifying substances that can interact with these targets and comprehending the underlying biological mechanisms of diseases. Subsequently, preclinical research

doi:10.1088/978-0-7503-4987-1ch4

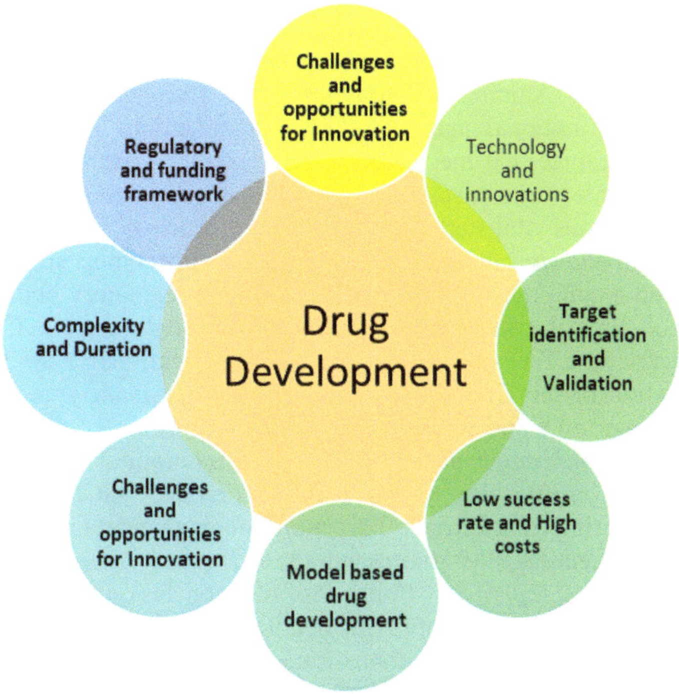

Figure 4.1. The development process of drug.

evaluates specific drugs' safety, effectiveness, and pharmacokinetics through laboratory and animal testing [1, 2].

If preclinical research shows promise, a drug candidate moves to clinical trials on human volunteers. Phases I, II, III, and occasionally IV of clinical trials aim to address questions regarding the medication's safety, effectiveness, and best use. Ultimately, before the medication is made available to the general public, it must pass a stringent regulatory approval process in which regulatory bodies examine data from clinical studies to guarantee the medication's efficacy and safety [3].

The process of developing new drugs is costly and time-consuming; it frequently takes over ten years and billions of dollars. Despite significant technological and methodological breakthroughs, the failure rate is still high. This emphasizes how complicated things are and how important it is to evaluate everything thoroughly at every step to ensure that only safe and effective medications are on the market [3, 4].

4.1.2 Importance of regulatory and clinical trials

Clinical trials and regulatory scrutiny are essential steps in the medication development process. They guarantee that novel medications are productive and safe before being released to the general population. The main goals of these phases are safeguarding public health and increasing trust in novel treatments [3].

4.1.3 Regulatory oversight

Regulatory organizations like the U.S. Drug Development is closely supervised by the Food and Drug Administration (FDA), the European Medicines Agency (EMA), and other national agencies. These organizations provide criteria and procedures to guarantee that medications are created and examined in a way that preserves patient safety and ensures the product's effectiveness [3, 5].

There are numerous vital steps in the regulatory process:

1. *Preclinical and clinical trial review:* Drug developers must submit preclinical data and a comprehensive clinical trial plan to regulatory bodies before the start of clinical trials. This submission, referred to as a Clinical Trial Application (CTA) in Europe and an Investigational New Drug (IND) application in the United States, is examined to make sure the suggested trials are morally and scientifically sound [3, 5, 6].
2. *Monitoring and compliance:* Regulatory bodies monitor continuing research projects to ensure that Good Clinical Practice (GCP) regulations are followed during clinical trials. This entails managing data integrity, informed consent procedures, and trial design [3, 6, 7].
3. *Evaluation and approval:* Following the conclusion of clinical studies, pharmaceutical companies provide detailed information to regulatory bodies for examination. This submission, sometimes called a Marketing Authorisation Application (MAA) or New Drug Application (NDA), contains all preclinical and clinical data and manufacturing and labeling details. Regulatory bodies examine this data to ascertain whether the medication satisfies safety and efficacy requirements [6, 7].
4. *Post-marketing surveillance:* Through post-marketing surveillance, regulatory bodies monitor a drug's safety even after it has been licensed and put on the market. This phase, known as Phase IV, entails continuous data gathering and analysis on the medication's long-term effects and infrequent adverse responses [6, 7].

Clinical trials

The foundation of drug development is clinical trials, which offer vital information on the efficacy and safety of novel medications. These experiments are carried out on human participants and are intended to provide answers to particular research queries [3, 5–7]. They are split up into various stages:

1. *Phase I studies:* The main goal is to assess a medication's safety in a few fit participants or patients. Researchers evaluate the medicine's pharmacodynamics, how the drug affects the body, pharmacokinetics, and how the drug is absorbed, distributed, metabolized, and eliminated. This stage aids in figuring out the correct dosage and locating any possible adverse effects.
2. *Phase II trials:* Patients with the ailment that the medicine is meant to treat make up a larger patient population in phase II trials. This phase's primary goal is to investigate the drug's safety and effectiveness further. Researchers watch for adverse side effects while searching for early indications of the drug's efficacy.

3. *Phase III studies:* Several sites and a sizable patient population are used to test the medication in Phase III studies. This stage tries to verify the medication's effectiveness, track any side effects, and contrast it with conventional therapies. Phase III trials are essential for proving the drug's benefit-risk profile and producing most of the data needed for regulatory approval.
4. *Phase IV studies:* Following a drug's approval and commercialization, Phase IV studies are carried out to get more data regarding the medication's long-term effects and general population performance. This stage aids in detecting any uncommon or persistent side effects and evaluates the efficacy of the medicines in practical situations [3, 5–7].

Clinical trials and regulatory monitoring are essential components of the drug development process to guarantee that novel treatments are high-quality, safe, and practical. By conducting thorough assessments and adhering to prescribed protocols, these procedures safeguard public health and foster the progress of medical science. To address new health issues and enhance patient care, continuous research, and innovation in clinical trial procedures and regulatory standards will be crucial as drug development changes [6, 7].

The complex drug development process aims to find, evaluate, and introduce novel pharmaceuticals to the market. Improving patient outcomes and furthering medical science depend on this process. Several crucial steps are involved in the complex process, from original medication discovery to market approval, including discovery, preclinical research, clinical trials, and regulatory approval [7, 8]. Usually, the discovery phase of the drug development process is where scientists find and evaluate possible therapeutic targets. Identifying substances that can interact with these targets and comprehending the underlying biological mechanisms of diseases are the main goals of this study phase. Subsequently, preclinical research evaluates specific drugs' safety, effectiveness, and pharmacokinetics through laboratory and animal testing [7, 9].

If preclinical research shows promise, a drug candidate moves to clinical trials on human volunteers. Phases I, II, III, and occasionally IV of clinical trials aim to address questions regarding the medication's safety, effectiveness, and best use. Lastly, before the medication is made available to the general public, it must pass a stringent regulatory approval process in which regulatory bodies examine data from clinical studies to guarantee the medication's efficacy and safety [7, 8, 10].

Developing new drugs is costly and time-consuming; it frequently takes tens of years and billions of dollars [11]. Despite major technological and methodological breakthroughs, the failure rate is still high. This emphasizes how complicated things are and how important it is to evaluate everything thoroughly at every step to ensure that only safe and effective medications are on the market [10, 11].

Clinical trials and regulatory scrutiny are essential steps in the medication development process. They are necessary to guarantee that novel medications are both productive and safe before being released into the general population. The main goals of these phases are to safeguard the public's health and increase trust in novel treatments. Regulatory organizations like the U.S. Drug Development is closely supervised by the Food and Drug Administration (FDA), the European

Medicines Agency (EMA), and other national agencies. These organizations set rules and recommendations to guarantee that medications are created and examined in a way that preserves patient safety and ensures the product's effectiveness [5, 7, 8, 12].

To guarantee that novel treatments are high-quality, safe, and practical, clinical trials and regulatory monitoring are essential components of the drug development process. By conducting thorough assessments and adhering to prescribed protocols, these procedures safeguard public health and foster the progress of medical science. To address new health issues and enhance patient care, continuous research, and innovation in clinical trial procedures and regulatory standards will be crucial as drug development changes.

4.2 The drug development process

4.2.1 Discovery and preclinical research

Drug discovery is the first step in drug development, where researchers find and validate biological targets and screen chemicals for possible therapeutic possibilities. Lead optimization is then carried out to improve efficacy and lower toxicity. In preclinical research, these candidates undergo a rigorous testing process, where their pharmacodynamics, pharmacokinetics, and safety profiles are assessed through *in vitro* (lab) and *in vivo* (animal) tests. Before moving further with human clinical trials, this stage is critical for comprehending how a medicine acts in the body and its possible harmful effects. Approval must be obtained from preclinical data to move forward with clinical testing.

4.2.2 Drug discovery

Finding new pharmacological agents is called drug discovery, and it involves several vital processes. The first step is target identification, in which scientists identify particular biological molecules or pathways connected to a disease. Usually, a protein, enzyme, or receptor essential to the illness's pathophysiology serves as this target [13, 14].

After discovering a target, compound screening involves testing a library of chemical compounds to see if they can interact with the target. High-throughput screening technologies are frequently used to quickly assess hundreds of chemicals for possible action [15]. 'Hits' are promising compounds found during this phase that are then subjected to additional testing to see if they will make good medication candidates. Lead optimization is the next step, in which the pharmacokinetic, selectivity, and effectiveness of the first hits are improved. Chemical alterations to the chemicals are made throughout this process to enhance their functionality and lessen any possible adverse effects [15]. The aim is to create a 'lead' compound with advantageous properties that can advance to the following stage of development.

4.2.3 Preclinical testing

Before beginning human trials, medication candidates go through a rigorous review process known as preclinical testing. *In vivo* and *in vitro* studies are conducted at this phase to evaluate several facets of the drug's characteristics. Drugs are tested in isolated cells or biological systems in *in vitro* research. These investigations offer preliminary information on the drug's pharmacodynamics, how the drug interacts with the body, and pharmacokinetics, how the body metabolizes the drug. Scientists evaluate variables including enzymatic activity, cellular toxicity, and receptor binding affinity [5, 16].

In vivo research uses animal models to assess a medication's safety, effectiveness, and possible adverse effects on a whole organism. Understanding the drug's pharmacokinetics, that is, its distribution, metabolism, excretion, and absorption, is aided by this phase. Studies on toxicology are conducted to find adverse effects and establish safe dosage ranges [15, 17].

4.2.4 Research on translation

Preclinical research and clinical trials are connected by translational research. This stage aims to apply research from animal models to people. As animal models may not always precisely anticipate human reactions, one challenge in translational research is ensuring that animal study findings apply to human conditions [5, 15, 18]. Translational research aims to optimize therapeutic formulations, develop suitable protocols for clinical trials, and determine whether large-scale manufacture is feasible. Successful translational research makes a smooth transition of potential drug candidates into human clinical trials possible, paving the way for additional safety and effectiveness testing [18].

4.3 Regulatory framework

4.3.1 International Regulatory Organisations

4.3.1.1 US FDA, or the Food and Drug Administration

One important regulatory agency in charge of guaranteeing the effectiveness and safety of medications in the US is the FDA. The FDA's responsibilities include approving drug applications, establishing standards for clinical trials, and monitoring the safety of drugs after they are marketed [19].

There are multiple steps in the FDA clearance process:

1. *Preclinical review:* Drug researchers must file an Investigational New Drug (IND) application before the start of clinical trials. Preclinical data, suggested clinical trial methods and manufacturing data are all included in this application [19].
2. *Phases of clinical trials:* The FDA supervises and ensures that Good Clinical Practice (GCP) regulations are followed. To assess the safety and effectiveness of the medication, the FDA examines data from Phase I, II, and III trials [19].
3. *New drug application (NDA):* An NDA is filed following the completion of fruitful clinical trials. The FDA examines this extensive data package when determining whether to approve a medicine for commercial use [19].

4.3.1.2 European Medicines Agency (EMA)

The EMA oversees pharmaceuticals' scientific assessment, oversight, and safety surveillance in the European Union. The FDA and EMA have comparable procedures, although EMA's are customized for the European regulatory environment [5, 19]. Important facets of the EMA's work consist of:

1. *Scientific evaluation:* The European Medicines Agency (EMA) uses its Committee for Medicinal Products for Human Use (CHMP) to evaluate new medications for quality, safety, and efficacy. Preclinical and clinical trial data are reviewed in the evaluation process [5, 19]. The CHMP reviews the Marketing Authorisation Application (MAA), submitted by pharmaceutical companies to the EMA. Based on this study, the EMA recommends marketing authorization [5, 19].
2. *Post-marketing surveillance:* The European Medicines Agency (EMA) conducts pharmacovigilance, gathering and evaluating information on side effects following a drug's release onto the market [5, 20].

4.3.1.3 Other agencies

Additional international regulatory organizations include The PMDA, or Japanese Pharmaceuticals and Medical Devices Agency, which is in charge of policing pharmaceuticals and medical devices in Japan. Its responsibilities include approving new medications, monitoring post-market safety, and assessing data from clinical trials [20]. World Health Organisation (WHO): The WHO offers global standards and guidelines for protecting and developing pharmaceuticals. It is essential for organizing responses to global health issues and guaranteeing the standard of medications across the board [21].

4.4 Regulatory submission

4.4.1 Investigational New Drug (IND) application

Before starting clinical trials, the United States requires submitting an Investigational New Drug (IND) application, an essential stage in drug development. The IND filing must include comprehensive data demonstrating the drug's safety and possible efficacy based on preclinical research. The application contains extensive details about the medicament's pharmacology, toxicity, manufacturing method, and composition [22]. The following are the main elements of an IND application:

Preclinical data: Outcomes of research conducted *in vivo* and *in vitro* show the medication's safety and effectiveness.

Clinical protocols: Comprehensive protocols that include research design, methodology, and statistical analysis for the clinical trials.

Details on the investigators: The qualifications and credentials of the clinical investigators who are leading the trials.

Manufacturing information: Specifics regarding the medication's manufacturing procedure, quality assurance protocols, and stability information [22].

The FDA examines the IND application to make sure the suggested clinical trials are supported by science and that the possible benefits outweigh the potential dangers to the participants. The sponsor may proceed with clinical testing if the FDA does not reject the IND within 30 days of receiving it [19, 22].

4.4.2 Clinical Trial Application (CTA)

A Clinical Trial Application (CTA) comparable to the IND in the United States must be submitted to start a clinical trial. The European Medicines Agency (EMA) oversees the CTA procedure, which entails submitting a thorough application that includes the following:

Study protocol: Details on the clinical study design's goals, procedures, and statistical analysis.

Preclinical data: Proof derived from research demonstrating the medication's effectiveness and safety. Documentation of informed consent processes and ethics committee clearances are two ethical considerations.

Manufacturing information: Specifics regarding the medication's manufacturing and quality control procedures.

Each EU member state's relevant national competent authorities and ethics committees assess the CTA. The application is approved if it satisfies all ethical and regulatory requirements, enabling the sponsor to start clinical testing [23].

4.4.3 New Drug Application (NDA) and Marketing Authorization Application (MAA)

The last stages in the drug approval process are the submission of the New Drug Application (NDA) in the United States and the Marketing Authorisation Application (MAA) in Europe, which are made following the conclusion of clinical trials. Comprehensive documentation and data from every stage of the clinical study are used in both applications [24]. NDA (FDA, 2020): The NDA contains manufacturing data, suggested labeling, and comprehensive clinical study results. The FDA examines the data to evaluate the drug's benefit-risk profile, safety, and effectiveness. There are various steps to the review process, such as advisory committee reviews and scientific examination. The FDA authorizes a medicine for marketing if it meets the necessary criteria.

The Committee for Medicinal Products for Human Use (CHMP) and other expert bodies evaluate the MAA. The EMA recommends marketing authorization based on its assessment of the drug's quality, safety, and efficacy [22, 24]. Both procedures entail a thorough examination of clinical data, and approval is subject to proving the medication has a considerable therapeutic benefit at a risk that can be tolerated [19, 22, 24].

4.5 Clinical investigations

4.5.1 Clinical trial phases

4.5.1.1 Phase I

A phase I trial is the initial step in evaluating a new human medication. Phase I studies are primarily concerned with determining the medicine's safety and pharmacokinetics or how it is absorbed, distributed, metabolized, excreted, and has a safe dosage range [12, 13]. Phase I trials usually involve healthy volunteers; however, occasionally, patients with the target ailment may be enrolled if it is anticipated that the medicine may be extremely hazardous. The primary goals are determining the maximum tolerable dose and finding any adverse effects. The drug's first safety profile must be ascertained during this phase to inform dose recommendations for later trials [12, 13].

4.5.1.2 Phase II

Phase II trials are designed to assess the safety and effectiveness of the medication in individuals with the intended condition. Compared to Phase I, this phase has a bigger sample size and seeks to offer preliminary information on the drug's efficacy [12, 13]. Phase II trials are commonly separated into two categories: Phase IIA, which concentrates on studies including dose range, and Phase IIB, which evaluates the drug's effectiveness in a more specific patient population. To improve treatment protocols and prepare for larger-scale studies, researchers gather information on the drug's therapeutic advantages, ideal dosage, and side effects [12, 13].

4.5.1.3 Phase III

Phase III trials are large-scale investigations to verify the medication's effectiveness and track side effects across various patient demographics. This step frequently involves thousands of participants to guarantee that the results are generalizable and are carried out at multiple sites [8, 12, 13]. Phase III trials assess the relative effectiveness of the new medication by comparing it to placebos or current therapies. This stage is essential for regulatory approval as it offers proof of the drug's benefit-risk profile. The NDA or MAA submission is based on the data gathered during Phase III studies [8, 12, 13].

4.5.1.4 Phase IV

Post-marketing studies, also known as phase IV trials, are carried out once a medicine has been approved for public use. Monitoring the drug's long-term effects and safety in a larger population is the primary goal of Phase IV trials [5, 12, 13]. These studies aid in detecting uncommon or persistent side effects that would not have been noticeable in previous stages. Additional details about the drug's efficacy in different subpopulations and its interactions with other medications are also provided by phase IV research. To ensure continuous drug safety and efficacy, real-world evidence obtained during this phase and ongoing pharmacovigilance are crucial [5, 8, 12, 13].

4.5.2 Clinical trial design

4.5.2.1 Randomized controlled trials (RCTs)

RCTs, or randomized controlled trials, are regarded as the gold standard in clinical trial design because of their exacting procedures and capacity to reduce bias. Randomization, or the process of randomly allocating individuals to the treatment or control group, is the fundamental idea behind randomized controlled trials (RCTs). By ensuring that the groups are comparable at the beginning of the trial, this random assignment helps lower the possibility of confounding variables and selection bias [8, 12, 13]. The existing standard treatment or a placebo may be administered to the control group, serving as a benchmark for assessing the efficacy of the new intervention. By uniformly allocating known and unknown confounding factors among the groups, randomization also improves the dependability of the results and enables a more precise evaluation of the treatment's impact [7, 8, 12, 13].

4.5.2.2 Blinding

Another crucial component of clinical trial design that lowers bias is blinding. In a single-masked study, the researchers are not blinded, but the participants are not aware of which group they are in (treatment or control). This lessens the possibility that participant expectations will affect how they behave throughout the trial or how they report the results [7, 8, 12, 13]. This is further enhanced by double-masked experiments, which guarantee that neither the volunteers nor the researchers are aware of who is receiving the treatment or a placebo. Because neither party's expectations can affect the outcome, this design reduces observer and participant bias [7, 8, 12, 13]. Blinding is essential to preserve the data's integrity and guarantee that the observed effects are due to the intervention and not biases or placebo effects.

4.5.2.3 Endpoints and outcomes

Endpoints and results are essential when assessing a drug's safety and effectiveness. Primary endpoints, which typically represent the most significant impact of the intervention, such as overall survival or a particular clinical improvement, are the primary outcomes that the study is intended to evaluate [12, 13, 25]. The primary endpoint selection is essential since it directly impacts the trial's design and statistical analysis. Secondary endpoints offer more details regarding the impact of the medication, such as unintended adverse effects or secondary advantages. These could include biomarker alterations, clinical outcomes, or quality-of-life metrics [25]. Secondary endpoints provide a more thorough comprehension of the drug's overall effects and possible therapeutic benefits.

4.5.3 Ethical considerations

4.5.3.1 Informed consent

A fundamental ethical need for clinical trials is informed consent. To enable participants to make an informed decision regarding their involvement entails giving them comprehensive information about the study, including its goals, methods, possible dangers, and advantages [7, 8, 12, 13]. The procedure guarantees that participants consent to the survey freely and are well-informed about its nature. Informed permission must be obtained continuously, and participants must be free to leave the experiment at any moment without incurring any fees. Ethics in study conduct and safeguarding participants' autonomy and well-being require that participants are aware of the information given to them and their rights [7, 8].

4.5.3.2 Ethics committees

Ethics committees, also known as Institutional Review Boards (IRBs) in the United States, greatly aid clinical trial supervision. Their primary duty is to check and approve trial procedures to ensure they adhere to moral principles and safeguard the welfare and rights of participants [7, 13, 26]. A trial's risk-to-benefit ratio, informed consent processes, and scientific validity are only a few of the factors that ethics committees assess. They also monitor ongoing experiments to address any ethical concerns that might surface throughout the study. Ethics committees assist in upholding high ethical standards and guarantee that studies are carried out honorably and with consideration for participants by offering an unbiased review [26].

4.6 Challenges and innovations

4.6.1 Challenges in drug development

4.6.1.1 High costs and long timelines

Drug development is a famously costly and time-consuming procedure. A new drug's introduction to the market can take ten to fifteen years and cost up to $2.6 billion on average [27]. Numerous factors contribute to this high cost, including the requirement for in-depth preclinical and clinical testing, regulatory approval, and significant research and development. Substantial financial resources are required at every stage of the process, and these expenses are made even more problematic by the high failure rate of drug candidates. The extensive testing necessary to guarantee drug safety and efficacy, which involves several stages of clinical trials and regulatory reviews, is another reason for the lengthy timescales [27].

4.6.1.2 Regulatory hurdles

One of the biggest obstacles to drug development is navigating the regulatory environment. Strict standards set by regulatory bodies such as the FDA and EMA to prove the safety and effectiveness of new medications might cause delays and higher expenses. Frequently encountered regulatory obstacles encompass the necessity of comprehensive paperwork, discrepancies in regulatory norms throughout nations, and the intricacy of fulfilling preclinical and clinical trial obligations. The requirement for further research or evidence sought by the regulatory bodies may also cause the approval process to take longer [5, 19, 27].

4.6.1.3 Patient recruitment

It might be challenging to find and keep clinical study participants. The pool of eligible participants may be limited by stringent inclusion and exclusion standards, the stress of participation on patients, and competition from other trials [28]. Furthermore, keeping trial participants for the whole term is essential for getting accurate data. However, this can be challenging because of things like the trial's length, potential side effects, and the requirement for frequent visits. Clinical trials must be completed, which requires effective recruitment and retention tactics [27, 28].

4.6.2 Innovations in drug development

4.6.2.1 Personalized medicine

Customizing medications based on patients' unique genetic profiles is a breakthrough in drug development known as personalized medicine. This method enables more targeted and efficient therapeutics by considering genetic variants that affect drug response and illness susceptibility [29]. Thanks to developments in genetics and biotechnology, targeted treatments that target specific genetic abnormalities or biomarkers can now be developed, improving patient outcomes and minimizing side effects [27, 29]. Pharmacogenomics, which investigates how genetic variants impact medication metabolism and efficacy, is another area of personalized medicine that contributes to increased treatment precision [29].

4.6.2.2 Adaptive trial designs

Clinical research can be more flexible when using adaptive trial designs, which enable trial alterations based on interim results. These designs can modify treatment regimens, sample sizes, or dose levels, allowing researchers to adapt to new information and maximize the trial's efficacy [30]. By lowering the number of participants exposed to failed medicines and identifying beneficial treatments more quickly, adaptive designs can improve the efficiency of clinical trials [7, 8, 30]. Adaptive approaches can also save costs and accelerate the time it takes to develop new drugs.

4.6.2.3 Digital health technologies

Drug development has been completely transformed by digital health technologies, which offer cutting-edge instruments for data gathering, tracking, and analysis. Real-time data gathering and enhanced patient monitoring are made possible by innovations, including wearable technology, mobile health applications, and electronic health records [31]. According to Nilsen *et al* these technologies improve patient participation, enable remote data collecting, and speed up and improve the accuracy of trial outcomes analysis, all of which increase the efficiency of clinical trials. By making it possible to follow patient outcomes and treatment reactions more precisely, digital health technologies also contribute to personalized medicine [32].

4.7 Case studies

4.7.1 Successful drug development examples

The creation of Imatinib (Gleevec), a targeted treatment for chronic myeloid leukemia (CML), is a noteworthy example of a successful drug development process. The development of imatinib entailed a significant amount of preclinical research, followed by rigorous clinical studies that proved the drug's safety and effectiveness in treating CML [33]. The medication's precise mode of action and adept handling of regulatory procedures contributed to its success. With its approval, imatinib represented a breakthrough in cancer treatment and demonstrated the promise of targeted therapies in medication development [33, 34].

4.7.2 Lessons learned from failures

The creation of the medication TGN1412 offers an insightful case study for comprehending the possible difficulties in drug development. During clinical studies, TGN1412, an immunomodulatory medication, caused patients to experience significant adverse responses, including potentially fatal cytokine storms [35]. This event made clear how crucial it is to conduct extensive preclinical testing and enhance safety assessments before starting human trials. The demise of TGN1412 highlights the vital need for improved safety evaluations and predictive models to avert such problems in subsequent medication development [36].

4.8 Future directions

4.8.1 Emerging trends

Clinical trials, regulatory procedures, and drug development are all changing quickly. The pharmaceutical industry's future is expected to be shaped by several new developments.

Biotechnology advances: As biotechnology develops, more advanced and focused treatments will be created. Advances in cellular therapies like CAR-T cell therapy and gene editing technologies like CRISPR/Cas9 are transforming the treatment choices available for diseases once thought incurable [37]. These biotechnology developments can potentially improve medication efficacy and offer individualized treatment plans based on each patient's unique genetic profile [37].

Combining machine learning and artificial intelligence: The methods involved in developing new drugs increasingly incorporate machine learning and artificial intelligence (AI). These technologies are applied to clinical trial design optimization, predictive modeling, and drug discovery. AI algorithms can analyze large-scale data to find promising drug candidates, forecast clinical results, and optimize the drug development process [38]. Additionally, machine learning helps to understand disease causes and find biomarkers, which may speed up the search for new drugs [39].

Extension of evidence from the real world (RWE): An increasing amount of real-world evidence derived from real-world data (RWD) is used to assess the safety and efficacy of pharmaceuticals. By offering insights into how medications function in regular clinical settings and across a range of demographics, RWE can supplement clinical trial data [40].

4.8.2 Regulatory reforms

Simplifying the regulatory procedures: Reforming regulations is essential to increasing the effectiveness of medication approval and development. Adopting more efficient and adaptable regulatory routes, such as the expedited approval procedure and conditional approvals for ground-breaking treatments, is one possible reform. The development of medications that meet unmet medical needs and show significant clinical benefits can be accelerated by following these routes. Regulatory bodies are also looking into ways to standardize practices and guidelines throughout various areas to cut down on red tape and boost the effectiveness of drug development worldwide [5].

Improving cooperation and information exchange: To advance medication development, regulatory bodies, pharmaceutical corporations, and research institutes must work together more. Research and development (R&D) productivity can be increased through partnerships and data sharing made possible by collaborative efforts. The Global Alliance for Genomics and Health (GA4GH) and the International Council for Harmonisation (ICH) are two initiatives that seek to advance international standardization and data exchange, which can expedite the drug development process and enhance regulatory results [41].

Developing patient-centric methods: Patient-centric methodologies are becoming increasingly popular in drug development. Recruitment, retention, and trial success can increase by including patient viewpoints in trial design and decision-making processes. Regulatory bodies are promoting patient-reported outcomes and preferences in clinical studies, acknowledging the growing significance of patient input. Improved patient involvement and ensuring clinical trials meet practical requirements will lead to more pertinent and successful treatment interventions [42].

4.9 Conclusion

This chapter has given a thorough overview of developing new drugs, emphasizing clinical trials and regulatory scrutiny's vital roles. We looked at the entire drug development process, from preclinical research and discovery to clinical trials, highlighting the role regulatory bodies play in guaranteeing the efficacy and safety of pharmaceuticals. We talked about the several stages of clinical trials, creative methods, and new developments influencing how drugs are developed in the future.

Drug development procedures must undergo ongoing improvement to progress medical knowledge and improve patient care. The pharmaceutical business must stay flexible and sensitive to new trends and regulatory changes as it navigates complex problems and adopts creative solutions. Global patient outcomes and therapy alternatives will eventually be enhanced by pursuing more effective and efficient drug development processes. Progress in the field and tackling global health issues will mostly depend on continued research, teamwork, and regulatory changes.

Abbreviations

CRO	Contract Research Organization
CTA	Clinical trial application
DNA	Deoxyribonucleic acid
EMA	European Medicines Agency
FDA	U.S. Food and Drug Administration
IND	Investigational new drug
IRB	Institutional Review Board
MAA	Marketing authorization application
NDA	New drug application
RCT	Randomized controlled trial

References

[1] Hughes J P, Rees S, Kalindjian S B and Philpott K L 2011 Principles of early drug discovery *Br. J. Pharmacol.* **162** 1239–49

[2] Deore A B, Dhumane J R, Wagh R and Sonawane R 2019 The stages of drug discovery and development process *Asian J. Pharm. Res. Dev.* **7** 62–7

[3] Piantadosi S 2024 *Clinical Trials: A Methodologic Perspective* (New York: Wiley)

[4] Sun D, Gao W, Hu H and Zhou S 2022 Why 90% of clinical drug development fails and how to improve it? *Acta Pharm. Sin. B.* **12** 3049–62

[5] Teixeira T, Kweder S L and Saint-Raymond A 2020 Are the European Medicines Agency, US Food and Drug Administration, and other international regulators talking to each other? *Clin. Pharmacol. Ther.* **107** 507–13

[6] Teicher B A and Andrews P A (ed) 2004 *Anticancer Drug Development Guide: Preclinical Screening, Clinical Trials, and Approval* (Berlin: Springer Science & Business Media)

[7] Allen M E and Vandenburg M J 1992 Good clinical practice: rules, regulations and their impact on the investigator *Br. J. Clin. Pharmacol.* **33** 463

[8] Padmanabhan S 2014 Clinical trials in pharmacogenomics and stratified medicine *Handbook of Pharmacogenomics and Stratified Medicine* (Academic) ch 15 pp 309–20

[9] Gad S C 2016 *Drug Safety Evaluation* (New York: Wiley)

[10] Roskoski J R 2020 Properties of FDA-approved small molecule protein kinase inhibitors: a 2020 update *Pharmacol. Res.* **152** 104609

[11] Taylor D 2015 The pharmaceutical industry and the future of drug development *Pharmaceuticals in the Environment* (Royal Society of Chemistry)

[12] Eskola S M, Leufkens H G M, Bate A, De Bruin M L and Gardarsdottir H 2022 Use of real-world data and evidence in drug development of medicinal products centrally authorized in Europe in 2018–2019 *Clin. Pharmacol. Ther.* **111** 310–20

[13] Chow S C and Liu J P 2008 *Design and Analysis of Clinical Trials: Concepts and Methodologies* **Vol 507** (New York: Wiley)

[14] Berry S M, Carlin B P, Lee J J and Muller P 2010 *Bayesian Adaptive Methods for Clinical Trials* (Boca Raton, FL: CRC Press)

[15] Collins F S and Varmus H 2015 A new initiative on precision medicine *New Engl. J. Med.* **372** 793–5

[16] Huang S M, Lertora J J, Vicini P and Atkinson A J (ed) 2021 *Atkinson's Principles of Clinical Pharmacology* (New York: Academic)

[17] Mukherjee P, Roy S, Ghosh D and Nandi S K 2022 Role of animal models in biomedical research: a review *Lab. Anim. Res.* **38** 18

[18] Begasse de Dhaem O, Wattiez A S, de Boer I, Pavitt S, Powers S W, Pradhan A, Gelfand A A and Nahman-Averbuch H 2023 Bridging the gap between preclinical scientists, clinical researchers, and clinicians: from animal research to clinical practice *Headache* **63** 25–39

[19] Fleming T R, Demets D L and McShane L M 2017 Discussion: the role, position, and function of the FDA—the past, present, and future *Biostatistics* **18** 417–21

[20] Labbé E 2010 Japanese regulations *Principles and Practice of Pharmaceutical Medicine* (Wiley) ch 38 pp 509–27

[21] Chattu V K, Singh B, Pattanshetty S and Reddy S 2023 Access to medicines through global health diplomacy *Health Promot. Perspect.* **13** 40

[22] Nugent P, Duncan J N and Colagiovanni D B 2017 Preparation of a preclinical dossier to support an investigational new drug (IND) application and first-in-human clinical trial *A Comprehensive Guide to Toxicology in Nonclinical Drug Development* (New York: Academic) pp 189–213

[23] Shamley D and Wright B (ed) 2017 *A Comprehensive and Practical Guide to Clinical Trials* (Academic)

[24] Ali J and Baboota S (ed) 2021 *Regulatory Affairs in the Pharmaceutical Industry* (New York: Academic)

[25] Rauch G, Schüler S and Kieser M 2017 *Planning and Analyzing Clinical Trials with Composite Endpoints* (Cham, Switzerland: Springer)

[26] Stryjewski T P, Kalish B T, Silverman B and Lehmann L S 2015 The impact of institutional review boards (IRBs) on clinical innovation: a survey of investigators and IRB members *J. Empir. Res. Hum. Res. Ethics* **10** 481–7

[27] Sinha M S 2021 Costly gadgets: barriers to market entry and price competition for generic drug-device combinations in the United States *Minn. JL Sci. Tech.* **23** 293

[28] Adams M, Caffrey L and McKevitt C 2015 Barriers and opportunities for enhancing patient recruitment and retention in clinical research: findings from an interview study in an NHS academic health science centre *Health Res. Policy Syst.* **13** 1–9

[29] Dugger S A, Platt A and Goldstein D B 2018 Drug development in the era of precision medicine *Nat. Rev. Drug Discov.* **17** 183–96

[30] Li Q, Lin J and Lin Y 2020 Adaptive design implementation in confirmatory trials: methods, practical considerations and case studies *Contemp. Clin. Trials* **98** 106096

[31] Stephenson D *et al* 2020 Precompetitive consensus building to facilitate the use of digital health technologies to support Parkinson disease drug development through regulatory science *Digit. Biomark.* **4** 28–49

[32] Nilsen P, Roback K, Broström A and Ellström P E 2012 Creatures of habit: accounting for the role of habit in implementation research on clinical behaviour change *Implement. Sci.* **7** 1–6

[33] Druker B J *et al* 2006 Five-year follow-up of patients receiving imatinib for chronic myeloid leukemia *New Engl. J. Med.* **355** 2408–17

[34] Jabbour E and Kantarjian H 2020 Chronic myeloid leukemia: 2020 update on diagnosis, therapy and monitoring *Am. J. Hematol.* **95** 691–709

[35] Broug E, Bland-Ward P A, Powell J and Johnson K S 2010 Fab-arm exchange *Nat. Biotechnol.* **28** 123–5

[36] Eastwood D, Findlay L, Poole S, Bird C, Wadhwa M, Moore M, Burns C, Thorpe R and Stebbings R 2010 Monoclonal antibody TGN1412 trial failure explained by species differences in CD28 expression on CD4+ effector memory T-cells *Br. J. Pharmacol.* **161** 512–26

[37] Tao R, Han X, Bai X, Yu J, Ma Y, Chen W, Zhang D and Li Z 2024 Revolutionizing cancer treatment: enhancing CAR-T cell therapy with CRISPR/Cas9 gene editing technology *Fron. Immunol.* **15** 1354825

[38] Vora L K, Gholap A D, Jetha K, Thakur R R S, Solanki H K and Chavda V P 2023 Artificial intelligence in pharmaceutical technology and drug delivery design *Pharmaceutics* **15** 1916

[39] Vora L K, Gholap A D, Jetha K, Thakur R R S, Solanki H K and Chavda V P 2023 Artificial intelligence in pharmaceutical technology and drug delivery design *Pharmaceutics* 2023**15** 1916

[40] Dang A 2023 Real-world evidence: a primer *Pharm. Med.* **37** 25–36
[41] Rehm H L *et al* 2021 GA4GH: International policies and standards for data sharing across genomic research and healthcare *Cell Genom* **1** 100029
[42] Årsand E and Demiris G 2008 User-centered methods for designing patient-centric self-help tools *Inform. Health Soc. Care* **33** 158–69

IOP Publishing

Viral Diseases

History and new developments in diagnostics and therapeutics

Arvind K Singh Chandel, Bhakti Tanna, Amisha Parmar, Gopal Patel and Neeraj S Thakur

Chapter 5

Molecular diagnostic techniques utilized in viral diseases

Raghawendra Kumar, Madhav Kumar, Bhakti Tanna and Bhavya Bhargava

The global human population has encountered different types of major issues of viral infections across the world. The recent outbreak of COVID-19 caused by SARS-CoV-2, monkeypox, H1N1, ebola, Nipah virus, etc serve as prime examples of how a viral infection could pose a extremely dangerous and negative impact on public health, world economy, and mental trauma. Thus, early and accurate diagnosis is the most important first step in the fight against the viral infection. Early and accurate diagnosis of viral samples is vital for the proper treatment, control, and prevention of the epidemic in society. The advancement of molecular techniques, such as polymerase chain reaction (PCR) has facilitated the accurate and efficient diagnosis of infections. Moreover, an advancement like real-time RT-PCR is sensitive and also quantifies viral infections. Molecular-based techniques such as Enzyme-Linked Immunosorbent (ELISA) and PCR are the backbone of viral assay. These techniques also serve as a platform for the development of other advances in the field, including biosensors, loop-mediated isothermal amplification (LAMP), polymerase spiral reaction (PSR), RT-PCR, microarrays and next-generation sequencing (NGS). In this chapter, we provide a summary of the features of commonly used viral infection diagnostic techniques, with an emphasis on the cutting-edge real-time PCR technique.

5.1 Introduction

Diagnosis is a vital part of addressing the repercussions of any fatal contagious diseases. Diagnostic procedures identify the presence or absence of an infectious agent. In the past, minimizing mortality caused by highly contagious and infectious diseases has been achieved by early and accurate diagnosis [1]. Diagnosis plays the most important role in such diseases that are caused by any unknown pathogen for which the community is not pre-immune before spreading in the population. The

doi:10.1088/978-0-7503-4987-1ch5

recent emergence of novel coronaviruses' nCOVID-19 has been highly infectious and deadly, resulting in extreme losses all over the world [2]. The epidemics have been associated with massive losses in both economic and social impact in several countries over the past 2.5 years. Most of the human and animal diseases are frequently brought on by viral infections. Worldwide, the hepatitis and human immunodeficiency viruses (HIV) kill millions of lives. The newly emerging or modified viruses in the human population are also causing serious health problems. Various viruses have trigerred multiple outbreaks across different countries, including avian influenza A (H5N1) in 1997, the 2002–03 outbreak of severe acute respiratory syndrome coronavirus (SARS-CoV), swine influenza A (H1N1) virus in 2009, the Ebola virus and Zika virus (ZIKV) in 2014, 2015, and most recently, pandemic SARS-CoV-2 outbreaks in 2019–20 worldwide. There has been demand for the establishment of strong and reliable new molecular-based diagnostic techniques to minimize the spread as well as early detection of such emergences as swine fever, highly virulent avian influenza, and COVID-19.

Through the constant advancement of various technologies, the laboratory-based diagnosis of viral infection has been improving throughout time to enhance objectivity, accuracy, and sensitivity [3]. Various techniques have been widely employed to identify viral infection in clinical samples. Higher throughputs have also been made possible by modifications to a few of these techniques. These methods are broadly classified as nucleic acid-based amplification assays, sequencing-based assays, and antigen–antibody based serological assays. Although cell culture-based approach is one of the 'gold standards' for diagnosing viral infection [3, 4], it takes a long time, has low sensitivity and specificity, and carries a high risk of contamination [5]. To get around these drawbacks, molecular biology techniques like the traditional PCR, quantitative real-time PCR (qRT-PCR), and next-generation sequencing (NGS), are currently being used for virus diagnosis. The qRT-PCR has a gold standard in diagnosis because of higher accuracy and sensitivity compared with conventional PCR. However, RT-PCR, which uses the threshold cycle as start the amplification point, can measure viral nucleic acids by validating the amplification. Nevertheless, in clinically suspected cases, a negative RT-PCR does not rule out the possibility of infection to avoid false-negative reporting, such results should be interpreted carefully [6, 7]. PCR-based diagnosis of viral infection is easy, fast, accurate, and suitable for the diagnostic disease progression treatment for the clinical trial.

New methods developed for the diagnosis of a viral infection include DNA microarray and NGS. Microarrays are suitable for the diagnosis of bulk samples surveillance of epidemics. A collection of spots affixed to a solid support, each containing one or more fragments of single-stranded DNA oligonucleotides, is known as a DNA array (DNA chip) [8]. In the microarray, fluorescently labeled nucleic acids of the virus are used for the test, while oligonucleotide probes are in microarray chips. These probes specifically hybridize with the target viral genome. Using fluorescently labeled viral nucleic acids in a test sample and DNA microarray diagnosis, various oligonucleotide probes immobilized on a solid surface (such as a glass slide) are screened. The oligonucleotide probes utilized here are unique to the target virus's genome. Immobilization of the target virus genome is in a microarray chip, after which there is hybridization between targeted sequences and probes and fluorescent light is emitted, which is detected and quantified by fluorescence-based detection. The microarray chip contains many probes so it is useful to diagnose multiple samples in a single reaction. The first application of microarray was to identify a mutation in the HIV genome, which is linked to resistance to antiretroviral drugs [9]. Subsequently, some researchers developed microarrays that detect several viruses such as respiratory viruses, hepatitis C virus, and central nervous system (CNS) infection caused by viruses [10–12]. High-throughput multiplex detection of gastrointestinal viruses, infections spread by small mammals, arthropods, herpesviruses, enteroviruses, flaviviruses, HIV-1, HIV-2, and hepatitis viruses, as well as double infections like dengue two virus serotype, have all been successfully detected using microarray technology [13–18]. DNA microarray is also used in the screening of mutation in hepatitis B virus (HBV) genotype associated with drug-resistant strains, determining the, lineage of influenza viruses, identifying the genotype of SARS coronavirus 2002 in china and is also helpful in detecting novel coronavirus family [19–21].

The NGS-based methods for the diagnosis of viruses are the most recent development and they can directly investigate viral infection by sequencing the DNA/RNA fragments from clinical samples [22, 23]. Usually, NGS-based detection involves several steps in test sample preparation such as fragmentation, library preparation, quantification of library, and sequencing of the target sequences. The sequencing platform is also important because different NGS instruments use different platform, methods, reagents and the most importantly the analysis tools. Therefore, it needs a suitable platform and bioinformatics tool for the data analysis [24, 25]. Kustin *et al* (2019) [26] used NGS for fast and thorough identification of respiratory viruses in clinical samples. It was successfully used for the tracking of influenza A (H1N1) pdm09 virus, drug resistance strain of HIV-1, and discovery of the Ebola virus [27–30].

5.1.1 Viral sampling, isolation, and purification of nucleic acids

Before the isolation of viral genetic material, the laboratory worker should be familiar with all techniques of both pre- and post-analytical methods. The detection of viruses in a clinical setting has a direct impact on patient treatment and outcomes. It also provides critical information about clinical judgment, hospital infection prevention and control, duration of patient stay in hospital, costs of treatment and laboratory efficiency [31]. Therefore, proper and timely diagnosis and treatment are essential for patient recovery. So proper accurate selection of diagnostic tests, along with timely collection, transportation, and storage of clinical patient specimens, is essential to ensure reliable virus detection and diagnosis [31]. From this point of view, professionals who work in a virology lab should be trained and have proper experience in molecular biology both practical and theoretical [32]. The World Health Organization (WHO) and the Centers for Disease Control and Prevention (CDC) are regularly updating the proper guidelines for collection and sampling of viral diseases. In fact, the approaches used for clinical sampling, storage, and transport are very important for diagnostic results. Apart from this, isolation of DNA/RNA from viruses is the most vital step in PCR, real-time PCR, microarray, and NGS technology. The isolation of nucleic acid from viral samples is broadly classified into five methods in both manual and commercial kits available in the market that use boiling of samples, an ion-exchange matrix, DNA precipitation, magnetic bead glass particles, and a silica membrane to purify the viral DNA/RNA [33, 34]. The extraction of viral genetic material should be executed according to protocol with respected methods to quantity and type of the specimen. The purity of nucleic acids also influences test results. After isolation, the 260/280 and 260/230 ratios should be close to 2 to ensure higher PCR efficiency and accuracy in other test methods.

5.1.1.1 PCR-based techniques

PCR is a model example of amplification of the target DNA/RNA. It has advanced the area of molecular biology developed by Mullis and Faloona [35]. The most crucial steps in PCR are the base purification of viral genetic material and the use of thermostable DNA polymerase and two particular oligonucleotide primers for exponential amplification of the target sequence. Since its beginning, PCR was used for the detection of viral infection in humans with a sensitivity range of 77.8%–100%, and clinical specificity of such samples is 89%–100% [36–39]. In the past, researchers used conventional PCR for diagnosis purposes and some laboratories worldwide still use it. PCR is an outstanding multilateral technique for the detection of viruses in many types of samples. For the development of technique, different types of conventional PCR technique have been developed. However, the most important and gold standard in molecular biology variants are RT-PCR and real-time PCR [40, 41].

5.1.1.1.1 Polymerase chain reaction (PCR)

PCR is a technique in which millions to billions of copies of a targeted nucleic acid sequence can be amplified rapidly. Short synthetic DNA fragments (primers) are involved in the PCR, which is specific to a segment of the genome to be amplified. DNA polymerase copies the DNA strand and after multiple rounds of synthesis, millions of copies of DNA are synthesized. The PCR reaction mixture consists of target DNA, two different oligonucleotide primers (specific for forward and reverse strands), a DNA polymerase (Taq polymerase is commonly used in normal PCR), a combination of Tris-HCL, $MgCl_2$, KCL and deoxy-ribonucleotide triphosphates (dNTPs). In a thermal cycler, the reaction mixture in PCR tubes is heated and cooled repeatedly, and after *n* cycles, the target DNA sequence can be amplified. After the PCR amplification, the amplified product can be detected using agarose gel electrophoresis [42]. The normal PCR technique is used for the detection of a wide range of DNA viruses, e.g., members of the same virus family or genus. To amplification of target viral sequences the primers are designed based on conserved regions of the virus genome [43]. This PCR technique is very valuable for diagnostic viral disease.

5.1.1.1.2 Reverse transcription-PCR

RT-PCR (reverse-transcription polymerase chain reaction) is a method used in RNA viruses by reverse transcription of RNA into DNA (cDNA) and then amplification of target DNA using PCR [44]. This technique is primarily used to amplify RNA targets. During the RT-PCR method, initially, RNA is converted into cDNA by using a reverse transcriptase enzyme and then the cDNA is amplified by PCR. In this process, a thermostable DNA polymerase from *Thermus thermophiles* (Tth polymerase) can be efficiently used as both an RT and a DNA polymerase [45]. There are commercial kits available in the market for dignosis of HCV RNA and HIV-1 (Roche Diagnostics, Indianapolis, IN). RT-PCR is an excellent method for the detection/diagnosis of human infection caused by RNA viruses. Some of the common examples of RNA viruses involved in human infection are Ebola, SARS-CoV-2, which is widely diagnosed by using RT-PCR technique [46–48]. In the detection of coronavirus, the RT-PCR technique played an important role globally.

5.1.1.1.3 Nested-PCR

In this PCR technique, two pairs of primers are used for the amplification in two rounds of PCR. In the first round of PCR, an initial primer pair is used for 15–30 cycles, depending on the specific PCR protocol. The amplified product from the first round then undergoes a second round of amplification using a different primer pair. This nested PCR technique enhances specificity and sensitivity, making it highly effective for detecting target sequences. [49]. The main drawback of this technique is associated with a high rate of non-specific amplification. The detection of Herpesviruses can be done using this technique.

5.1.1.1.4 Multiplex PCR

In the multiplex PCR technique, more than one primer pair (each primer pair is designed for the amplification of a different gene) in the same reaction mixture allows the amplification of distinct targets at the same time [50]. The main advantage of this technique is that multiple targets can be co-amplified in a single tube without the wastage of the PCR reaction mixture. However, care must be taken for the selection of primers because all the primer sets to be used should have similar annealing temperatures and there should be a lack of complementarity between/within the primers. Multiplex PCR is less sensitive than other PCR techniques that use a single primer set. Multiplex PCR tests have been developed and commercialized for detecting different diseases such as viral respiratory pathogens, CNS infections, Herpesviruses, respiratory viruses, etc [51, 52].

5.1.1.1.5 Real-time PCR

Real-time PCR, also known as qPCR, is a technique that combines simultaneous target amplification and detection. In this method, a special thermal cycler is used which can detect the fluorescence emission from the sample [53]. Specially created software that is compatible with a thermal cycler tracks the data at each cycle and creates an amplification plot. The qPCR approach has gained immense popularity in the field of molecular diagnostics due to its remarkable sensitivity, specificity, huge dynamic range, and minimal or no post-amplification processing (e.g., gel electrophoresis or nanodrop reading) [54]. Fluorescence resonance energy transfer (FRET) probes can be used to boost the specificity of qPCR [55]. In another approach dual hybridization probes that can use two specially designed sequence-specific probes can be used. Finally, molecular beacons can be used to detect and quantify amplification products. The main advantage of qPCR is the reduction of contamination and the possibility of quantitative applications. Several variants of qPCR methods and chemistries, such as TaqMAN, dye-labelled oligonucleotide ligation molecular beacons (MB), scorpion primers, and primer–probe energy tansfer system, are used today. Most viruses carrying DNA as their genetic materials can be detected using this technique.

5.1.1.1.6 Loop-mediated isothermal amplification (LAMP)

The main disadvantage of nucleic acid amplification methods is a requirement of an expensive thermal cycler. To overcome this problem, isothermal techniques were introduced as viral diagnostic tools because of their easy operation, fast reaction, and simple detection. These isothermal techniques do not require the precision thermal cycler and can use water baths and/or heating blocks. LAMP is a simple low-cost single isothermal tube technique for the amplification of DNA to detect certain diseases [56]. This is an improved classical PCR because of its increased amplification efficiency and accuracy. This method is very fast and can be accomplished within an hour. The process of LAMP can be carried out either with a heating block or water bath so there is no need for expensive thermal cyclers. It is a one-step amplification process that operates at isothermal temperatures. The strand displacement principle is the foundation of LAMP chemistry [57]. LAMP basically operates in a three-step process: a non-cycling step, a cyclic amplification step and a final elongation step. Reverse transcriptase enzyme (RT-LAMP) is a tool that can be used for amplification of cDNA from RNA. The method of LAMP has been widely used for viral infections such as Dengue and SARS viruses [58, 59]. The RT-LAMP approach has been developed to identify HSV, VZV, CMV, HPV, and BK viruses in addition to influenza A and B viruses [60–65].

5.1.1.1.7 Transcription-based amplification methods

Transcription-based amplification method is a combination of two procedures for viral diagnosis, the first is nucleic acid sequence-based amplification (NASBA), and the second is transcription-mediated amplification (TMA). It is a two-step process: the first step is denaturation of the nucleic acid, and the second step is temperature-based isothermal amplification [66]. The whole amplification procedure is carried out at 41 °C. In the first step, viral RNA is reverse transcribed into cDNA using reverse transcriptase (RT) in both methods, after that multiple copies of viral RNA are produced with the help of RNA polymerase. Fluorochrome labeled probes are added to the PCR reaction for real-time monitoring. In the amplification process, the only distinction between TMA and NASBA is the existence of two enzymes RT and RNA polymerase. TMA uses two enzymes, while NASBA uses three different enzymes RNase H, T7 RNA polymerase and avian myeloblastosis virus reverse transcriptase (AMV-RT) [67]. Multiplex real-time nucleic acid sequence-based amplification (RT-NASBA) has been developed to detect infections caused by Rotavirus A and Norovirus Geno group II/Astrovirus [68].

Transcription-based amplification methods have numerous advantages such as not needing a PCR machine such that those countries on limited budget can use this method for dignosis purposes. It is fast and time less time consuming and produces single-stranded RNA (ssRNA) [69, 70]. This RT-NASBA multiplex is more sensitive compared to normal multiplex RT-PCR and the advantage is that it detects multiple infections at the same time. The RNA virus infection in human transcription-based amplification methods is appropriate for the diagnosis.

5.1.1.2 Microarray

In this technique thousands to millions of known single-stranded DNA fragments (oligonucleotide) are attached to a solid support (DNA array or DNA chip). High-density arrays, which allow the attachment of hundreds to thousands of oligonucleotides, are known as microarrays. The DNA chip is then bathed with labeled amplified DNA or RNA products isolated from the sample. In this way, complementary base pairing between the amplified product and DNA chip immobilized fragment (hybridization) occurs. The hybridization signals generated during the hybridization process are mapped to several locations within the array. The PCR sequences can be identified by the pattern of hybridization (in the case of large probes). The hybridization results are revealed by scanning the DNA array surface. Fluorescent signals from the array surface are detected using confocal microscopy and precise locations of hybridization on the chip are observed. Based on the variations of multiple DNA sequences present on the chip, multiple viruses can be analysed simultaneously. Microarrays have been used in diagnostic virology for the detection of viral mutations associated with antiretroviral drug resistance [9]. Some researchers developed the microarrays that can detect numerous viruses' infection such as hepatitis C virus, respiratory viruses [10] and virus-causing CNS infection [12].

5.1.1.3 Next-generation sequencing

NGS is very useful for the diagnosis/identification of viruses in clinical samples. It is a revolution in molecular biology and increases understanding about transmission, characterization, and molecular epidemiology of pathogens. As a substitute for each analysis, because a large number of gene sequences are deposited in the public database in the clinical sample which can be identified in a single run. NGS applications are most useful and resourceful in molecular biology and are commonly acknowledged as a diagnostic tool. Different modifications and improvements will make it more practical and allow large changes in the sequencing and identification of viral genomes. NGS involves several steps starting from isolation of viral genetic material from a clinical specimen sample, fragmentation or PCR amplification of targeted sequences. This is followed by library preparation, and quantification of the library followed by sequencing using suitable platforms [24, 25]. However, different companies provide different platforms and machines, using different reagent methods for sequencing (single end or pair end) and most important data analysis with suitable bioinformatics tools [23].

The NGS instrument started with pyrosequencing on the Roach 454 platform, detecting a pyrophosphate that is released during DNA polymerization. The Illumina platform provides paired-end production and detection process with fluorescently labeled nucleotides added during DNA polymerization. The third-generation sequencing platforms are PacBio and Oxford nanopore (MinION), produce long-read sequences, allowing for more comprehensive genomic analysis. The detection is based on sensing of ionic current of nucleic acid either DNA/RNA which is passed through the nanopores [23–25]. The main problem in the MinION nanopore sequencer is in terms of error rate and analysis software. However, each improvement in the sequencing platform has increased the efficiency, read length, and read size and, most importantly, reduced the error rate [71, 72]. Third-generation sequencers have the benefit of being quick and inexpensive enough to sequence an entire virus' genome, making them particularly accessible in low- and middle-income nations [71, 73]. The advantage of NGS in diagnostics does not require prior knowledge of genome sequences of any unknown viruses [74, 75]. However, it comes with limitations in clinical laboratories due to the time consumption, required large number of samples to run the cost of sequencers, and most importantly bioinformatics analysis with skilled person [76].

5.1.1.4 Viral genotyping

In biology, medicine, and agriculture, the detection of viral pathogens is essential. Unfortunately, existing methods for screening for a wide range of viruses have significant limitations [77]. Virus genotyping is most important for epidemiology studies and development of effective vaccines for treatment of major viral diseases such as HIV and hepatitis. The use of antiviral drugs to treat reactive herpesvirus infection, as well as the combinations of drugs to reduce or inactivate the viral replication in HIV infection, has been selected for drug resistance mutations. For example, genotypes of HIV-1 in clinical samples correlation with available clinical data is vital for identifying and quantification in AIDS patients regarding viral drug resistance [78, 79]. Hepatitis B virus (HBV) genotyping is used to screen epidemiology research, and various genotypes of the hepatitis virus have been linked to varying degrees of acute liver damage and chronic disease in some recent studies on the severity of hepatitis [80]. For hepatitis C virus (HCV), effective treatment is based on the viral genotype [81]. A drug-resistant viral strain can quickly become the dominant phenotype under selective pressure. However, molecular-based diagnosis has improved the clinical management of such patients by making it easier to identify mutations conferring resistance [82]. Although these techniques have been employed in the past to identify resistance to a family of antiviral drugs known as reverse transcriptase inhibitors, they are likely to be applied to additional phenotypic factors due to their speed and affordability. The same method has been used to genotype HCV infection for treatment progression and epidemiological studies [83].

Tracking and treatment of viruses of genetic variable strain is most important to assess how many particular virus variants are circulating in the country. Today, NGS technology solves this issue with rapid sequencing and analysis of viruses' genomes giving proper information about genotypes. For example, the genotype of

HCV strain of the virus identifies when people were infected or tested in a particular location. The ‘genotype’ of HCV that each patient with chronic infection with the hepatitis C virus carries is a crucial factor. Frequently, a clinical sample was tested in blood tests but did not give information about which genotypes were in circulation in a particular country. Due to selective pressure, environmental conditions, and the immune system, the genotypes of HCV are genetically different groups, that is, they evolve with slight modifications of their genome. Nearly 75% of Americans infected with HCV genotype 1 subtypes of viruses were 1a or 1b, and around 20%–25% of populations infected with either genotype 2 or 3, and genotype 4, but genotype 5 infects the population much less [84]. The majority of patients infected with HCV are found to contain genotype 1, other genotype-infected patients are quite unlikely to be infected with multiple genotypes [85]. In Africa and other parts of the world, HCV genotype 4 is common, and genotype 6 is common in Southeast Asia. The distribution of HCV genotype in each area of the world is unique and depends upon several factors [86]. Another illustration of the genotyping of the Measles virus can be useful for treatment, tracking and identifying transmission pathways during investigations. The genotyping results can help refute, confirm, or distinguish links between cases. If two cases have identical N-450 sequences, they may be linked even if the link is not noticeable. Genotyping can also tell the difference between a wild-type measles virus infection and an infection caused by vaccination, because due to vaccination few people show rash and fever 10–14 days after the vaccination. For control, with measles outbreaks in particular regions or countries a large population is vaccintated to control the outbreaks. In such cases, a vaccine reaction could potentially be misinterpreted as a measles infection. Therefore, in that situation virus genotyping is most important to distinguish the genotype of the clinical sample [87]. The recent emerging global COVID-19 infection caused by SARS novel Coronavirus (SARS-nCoV-2) was a serious public global threat. Viruses evolve quickly with modification of their own genome. The genotyping of virus isolates in clinical samples is critical for understanding the evolution and transmission of SARS-CoV-2. The genotyping of SARS-CoV-2 used multiple sequences alignment method of isolated genome with reference genome. The single nucleotide polymorphism (SNP) difference was measured by Jaccard distances to identify the evolutionary history and relationship with the reference strain. The genotyping of SARS-CoV-2 isolates from around the world reveals the specific most common mutation or multiple nucleotide polymorphism (MNP) during the current epidemic. The analysis of SARS-CoV-2 genome shows most mutations occur in S proteins and RNA polymerase, RNA primase, and nucleoprotein. These mutations are crucial for the control of outbreaks and vaccine development [88].

5.1.1.5 Enzymatic-based methods

The capability to recognize disease with high specificity and sensitivity is a vital part of any healthcare system and a valuable tool in biomedical research. *In vitro* diagnostics (IVDs) using the enzymes with an incredible variety of mechanisms and a wide range of biochemical processes plays a significant role in identifying the disease at both individual and population levels. This is predominantly important for viral infectious diseases, where IVDs aid in disease tracing and provide crucial data for epidemiological models, which helps to slow down or stop the spread of disease. Enzyme-based processes are easily exploitable for signal generation in the presence of disease biomarkers. In this section, we will look at some of the more popular approaches.

5.1.1.6 CRISPR-Cas enzyme-based detection

Nucleases are enzymes that catalyse the chemical reaction for nucleic acid degradation and have been widely used for several decades for nucleic acid amplification, also known as enzyme-assisted nucleic acid amplification. Various nucleases have recently found use as tools for gene editing; several research groups are now exploring their potential for diagnostic applications. One of the most important proteins, effector proteins, known as Cas proteins, are crucial to the clustered regularly interspaced short palindromic repeats (CRISPR)-Cas system. Cas effector proteins are capable of cleaving DNA or RNA. The cleavage activity of the Cas proteins is regulated by guide-RNAs, which point them to the appropriate cutting spot on the target nucleic acid. In the CRISPR-Cas system's guide, RNA guides the sequences' specific modification for nucleic acid detection [89]. Different nucleases have recently been identified by several researchers to be useful for the gene tool and, further, this tool is used for diagnostic applications. The working procedure of these CRISPR-Cas systems is different from other molecular techniques. First, they are integrated with the specific sequences, which cause pathogenicity, transcribed, and processed into small non-coding RNAs. After that, the Cas nuclease binds with guided sequences and follows selective degradation.

5.1.1.7 Biosensors-based detection

Biosensors-based diagnosis of the viral disease is rapid for diagnosis of viruses in different samples. Biosensors are analytical tools that convert biological responses into measurable signals [90]. Choosing the appropriate type of membrane is a crucial step in the building of biosensors. Numerous researchers have employed both organic and inorganic materials, such as nylon, sodium azide, nitrocellulose, and polyether-sulfonate. The detection limit is the primary goal of all biosensors, although any protein or the entire virus can be detected [91].

The transducer subsequently converts this biological response into a signal that the digital detector module can measure [92, 93]. The three primary types of transducing systems are piezoelectric, optical, and electrochemical. Electrochemical biosensors use potentiometric, amperometric, or impedimetric measurements to detect changes in charge distribution over the transducer surface transduction principles [94–98]. Because optical biosensors provide multiplexed detection within a single device, they are adaptable and flexible tools for analytical purposes. When an analyte interacts with a recognition element, these devices focus on measuring the optical properties and surface characteristics of the transducer [99–101]. Transducers used in piezoelectric biosensors react to an applied external alternating electrical field. Their foundation lies in the identification of resonance frequency fluctuations caused by immobilized biological material and crystal mass. Based on the corresponding change in electrical signal upon contact with the analytic medium, the mass difference can be calculated. These biosensors have a wide range uses in medicine, including the detection of targets in biological systems [102–104].

Biosensor-based detection of viruses is fast and plays a vital role in diagnosing the infection and preventing the spread of diseases and pathologies [105]. Compared to traditional methods like biochemical tests and immunoassays, biosensors deliver results that are more precise, sensitive, quick, and repeatable. They have found extensive use in the field of medical diagnostics [106]. Because they are portable and may be used for point-of-care testing (POCT) that can assess actual biological samples in typical clinical settings, biosensors are being used in clinical analysis more and more [107]. The detection of biological specimens has increased when using nanotechnology to develop improved biosensors, and creation of self-assembled monolayer (SAM) biointerfaces that increase biocompatibility and resistance to non-specific adsorption [108, 109]. POCT is one of the most valuable and effective techniques of biosensors for the identification of viral infection. POCT measurement is the process of doing a diagnostic test close to the patient resulting in quick findings without requiring the assistance of a particular lab. This testing provides accurate, convenient, and, more importantly, effective and quick treatment for when viral infection spreads rapidly in the community. Additionally, these devices don't need expensive instruments to diagnose viral infections [110, 111]. Initial and correct diagnosis is important for determining the true origin and nature of any disease. Currently, the emphasis is on early detection of COVID-19 disease. Saliva plays an important role in non-invasive salivary diagnostics, which offer a practical and affordable POCT platform for quick diagnosis and may be an effort to increase the likelihood of survival of patients with COVID-19 disease [111, 112].

5.1.1.8 Nucleic acid-based biosensors

5.1.1.8.1 Polymerase chain reaction (PCR) biosensors

PCR biosensors are designed to detect viral genetic material (RNA or DNA) through amplification. Real-time PCR biosensors can provide quantitative results, allowing for the determination of viral load.

5.1.1.8.2 Loop-mediated isothermal amplification (LAMP) biosensors

LAMP biosensors offer isothermal amplification of nucleic acids, making them suitable for field applications. They are used to detect viral RNA or DNA rapidly and sensitively.

5.1.1.8.3 CRISPR-Cas biosensors

These biosensors use the CRISPR-Cas system to target and cleave specific viral nucleic acids. They can provide rapid and specific detection of viral genomes.

5.1.1.8.4 Antibody-based biosensors

ELISA: ELISA-based biosensors use antibodies to detect viral proteins or antigens in patient samples, such as blood or saliva. They are widely used for the detection of viral infections like HIV, hepatitis, and COVID-19.

5.1.1.8.5 Surface plasmon resonance (SPR) biosensors

SPR biosensors measure changes in refractive index caused by antibody-antigen binding. They are highly sensitive and can be used to detect viral proteins at low concentrations.

5.1.1.8.6 Lateral flow assays (LFAs)

LFAs are simple, paper-based biosensors that use antibodies to capture viral antigens. They are commonly used for rapid, POCT for viruses like HIV and influenza.

5.1.1.8.7 Virus-integrated biosensors

(a) **Virus-based biosensors:** Some biosensors incorporate modified viruses that are engineered to interact with specific target molecules, making them highly specific and versatile for various viral detections.

5.1.1.8.8 Microfluidic biosensors

(a) **Lab-on-a-chip biosensors:** These miniaturized biosensors integrate various detection methods into a small chip. They are often used for point-of-care diagnostics, enabling rapid and automated viral disease detection.

(b) **Smartphone-based biosensors:** Mobile Health (mHealth) Biosensors: Some biosensors are designed to work with smartphones, allowing users to perform viral disease tests at home or in resource-limited settings. Results can be transmitted digitally to healthcare providers for remote monitoring.

(c) **Biosensors for emerging viruses:** Biosensors can be quickly adapted for the detection of emerging viral diseases. For instance, biosensors were rapidly developed and deployed for the detection of SARS-CoV-2 during the COVID-19 pandemic.

5.1.2 Conclusion

In recent years, molecular tools for diagnostics of viral infection have been important for global public health. The use of molecular diagnostics provides crucial information based on the early discovery of infections and minor alterations in their patients' genes and chromosomes. Assisting earlier diagnosis, the choice of suitable treatments, and the tracking of illness development. Using molecular tools such as PCR, real-time PCR, FISH, microarrays biosensor and sequencing technologies, a large number of molecular assays are available to assess DNA/RNA to identify the alteration, mutation, or gene silencing changes in gene expression. However, there are several obstacles to overcome before these tests are carried out in the clinical laboratory, like which test is suitable, selection of technology, equipment, cost effectiveness, reproducibility, accuracy and proper training of testing staff. Currently, conventional PCR-based testing is successful but different technology needs to explore the genome complexity and also incorporate the sequencing technology to be more robust. Furthermore, the development of nanobiotechnology and integrated silicon base chip coating with biomolecules specific nucleic acid or protein will change the traditional lab-based test concept.

Thus it is possible to analyze thousands of genes and proteins in a short time with a low amount of sample. The usage of commercial electrodes, such as screen-printed electrodes, and equipment that can simultaneously detect many respiratory viruses provides some perspective.

Abbreviations

AMV-RT	Avian myeloblastosis virus reverse transcriptase
CDC	Centers for Disease Control Prevention
cDNA	complementary DNA
CMV	Cytomegalovirus
CNS	Central nervous system
COVID-19	Coronavirus disease 2019
DNA	Deoxyribonucleic acid
ELISA	Enzyme-linked immunoassay
FISH	Fluorescence *in situ* hybridization
FRET	Fluorescence resonance energy transfer
H1N1	Swine influenza A (H1N1)
HCV	hepatitis C virus
HIV	Human immunodeficiency virus
HPV	Human papillomavirus
HSV	Herpes simplex virus
IVDs	*In vitro* diagnostics
LAMP	loop mediated isothermal amplification
LFAs	Lateral flow assays
MB	Molecular beacons
MNP	Multiple nucleotide polymorphism
NASBA	Nucleic acid sequence-based amplification
NGS	Next generation sequencing
PCR	Polymerase chain reaction
POCT	Point-of-care testing
PSR	Polymerase spiral reaction
qRT-PCR	Quantitative real-time reverse-transcription PCR
RNA	Ribonucleic acid
RT-PCR	Reverse transcription polymerase chain reaction
SARS-CoV-2	Severe acute respiratory syndrome coronavirus 2
SAM	Self-assembled monolayer
VZV	Varicella zoster virus
WHO	World Health Organization

References

[1] Caliendo A M *et al* 2013 Better tests, better care: improved diagnostics for infectious diseases *Clin. Infect. Dis* **57** S139–70

[2] Cascella M, Rajnik M, Aleem A, Dulebohn S C and Di Napoli R 2018 Features, evaluation, and treatment of coronavirus (COVID-19) *StatPearls* (Treasure Island, FL: StatPearls)

[3] Hwang K A, Ahn J H and Nam J H 2018 Diagnosis of viral infection using real-time polymerase chain reaction *J. Bacteriol. Virol.* **48** 1–3

[4] Malik Y S *et al* 2019 Advances in diagnostic approaches for viral etiologies of diarrhea: from the lab to the field *Front. Microbiol.* **10** 1957

[5] Dohla M *et al* 2020 Rapid point-of-care testing for SARS-CoV-2 in a community screening setting shows low sensitivity *Public Health* **182** 170–2

[6] Wang Y *et al* 2019 A sandwich-type electrochemical immunosensor for ultrasensitive detection of tumor markers using NH2-MIL-125(Ti) and NH2-MIL-125(Ti)-AuPt nanocomposites as signal tags *Biosens. Bioelectron.* **127** 50–7

[7] Kucirka L M, Lauer S A, Laeyendecker O, Boon D and Lessler J 2020 Variation in false-negative rate of reverse transcriptase polymerase chain reaction–based SARS-CoV-2 tests by time since exposure *Ann. Intern. Med.* **173** 262–7

[8] Hackett J L, Archer K J, Gaigalas A K, Garrett C T, Joseph L J, Koch W H, Kricka L J, McGlennen R C, Van Deerlin V and Vasquez G B 2006 *Diagnostic Nucleic Acid Microarrays; Approved Guideline* (Wayne, PA: Clinical and Laboratory Standards Institute)

[9] Kozal M J *et al* 1996 Extensive polymorphisms observed in HIV–1 clade B protease gene using high–density oligonucleotide arrays *Nat. Med.* **2** 753–9

[10] Coiras M T, López-Huertas M R, López-Campos G, Aguilar J C and Pérez-Breña P 2005 Oligonucleotide array for simultaneous detection of respiratory viruses using a reverse-line blot hybridization assay *J. Med. Virol* **76** 256–64

[11] Xu Z, Qiao J, Sheng Y, Liu Y, Li Z, Wei L, Pan H and Xiao F 2019 Development of a lateral flow biosensor for visual detection of enterovirus 71 using a pair of sandwich-type aptamers *Anal. Chim. Acta* **1055** 140–8

[12] Leveque N, Van Haecke A, Renois F, Boutolleau D, Talmud D and Andreoletti L 2011 Rapid virological diagnosis of central nervous system infections by use of a multiplex reverse transcription-PCR DNA microarray *J. Clin. Microbiol.* **49** 3874–9

[13] Díaz-Badillo A, de Lourdes Muñoz M, Perez-Ramirez G, Altuzar V, Burgueño J, Mendoza-Alvarez J G, Martínez-Muñoz J P, Cisneros A, Navarrete-Espinosa J and Sanchez-Sinencio F 2014 A DNA microarray-based assay to detect dual infection with two dengue virus serotypes *Sensors* **14** 7580–601

[14] Masimba P, Gare J, Klimkait T, Tanner M and Felger I 2014 Development of a simple microarray for genotyping HIV-1 drug resistance mutations in the reverse transcriptase gene in rural T anzania *Trop. Med. Int. Health* **19** 664–71

[15] Martínez M A, Soto-del Río M D, Gutiérrez R M, Chiu C Y, Greninger A L, Contreras J F, López S, Arias C F and Isa P 2015 DNA microarray for detection of gastrointestinal viruses *J. Clin. Microbiol.* **53** 136–45

[16] Khan M J, Trabuco A C, Alfonso H L, Figueiredo M L, Batista W C, Badra S J, Figueiredo L T, Lavrador M A and Aquino V H 2016 DNA microarray platform for detection and surveillance of viruses transmitted by small mammals and arthropods *PLoS Negl. Trop. Dis.* **10** e0005017

[17] Martín V *et al* 2016 An efficient microarray-based genotyping platform for the identification of drug-resistance mutations in majority and minority subpopulations of HIV-1 quasispecies *PLoS One* **11** e0166902

[18] Granade T C, Kodani M, Wells S K, Youngpairoj A S, Masciotra S, Curtis K A, Kamili S and Owen S M 2018 Characterization of real-time microarrays for simultaneous detection of HIV-1, HIV-2, and hepatitis viruses *J. Virol. Methods* **259** 60–5

[19] Wang D *et al* 2003 Viral discovery and sequence recovery using DNA microarrays *PLoS Biol.* **1** e2

[20] Dankbar D M, Dawson E D, Mehlmann M, Moore C L, Smagala J A, Shaw M W, Cox N J, Kuchta R D and Rowlen K L 2007 Diagnostic microarray for influenza B viruses *Anal. Chem.* **79** 2084–90

[21] Guo X, Geng P, Wang Q, Cao B and Liu B 2014 Development of a single nucleotide polymorphism DNA microarray for the detection and genotyping of the SARS coronavirus *J. Microbiol. Biotechnol.* **24** 1445–54

[22] Lefterova M I, Suarez C J, Banaei N and Pinsky B A 2015 Next-generation sequencing for infectious disease diagnosis and management: a report of the Association for Molecular Pathology *J. Mol. Diagn.* **17** 623–34

[23] Vemula S V, Zhao J, Liu J, Wang X, Biswas S and Hewlett I 2016 Current approaches for diagnosis of influenza virus infections in humans *Viruses* **8** 96

[24] Souf S 2016 Recent advances in diagnostic testing for viral infections *Biosci. Horizons* **9** hzw010

[25] Deurenberg R H *et al* 2017 Application of next generation sequencing in clinical microbiology and infection prevention *J. Biotechnol.* **243** 16–24

[26] Kustin T, Ling G, Sharabi S, Ram D, Friedman N, Zuckerman N, Bucris E D, Glatman-Freedman A, Stern A and Mandelboim M 2019 A method to identify respiratory virus infections in clinical samples using next-generation sequencing *Sci. Rep.* **9** 2606

[27] Towner J S *et al* 2008 Newly discovered ebola virus associated with hemorrhagic fever outbreak in Uganda *PLoS Pathog.* **4** e1000212

[28] Baillie G J *et al* 2012 Evolutionary dynamics of local pandemic H1N1/2009 influenza virus lineages revealed by whole-genome analysis *J. Virol* **86** 11–8

[29] Dessilly G, Goeminne L, Vandenbroucke A T, Dufrasne F E, Martin A and Kabamba-Mukabi B 2018 First evaluation of the next-generation sequencing platform for the detection of HIV-1 drug resistance mutations in Belgium *PLoS One* **13** e0209561

[30] Bhoyar R C *et al* 2021 High throughput detection and genetic epidemiology of SARS-CoV-2 using COVIDSeq next-generation sequencing *PLoS One* **16** e0247115

[31] Baron K G, Reid K J and Zee P C 2013 Exercise to improve sleep in insomnia: exploration of the bidirectional effects *J. Clin. Sleep Med.* **9** 819–24

[32] Fernando K 2012 Training in molecular virology *Methods Mol. Biol.* **903** 3–10

[33] Van Tongeren S P, Degener J E and Harmsen H J 2011 Comparison of three rapid and easy bacterial DNA extraction methods for use with quantitative real-time PCR *Eur. J. Clin. Microbiol. Infect. Dis* **30** 1053–61

[34] Sun Y, Zhao L, Zhao M, Zhu R, Deng J, Wang F, Li F, Ding Y, Tian R and Qian Y 2014 Four DNA extraction methods used in loop-mediated isothermal amplification for rapid adenovirus detection *J. Virol. Methods* **204** 49–52

[35] Mullis K B and Faloona F A 1987 [21] Specific synthesis of DNA *in vitro* via a polymerase-catalyzed chain reaction *Methods Enzymol.* **155** 335–50

[36] Demmler G J, Buffone G J, Schimbor C M and May R A 1988 Detection of cytomegalovirus in urine from newborns by using polymerase chain reaction DNA amplification *J. Infect. Dis.* **158** 1177–84

[37] Myerson D, Lingenfelter P A, Gleaves C A, Meyers J D and Bowden R A 1993 Diagnosis of cytomegalovirus pneumonia by the polymerase chain reaction with archived frozen lung tissue and bronchoalveolar lavage fluid *Am. J. Clin. Pathol* **100** 407–13

[38] Sundaramurthy R, Dhodapkar R, Kaliaperumal S and Harish B N 2018 Investigational approach to adenoviral conjunctivitis: comparison of three diagnostic tests using a Bayesian latent class model *J. Infect. Dev. Ctries* **12** 43–51

[39] Hassan R, White L R, Stefanoff C G, de Oliveira D E, Felisbino F E, Klumb C E, Bacchi C E, Seuánez H N and Zalcberg I R 2006 Epstein–Barr virus (EBV) detection and typing by PCR: a contribution to diagnostic screening of EBV-positive Burkitt's lymphoma *Diagn. Pathol* **1** 1–7

[40] Cobo F, Talavera P and Concha A 2006 Diagnostic approaches for viruses and prions in stem cell banks *Virology* **347** 1–0

[41] Reta D H, Tessema T S, Ashenef A S, Desta A F, Labisso W L, Gizaw S T, Abay S M, Melka D S and Reta F A 2020 Molecular and immunological diagnostic techniques of medical viruses *Int. J. Microbiol.* **2020** 8832728

[42] Osawa Y, Ikebukuro K, Motoki H, Matsuo T, Horiuchi M and Sode K 2008 The simple and rapid detection of specific PCR products from bacterial genomes using Zn finger proteins *Nucleic Acids Res.* **36** e68

[43] Jailani A A, Chattopadhyay A, Kumar P, Singh O W, Mukherjee S K, Roy A, Sanan-Mishra N and Mandal B 2023 Accelerated long-fragment circular PCR for genetic manipulation of plant viruses in unveiling functional genomics *Viruses* **15** 2332

[44] Freeman W M, Walker S J and Vrana K E 1999 Quantitative RT-PCR: pitfalls and potential *Biotechniques* **26** 112–25

[45] Myers T W and Gelfand D H 1991 Reverse transcription and DNA amplification by a *Thermus thermophilus* DNA polymerase *Biochemistry* **30** 7661–6

[46] Cherpillod P, Schibler M, Vieille G, Cordey S, Mamin A, Vetter P and Kaiser L 2016 Ebola virus disease diagnosis by real-time RT-PCR: a comparative study of 11 different procedures *J. Clin. Virol* **77** 9–14

[47] Wang W, Xu Y, Gao R, Lu R, Han K, Wu G and Tan W 2020 Detection of SARS-CoV-2 in different types of clinical specimens *JAMA* **323** 1843–4

[48] Munne K, Bhanothu V, Bhor V, Patel V, Mahale S D and Pande S 2021 Detection of SARS-CoV-2 infection by RT-PCR test: factors influencing interpretation of results *Virusdisease* **32** 187–9

[49] Haqqi T M, Sarkar G, David C S and Sommer S S 1988 Specific amplification with PCR of a refractory segment of genomic DNA *Nucleic Acids Res.* **16** 11844

[50] Chamberlain J S, Gibbs R A, Rainer J E, Nguyen P N and Thomas C 1988 Deletion screening of the Duchenne muscular dystrophy locus via multiplex DNA amplification *Nucleic Acids Res.* **16** 11141–56

[51] Boriskin Y S, Rice P S, Stabler R A, Hinds J, Al-Ghusein H, Vass K and Butcher P D 2004 DNA microarrays for virus detection in cases of central nervous system infection *J. Clin. Microbiol.* **42** 5811–8

[52] Templeton K E, Scheltinga S A, Beersma M F, Kroes A C and Claas E C 2004 Rapid and sensitive method using multiplex real-time PCR for diagnosis of infections by influenza A and influenza B viruses, respiratory syncytial virus, and parainfluenza viruses 1, 2, 3, and 4 *J. Clin. Microbiol.* **42** 1564–9

[53] Mackay I M, Arden K E and Nitsche A 2004 Real-time fluorescent PCR techniques to study microbial–host interactions *Methods Microbiol.* **34** 255–330

[54] Kralik P and Ricchi M 2017 A basic guide to real time PCR in microbial diagnostics: definitions, parameters, and everything *Front. Microbiol.* **8** 239909

[55] Mens P F, van Overmeir C, Bonnet M, Dujardin J C and d'Alessandro U 2008 Real-time PCR/MCA assay using fluorescence resonance energy transfer for the genotyping of resistance related DHPS-540 mutations in *Plasmodium falciparum Malar. J.* **7** 1–7

[56] Sidoti F, Bergallo M, Costa C and Cavallo R 2013 Alternative molecular tests for virological diagnosis *Mol. Biotechnol.* **53** 352–62

[57] Notomi T, Okayama H, Masubuchi H, Yonekawa T, Watanabe K, Amino N and Hase T 2000 Loop-mediated isothermal amplification of DNA *Nucleic Acids Res.* **28** e63

[58] Parida M, Horioke K, Ishida H, Dash P K, Saxena P, Jana A M, Islam M A, Inoue S, Hosaka N and Morita K 2005 Rapid detection and differentiation of dengue virus serotypes by a real-time reverse transcription-loop-mediated isothermal amplification assay *J. Clin. Microbiol.* **43** 2895–903

[59] Thai H T, Le M Q, Vuong C D, Parida M, Minekawa H, Notomi T, Hasebe F and Morita K 2004 Development and evaluation of a novel loop-mediated isothermal amplification method for rapid detection of severe acute respiratory syndrome coronavirus *J. Clin. Microbiol.* **42** 1956–61

[60] Ito M, Watanabe M, Nakagawa N, Ihara T and Okuno Y 2006 Rapid detection and typing of influenza A and B by loop-mediated isothermal amplification: comparison with immunochromatography and virus isolation *J. Virol. Methods* **135** 272–5

[61] Okamoto S, Yoshikawa T, Ihira M, Suzuki K, Shimokata K, Nishiyama Y and Asano Y 2004 Rapid detection of varicella–zoster virus infection by a loop-mediated isothermal amplification method *J. Med. virol* **74** 677–82

[62] Enomoto Y *et al* 2005 Rapid diagnosis of herpes simplex virus infection by a loop-mediated isothermal amplification method *J. Clin. Microbiol.* **43** 951–5

[63] Suzuki R, Yoshikawa T, Ihira M, Enomoto Y, Inagaki S, Matsumoto K, Kato K, Kudo K, Kojima S and Asano Y 2006 Development of the loop-mediated isothermal amplification method for rapid detection of cytomegalovirus DNA *J. Virol. Methods* **132** 216–21

[64] Bista B R, Ishwad C, Wadowsky R M, Manna P, Randhawa P S, Gupta G, Adhikari M, Tyagi R, Gasper G and Vats A 2007 Development of a loop-mediated isothermal amplification assay for rapid detection of BK virus *J. Clin. Microbiol.* **45** 1581–7

[65] Hagiwara M, Sasaki H, Matsuo K, Honda M, Kawase M and Nakagawa H 2007 Loop-mediated isothermal amplification method for detection of human papillomavirus type 6, 11, 16, and 18 *J. Med. Virol* **79** 605–15

[66] Compton J 1991 Nucleic acid sequence-based amplification *Nature* **350** 91–2

[67] Fakruddin M, Mazumdar R M, Chowdhury A and Mannan K B 2012 Nucleic acid sequence based amplification (NASBA)-prospects and applications *Int. J. Life Sci. Pharma. Res.* **2** 106–21

[68] Mo Q H, Wang H B, Dai H R, Lin J C, Tan H, Wang Q and Yang Z 2015 Rapid and simultaneous detection of three major diarrhea-causing viruses by multiplex real-time nucleic acid sequence-based amplification *Arch. Virol* **160** 719–25

[69] Mohammadi-Yeganeh S, Paryan M A, Samiee S M, Kia V and Rezvan H 2012 Molecular beacon probes–base multiplex NASBA Real-time for detection of HIV-1 and HCV *Iran. J. Microbiol.* **4** 47

[70] Yu A C *et al* 2012 Nucleic acid-based diagnostics for infectious diseases in public health affairs *Front. Med.* **6** 173–86

[71] Laver T, Harrison J, O'neill P A, Moore K, Farbos A, Paszkiewicz K and Studholme D J 2015 Assessing the performance of the Oxford Nanopore Technologies MinION *Biomol. Detect. Quantif.* **3** 1–8
[72] Jain M *et al* 2018 Nanopore sequencing and assembly of a human genome with ultra-long reads *Nat. Biotechnol.* **36** 338–45
[73] Ji W A, Ke Y H, Zhang Y, Huang K Q, Lei W A, Shen X X, Dong X P, Xu W B and Jun X 2017 Rapid and accurate sequencing of enterovirus genomes using MinION nanopore sequencer *Biomed. Environ. Sci.* **30** 718–26
[74] Lin Z, Farooqui A, Li G, Wong G K, Mason A L, Banner D, Kelvin A A, Kelvin D J and León A J 2014 Next-generation sequencing and bioinformatic approaches to detect and analyze influenza virus in ferrets *J. Infect. Dev. Ctries* **8** 498–509
[75] Kustin T, Ling G, Sharabi S, Ram D, Friedman N, Zuckerman N, Bucris E D, Glatman-Freedman A, Stern A and Mandelboim M 2019 A method to identify respiratory virus infections in clinical samples using next-generation sequencing *Sci. Rep.* **9** 2606
[76] Dron J S, Wang J, McIntyre A D, Iacocca M A, Robinson J F, Ban M R, Cao H and Hegele R A 2020 Six years' experience with LipidSeq: clinical and research learnings from a hybrid, targeted sequencing panel for dyslipidemias *BMC Med. Genet.* **13** 1–5
[77] Wang D, Coscoy L, Zylberberg M, Avila P C, Boushey H A, Ganem D and DeRisi J L 2002 Microarray-based detection and genotyping of viral pathogens *Proc. Natl. Acad. Sci.* **99** 15687–92
[78] Sturmer M, Doerr H W and Preiser W 2003 Variety of interpretation systems for human immunodeficiency virus type 1 genotyping: confirmatory information or additional confusion? *Curr. Drug Targets-Infect. Disord* **3** 373–82
[79] Parkin N T and Schapiro J M 2004 Antiretroviral drug resistance in non-subtype B HIV-1, HIV-2 and SIV *Antivir. Ther.* **9** 3–12
[80] Tsubota A, Arase Y, Ren F, Tanaka H, Ikeda K and Kumada H 2001 Genotype may correlate with liver carcinogenesis and tumor characteristics in cirrhotic patients infected with hepatitis B virus subtype adw *J. Med. Virol* **65** 257–65
[81] Boyer J L *et al* 2003 National Institutes of Health Consensus Development Conference Statement-Management of Hepatitis C: 2002-June 10–12, 2002 *HIV Clin. Trials* **4** 55–75
[82] Read S J, Burnett D and Fink C G 2000 Molecular techniques for clinical diagnostic virology *J. Clin. Pathol* **53** 502–6
[83] Picciotto A, Campo N, Brizzolara R, Sinelli N, Poggi G, Grasso S and Celle G 1997 HCV-RNA levels play an important role independently of genotype in predicting response to interferon therapy *Eur. J. Gastroenterol. Hepatol* **9** 67–9
[84] Ott J J, Stevens G A, Groeger J and Wiersma S T 2012 Global epidemiology of hepatitis B virus infection: new estimates of age-specific HBsAg seroprevalence and endemicity *Vaccine* **30** 2212–9
[85] Messina J P, Humphreys I, Flaxman A, Brown A, Cooke G S, Pybus O G and Barnes E 2014 Global distribution and prevalence of hepatitis C virus genotypes *Hepatology* **61** 77–87
[86] Poovorawan Y 2012 Epidemiology of hepatitis C virus-Genotypes 1 through 6 in Asia and the world *Int. J. Infect. Dis* **16** e33
[87] Rota J S, Rota P A, Redd S B, Redd S C, Pattamadilok S and Bellini W J 1998 Genetic analysis of measles viruses isolated in the United States, 1995–1996 *J. Infect. Dis.* **177** 204–8
[88] Yin C 2020 Genotyping coronavirus SARS-CoV-2: methods and implications *Genomics* **112** 3588–96

[89] Sharma G, Sharma A R, Bhattacharya M, Lee S S and Chakraborty C 2021 CRISPR-Cas9: a preclinical and clinical perspective for the treatment of human diseases *Mol. Ther.* **29** 571–86

[90] Ribeiro B V, Cordeiro T A, e Freitas G R, Ferreira L F and Franco D L 2020 Biosensors for the detection of respiratory viruses: a review *Talanta Open* **2** 100007

[91] Naresh V and Lee N A review on biosensors and recent development of nanostructured materials-enabled biosensors *Sensors (Switzerland)* **21** 1–35

[92] Goode J A, Rushworth J V and Millner P A 2015 Biosensor regeneration: a review of common techniques and outcomes *Langmuir* **31** 6267–76

[93] Yang F, Ma Y, Stanciu S G and Wu A 2020 Transduction process-based classification of biosensors *Nanobiosensors: From Design to Applications* (Wiley) pp 23–44

[94] Saeedfar K, Heng L Y and Rezayi M 2017 Fabricating long shelf life potentiometric urea biosensors using modified MWCNTs on screen printed electrodes *Sens. Lett.* **15** 97–103

[95] German N, Ramanavicius A and Ramanaviciene A 2017 Amperometric glucose biosensor based on electrochemically deposited gold nanoparticles covered by polypyrrole *Electroanalysis* **29** 1267–77

[96] Chakraborty A, Tibarewala D N and Barui A 2019 Impedance-based biosensors *Bioelectronics and Medical Devices* (Cambridge: Woodhead Publishing) pp 97–122

[97] Cordeiro T A, Gonçalves M V, Franco D L, Reis A B, Martins H R and Ferreira L F 2019 Label-free electrochemical impedance immunosensor based on modified screen-printed gold electrodes for the diagnosis of canine visceral leishmaniasis *Talanta* **195** 327–32

[98] Ding J and Qin W 2020 Recent advances in potentiometric biosensors *TrAC, Trends Anal. Chem.* **124** 115803

[99] Soni A, Surana R K and Jha S K 2018 Smartphone based optical biosensor for the detection of urea in saliva *Sens. Actuators* B **269** 346–53

[100] Masson J F 2017 Surface plasmon resonance clinical biosensors for medical diagnostics *ACS Sens.* **2** 16–30

[101] Dimitrusev N, Nedeljko P, Mabes Raj A A and Lobnik A 2023 Comparison of surface and spectral properties of optical sensor layers prepared by spin/spray coating and printing techniques *Chemosensors* **11** 136

[102] Pohanka M 2018 Piezoelectric biosensor for the determination of tumor necrosis factor alpha *Talanta* **178** 970–3

[103] Chorsi M T, Curry E J, Chorsi H T, Das R, Baroody J, Purohit P K, Ilies H and Nguyen 2019 TD. Piezoelectric biomaterials for sensors and actuators *Adv. Mater.* **31** 1802084

[104] Jeffree A I, Karman S, Ibrahim S, Karim M S and Rozali S 2020 Biosensors approach for lung cancer diagnosis—a review *RITA 2018: Proceedings of the 6th International Conference on Robot Intelligence Technology and Applications* (Singapore: Springer) pp 425–35

[105] Ricci F, Adornetto G and Palleschi G 2012 A review of experimental aspects of electrochemical immunosensors *Electrochim. Acta* **84** 74–83

[106] Saylan Y, Yilmaz F, Özgür E, Derazshamshir A, Yavuz H and Denizli A 2017 Molecular imprinting of macromolecules for sensor applications *Sensors* **17** 898

[107] Justino C I, Duarte A C and Rocha-Santos T A 2016 Immunosensors in clinical laboratory diagnostics *Adv. Clin. Chem.* **73** 65–108

[108] Acosta S, Quintanilla L, Alonso M, Aparicio C and Rodríguez-Cabello J C 2019 Recombinant AMP/polypeptide self-assembled monolayers with synergistic antimicrobial properties for bacterial strains of medical relevance *ACS Biomater. Sci. Eng* **5** 4708–16

[109] Lan W C, Huang T S, Cho Y C, Huang Y T, Walinski C J, Chiang P C, Rusilin M, Pai F T, Huang C C and Huang M S 2020 The potential of a nanostructured titanium oxide layer with self-assembled monolayers for biomedical applications: surface properties and biomechanical behaviors *Appl. Sci.* **10** 590

[110] Baryeh K, Takalkar S, Lund M and Liu G 2017 Introduction to medical biosensors for point of care applications *Medical Biosensors for Point of Care (POC) Applications* (Cambridge: Woodhead Publishing) pp 3–25

[111] Brazaca L C, Ribovski L, Janegitz B C and Zucolotto V 2017 Nanostructured materials and nanoparticles for point of care (POC) medical biosensors *Medical Biosensors for Point of Care (POC) Applications* (Cambridge: Woodhead Publishing) pp 229–54

[112] Sabino-Silva R, Jardim A C and Siqueira W L 2020 Coronavirus COVID-19 impacts to dentistry and potential salivary diagnosis *Clin. Oral Investig.* **24** 1619–21

IOP Publishing

Viral Diseases

History and new developments in diagnostics and therapeutics

Arvind K Singh Chandel, Bhakti Tanna, Amisha Parmar, Gopal Patel and Neeraj S Thakur

Chapter 6

Variant identification techniques targeting viral infections

Urvi Budhbhatti and Bhakti Tanna

The advancements in virus detection and discovery through high throughput sequencing (HTS) and bioinformatics have indeed been significant, especially highlighted by the emergence of the SARS-CoV-2 pandemic. However, challenges persist, particularly regarding the availability of high-performance computing (HPC) facilities and specialized bioinformatics tools. The limited accessibility to such resources hampers the efficient processing of the complex computational steps involved in virus identification and discovery. Currently, there's a notable absence of dedicated tools specifically tailored for virus identification and discovery. Additionally, the absence of a centralized virus sequence database poses a challenge, necessitating bioinformaticians to manually extract viral sequences from various sources such as GenBank. This process is often time-consuming and inefficient. The existing tools for virus discovery primarily consist of generic bioinformatics tools designed for sequence mapping (e.g., BWA, bowtie), *de novo* assembly (e.g., Trinity, SPAdes, Velvet), and National Center for Biotechnology Information Basic Local Alignment Search Tool (NCBI BLAST). While these tools serve their purpose, they may not be optimized for the specific requirements of virus identification and discovery.

6.1 Introduction

Viruses are tiny entities that depend heavily on host cells to reproduce their genome and disseminate their infectious progeny. Specifically, they lack efficient intravital biochemical networks and processes that enable their existence [1]. Viruses pose a formidable public health issue due to their diverse structure and rapid adaptability. The 21st century has already encountered a series of epidemics, beginning with the severe acute respiratory syndrome coronavirus, subsequently followed by the 2009 swine flu pandemic, the 2012 Middle East respiratory syndrome coronavirus outbreak, the 2013–16 Ebola virus disease epidemic in West Africa, the 2015 Zika

doi:10.1088/978-0-7503-4987-1ch6

virus disease, and, finally, the COVID-19 pandemic, that have had a catastrophic impact on lives and livelihoods across the globe [2]. Emerging contagious ailments have become more common in people recently, or they appear to be getting worse lately. In the past three decades, more than 30 novel infectious agents have been found worldwide, with 60% of them having zoonotic origins [3].

Advances in socioeconomic conditions, cleanliness, and literacy have helped decrease the spread of several prevalent illnesses among children, resulting in many infections occurring later in life. Some viruses produce more clinical disease in older age groups; therefore, these improvements may result in an unexpected rise in the cases of clinical disease [4]. Pathogens from wild or domesticated livestock reservoirs have frequently erupted in human populations in recent decades, including human immunodeficiency virus (HIV)-1 and HIV-2, the 1918 influenza virus, Middle East respiratory syndrome coronavirus, and severe acute respiratory syndrome coronavirus 2 (SARS-CoV-2). To pose an imminent risk to human populations, a novel pathogen must initially come into proximity with the animal reservoir; the infectious agent must either possess or adapt an ability for human-to-human transfer; and subsequently, human-to-human transmission must enable the pathogen's geographical range to expand beyond the zone of spill-over. Recent worldwide changes have had an impact on all of these processes [2].

The vast genetic diversity of viruses contributes to the incomplete understanding of total viral diversity in various environments [5]. Limited knowledge of host–virus interactions can lead to unforeseen consequences, where viral infections may not always harm the host due to gaps in understanding the full host range of viruses [6].

6.2 Evolving nature of viruses

Viruses evolve at a faster rate than other living organisms, alterations can be easily seen over time when compared to collected isolates of the same virus species. The rapid rate of virus mutation poses a persistent threat in a variety of ways, including the development of medication resistance, pathogenesis, the success of antiviral treatment, vaccination efficacy, and the potential of the creation of new diseases or an increase in the virulence of an existing disease. Mutations are rarely caused via replication, but they can occur as a result of editing or continual damage to genetic material. Normally, viruses with a high mutation rate can efficiently prevent immune defense [7].

Advances in biotechnology over the last year have resulted in the creation of several methods. There are two general categories for virus detection techniques: direct and indirect.

The mainstay of indirect approaches is monitoring the effect of the virus on host cells. For example, methods like cell culture concentrate on identifying cytopathic effect (CPE) or pre-cytopathic effect (pre-CPE). These techniques are thought to be conventional and somewhat slow for diagnostic purposes, but they offer insights into propagation and characterization [8].

Conversely, direct approaches require the virus to be found right away. These approaches frequently make use of nucleic acid-based procedures, like amplification or hybridization of particular genomic regions. Furthermore, polyclonal or monoclonal antibodies that have an affinity for particular viral antigens are used in enzyme-linked immunosorbent assay (ELISA)-based procedures [9]. Mutation can significantly affect diagnostic assays. Polymerase chain reaction (PCR) depends on the specific sequence of primer or probe binding. The mismatches due to mutations at the primer or probe binding site will significantly influence the diagnostic assay's specificity and sensitivity [10].

6.2.1 Variant calling

Variant calling is the technique of determining variations between the sequencing reads produced by next-generation sequencing (NGS) experiments and a reference genome [11]. Accurate variant identification in NGS data is a crucial element that underpins almost all subsequent analysis and interpretation methods [12].

Viruses evolve within hosts throughout time, often undermining the efficacy of host immunity and therapeutic approaches, and in order to develop effective vaccines and therapies, it is necessary to first understand viral diversification, which includes fully defining the genetic variants in viral intra-host populations and modeling changes from transmission to infection [13]. The sequencing of the viral genome will be critical for the advancement of vaccines, epidemiology, and genomics. Furthermore, through analyzing the variants, we can detect low-level drug-resistant mutations and that will enable us to have extra measures to engage before such variants emerge as clinically prominent [14]. With the advance in massive sequencing technologies, viral populations can be studied with unprecedented (extreme) precision. However, the most crucial issue is to distinguish the biological variants from the sequencing-related error to interpret the sequencing data [13].

For the identification of short variants, probabilistic and heuristic-based algorithms are widely used. The probabilistic method represents the actual data distribution. After that, Bayesian statistics is utilized to derive the genetic probability. The heuristic approach is based on factors like minimum allelic counts, read quality threshold, read depth, and several other heuristic factors. While heuristic-based algorithms are less common, they can be resistant to outlier data that violates the principles of probabilistic models [11]. Those variants that surpass the error rate predicted by the statistical algorithms are considered true variants [15].

However, there is a major challenge to differentiate between the rare variant with the sequencing errors, especially when sequencing in the case of viral pathogen sequencing from the clinical samples. There is intra-host viral diversity, especially in the case of ribonucleic acid (RNA) virus which is prone to high replicative error [16].

In deep sequencing data, many filtering criteria are applied. Before aligning the sequence to the reference genome, it is necessary to trim the adaptors and bad sequences. Variant calling software also distinguishes between the variant and artifact by using different approaches. For example, VarScan takes into account the read quality, total coverage, and variant frequency. One other method includes the statistical approach which takes into account the position error model for the detection of the variants. Position error is modelled using either the Bayesian approach which takes into account sequencing depth and other parameters, or the hidden Markov model which uses a machine learning algorithm to detect the variants. The v-phaser variant calling tool takes into account the covariance between the variants [17]. Another tool called ShoRAH (Short Read Assembly into Haplotype) identifies variants by combining all reads that overlap a common region and are aligned together and consensus is generated [18]. The most widely used variant callers include LoFreq [19], DeepSNV [15], V-Phazer [13], and many other variant callers are widely used for the detection of the variants each using a different variant calling algorithm. Although being applied to several NGS-based viral research variations, few of these approaches have been tested using predefined viral samples. The accuracy and selectivity of the rare variant detection are greatly affected by the nucleic acid titer that varies substantially in the patient-derived samples and also in the experimental setup and sample processing [15].

Nevertheless, since no single variant caller employs all the different algorithms, aggregation of variants called from multiple variant callers has the ultimate strategy [20].

6.2.2 Variant annotation

Assigning functional details to a variant, such as the type of mutation—coding or noncoding—or the change in amino acid, sequence conservation, etc—is known as variant annotation [21]. Following the sequencing of new variants, there is unusual desire because researchers want to acquire knowledge more about how rapidly they disseminate, whether they facilitate virus spread, whether they have been linked to more severe or less severe diseases, and whether they could reduce the efficacy of both currently available and potential vaccines [22]. VirVarSeq is a software package for variant calling and it performs pileup, i.e. it constructs a codon table where with reference to the genome it reports the different codons detected along with the Qs score of all three nucleotides within the codon [23]. The snpEff is a tool that is frequently used for variant annotation. Along with the viral genome, it is the open-source programme that is utilized for more than 320 genomes for various species. The user has the option to add more genomes or request them [24].

Although there are several tools for annotating human and other species' variants, there are relatively few tools for annotating viral variants and their anticipated functionality. However, the SARS-CoV2 pandemic highlighted that it was crucial to develop the tool for the various viral species since they continue to pose a severe threat to people and because precise and thorough annotation of the viral variants is constantly required.

6.3 Validation by Sanger's (metagenomics) or polymerase chain reaction-restriction fragment length polymorphism PCR-RFLP

Sanger's sequencing is the 'gold standard' for sequencing in clinical research with an accuracy of 99.99%. Sanger's sequencing for the successful determination of pathogen requires primer availability as it targets the specific pathogen and does not allow sequencing of another pathogen or host genome. It can also provide a facility for whole genome generation for the laboratories where NGS is not available. Development of diagnostics and vaccines, understanding of the evolutionary path, study of the association between virus and their hosts, and studying virulence require information on complete genome sequencing of viruses [25]. Sanger's sequencing is considered first-generation sequencing and can process 96 to even 384 samples at a time with read length up to 600–1000 nucleotides.

Sanger's sequencing is an older sequencing technique than NGS and has a lower throughput, it is more expensive when many samples need to be processed together and has a huge genome size. The extreme sites where primers bind doesn't provide high-quality sequences. Nonetheless, the quality of sequence obtained between 500–900 bp in Sanger's is very high and thus it tends to reduce chances of error when compared to NGS [25]. Virus detection using Sanger's sequencing is simpler than next-generation data analysis. For its analysis, first the quality of sequences is verified using its chromatogram peaks and then the sequences are compared with the databases available for the final identification [26]. Sanger's sequencing is used for COVID-19 identification using its primers for spike gene [27]. In one study, the whole genome of SARS-CoV-2 with a length of 29,760 was analyzed using Sanger's sequencing, and their variations were observed in samples collected from the Nigerian population, and the sequences were submitted to GenBank [25]. They observed 99.97% similarity with the reference sequence in BLAST. The BigDye XTerminator v. 3.1 kit was used in their analysis, which is most widely used for Sanger's sequence analysis. In another study, confirmation of Grapevine virus H was done using Sanger's analysis where initially sequencing was performed using the NovSeq6000 platform, and confirmation of its open reading frame 1 (ORF1) was done using Sanger's, which provided 97.5% identity with corresponding graft-versus-host disease (GVH)-like *de novo* contig (GeA-9) and 97.1% identical to GVH reported in US and Portugal [28]. Identification of anellovirus from human blood metagenomics was performed and validation was done using Sanger's sequencing for the removal of artifacts [29].

Identification of various viruses has required the use of sequencing techniques which mainly involves confirmation with Sanger's sequencing. Identification of mutations in cytomegalovirus which caused antiviral resistance was evaluated with the help of NGS utilizing MinION (amplicon-based nanopore sequencing technology) technology and it was compared using Sanger's sequencing method. They were able to identify two additional mutations (UL97 and/or UL54) in 62% [8/13] of their selected population [30]. Sanger's can also be used when NGS has not been able to produce sequences or has missing sequences. One such study includes when samples with SARS-CoV-2 infection had shown missing fragments for key mutations in RBD (receptor binding domain). The identification of key mutations was successful and beta variations were observed in samples with 13.85–37.47 Ct scores [31]. Epidemiology and phenotype understanding of HEV (Hepatitis E Virus) was evaluated by targeted genome sequencing and Sanger's. The genotyping was done using partial genome sequences obtained by Sanger's sequencing and by combining its results with deep targeted sequencing, the development of phylogenetic analysis of the virus could be done [32].

Identification and pathotyping of avian IAV (influenza A viruses) has also been done using MinION technique as well as Sanger's sequencing [33].

6.4 Concluding remarks and outlook

Virus detection and discovery using HTS and bioinformatics tools have improved over the years, specifically with the introduction of SARS-CoV-2 pandemic condition. However, there are few laboratories in the world that can process the steps reported in this chapter as HPC facilities and bioinformatics are limited which can effectively run the computer scripts.

To date there has been no crucial tool specifically written for virus identification and discovery, and even a centralized virus sequence database is required. At present, for the comparison, bioinformaticians need to extract viral sequences from GenBank, nr for amino acids, and nt for nucleotides. The tools for the pipeline of virus discovery are mostly generic tools written for sequence mapping (e.g., BWA, bowtie), *de novo* assembly (e.g., Trinity, SPAdes, Velvet, etc), and NCBI BLAST [26]. Identification of viruses will become more vigorous with an increase in new database and algorithm developments. However, to have new technologies, they would have to clear meticulous tests and prove their capabilities to current standards before they get approved.

Abbreviations

CPE	Cytopathic effect
ELISA	Enzyme-linked immunosorbent assay
HIV	Human immunodeficiency virus
NGS	Next-generation sequencing
PCR	Polymerase chain reaction
RNA	Ribonucleic acid
SARS-CoV-2	Severe acute respiratory syndrome coronavirus 2

References

[1] Barroso-González J, García-Expósito L, Puigdomènech I, de Armas-Rillo L, Machado J-D, Blanco J *et al* 2011 Viral infection: moving through complex and dynamic cell-membrane structures *Commun. Integr. biol.* **4** 398–408

[2] Baker R E, Mahmud A S, Miller I F, Rajeev M, Rasambainarivo F, Rice B L *et al* 2022 Infectious disease in an era of global change *Nat. Rev. Microbiol.* **20** 193–205

[3] Dikid T, Jain S K, Sharma A, Kumar A and Narain J P 2013 Emerging and re-emerging infections in India: an overview *Indian J. Med. Res.* **138** 19–31

[4] Burrell C J, Howard C R and Murphy F A 2017 Epidemiology of viral infections *Fenner and White's Medical Virology* (Academic) pp 185–203

[5] Coclet C, Sorensen P O, Karaoz U, Wang S, Brodie E L, Eloe-Fadrosh E A *et al* 2023 Virus diversity and activity is driven by snowmelt and host dynamics in a high-altitude watershed soil ecosystem *Microbiome* **11** 1–19

[6] Olo Ndela É, Cobigo L-M, Roux S and Enault F 2022 A better understanding of Earth's viruses thanks to metagenomes *Med. Sci. (Paris)* **38** 999–1007

[7] Khan Z M I, Nazli A, Khan D, Shah J and Farooq M A 2022 An overview of viral mutagenesis and the impact on pathogenesis of SARS-CoV-2 variants *Front. Immunol.* **13** 1034444

[8] Louten J 2016 Detection and diagnosis of viral infections *Essential Human Virology* (Academic) pp 111–32

[9] Cassedy A, Parle-McDermott A and O'Kennedy R 2021 Virus detection: a review of the current and emerging molecular and immunological methods *Front. Mol. Biosci.* **8** 1–21

[10] Alkhatib M, Carioti L, D'Anna S, Ceccherini-Silberstein F, Svicher V and Salpini R 2022 SARS-CoV-2 mutations and variants may muddle the sensitivity of COVID-19 diagnostic assays *Microorganisms* **10** 1–10

[11] Ugur Sezerman O, Ulgen E, Seymen N and Melis Durasi I 2019 Bioinformatics workflows for genomic variant discovery, interpretation and prioritization *Bioinformatics Tools Detection an Clinical Interpretation of Genomic Variations* (Books on Demand)

[12] Koboldt D C 2020 Best practices for variant calling in clinical sequencing *Genome Med.* **12** 1–13

[13] Macalalad A R, Zody M C, Charlebois P, Lennon N J, Newman R M, Malboeuf C M *et al* 2012 Highly sensitive and specific detection of rare variants in mixed viral populations from massively parallel sequence data *PLoS Comput. Biol.* **8** 1002417

[14] Houldcroft C J 2019 Human herpesvirus sequencing in the genomic era: The growing ranks of the herpetic legion *Pathogens* **8** 186

[15] McCrone J T and Lauring A S 2016 Measurements of intrahost viral diversity are extremely sensitive to systematic errors in variant calling *J. Virol* **90** 6884–95

[16] Mccrone J T and Lauring S 2016 Measurements of intrahost viral diversity are extremely sensitive to *J. Virol* **90** 6884–95

[17] McElroy K, Thomas T and Luciani F 2014 Deep sequencing of evolving pathogen populations: applications, errors, and bioinformatic solutions *Microb. Inform. Exper.* **4** 1–14

[18] Zagordi O, Bhattacharya A, Eriksson N and Beerenwinkel N 2011 ShoRAH: estimating the genetic diversity of a mixed sample from next-generation sequencing data *BMC Bioinform.* **12** 119

[19] Wilm A, Aw P P K, Bertrand D, Yeo G H T, Ong S H, Wong C H *et al* 2012 LoFreq: a sequence-quality aware, ultra-sensitive variant caller for uncovering cell-population heterogeneity from high-throughput sequencing datasets *Nucleic Acids Res.* **40** 11189–201

[20] Zverinova S and Guryev V 2022 Variant calling: considerations, practices, and developments *Hum. Mutat* **43** 976–85

[21] McCarthy D J, Humburg P, Kanapin A, Rivas M A, Gaulton K, Cazier J-B *et al* 2014 Choice of transcripts and software has a large effect on variant annotation *Genome Med.* **6** 26

[22] Bernasconi A, Gulino A, Alfonsi T, Canakoglu A, Pinoli P, Sandionigi A *et al* 2021 VirusViz: comparative analysis and effective visualization of viral nucleotide and amino acid variants *Nucleic Acids Res.* **49** e90

[23] Verbist B M P, Thys K, Reumers J, Wetzels Y, Van Der Borght K, Talloen W *et al* 2015 VirVarSeq: a low-frequency virus variant detection pipeline for Illumina sequencing using adaptive base-calling accuracy filtering *Bioinformatics* **31** 94–101

[24] Cingolani P, Platts A, Wang L L, Coon M, Nguyen T, Wang L *et al* 2012 A program for annotating and predicting the effects of single nucleotide polymorphisms, SnpEff: SNPs in the genome of *Drosophila melanogaster* strain w1118; iso-2; iso-3 *Fly (Austin)* **6** 80–92

[25] Shaibu J O, Onwuamah C K, James A B, Okwuraiwe A P, Amoo O S, Salu O B *et al* 2021 Full length genomic sanger sequencing and phylogenetic analysis of Severe Acute Respiratory Syndrome Coronavirus 2 (SARS-CoV-2) in Nigeria *PLoS One* **16** e0243271

[26] Villamor D E V, Ho T, Al Rwahnih M, Martin R R and Tzanetakis I E 2019 High throughput sequencing for plant virus detection and discovery *Phytopathology* **109** 716–25

[27] Daniels R S, Harvey R, Ermetal B, Xiang Z, Galiano M, Adams L *et al* 2021 A sanger sequencing protocol for SARS-CoV-2 S-gene *Influenza Other Respir. Viruses* **15** 707–10

[28] Panailidou P, Lotos L, Sassalou C-L, Gagiano E, Pietersen G, Katis N I *et al* 2021 First report of grapevine virus H in grapevine in greece *Plant Dis.* **105** 2738

[29] Cebriá-Mendoza M, Arbona C, Larrea L, Díaz W, Arnau V, Peña C *et al* 2021 Deep viral blood metagenomics reveals extensive anellovirus diversity in healthy humans *Sci. Rep.* **11** 6921

[30] Chorlton S D, Ritchie G, Lawson T, McLachlan E, Romney M G, Matic N *et al* 2021 Next-generation sequencing for cytomegalovirus antiviral resistance genotyping in a clinical virology laboratory *Antivir. Res.* **192** 105123

[31] Singh L, San J E, Tegally H, Brzoska P M, Anyaneji U J, Wilkinson E *et al* 2022 Targeted Sanger sequencing to recover key mutations in SARS-CoV-2 variant genome assemblies produced by next-generation sequencing *Microb. Genom* **8** 000774

[32] Davis C A, Haywood B, Vattipally S, Filipe A D S, AlSaeed M, Smollet K *et al* 2021 Hepatitis E virus: whole genome sequencing as a new tool for understanding HEV epidemiology and phenotypes *J. Clin. Virol* **139** 104738

[33] Crossley B M, Rejmanek D, Baroch J, Stanton J B, Young K T, Killian M L *et al* 2021 Nanopore sequencing as a rapid tool for identification and pathotyping of avian influenza A viruses *J. Vet. Diagn. Investig* **33** 253–60

IOP Publishing

Viral Diseases

History and new developments in diagnostics and therapeutics

Arvind K Singh Chandel, Bhakti Tanna, Amisha Parmar, Gopal Patel and Neeraj S Thakur

Chapter 7

Next generation sequencing: disease detection, research, and treatment

Priyambada Singh and Bhakti Tanna

NGS (next-generation sequencing) has revolutionized our ability to study viral infections and populations within hosts, offering insights crucial for guiding treatment strategies, preventive measures, and outbreak containment efforts. In diagnostic virology, NGS has proven invaluable in several key areas: (1) Identification and genomic characterization of several novel and rare viruses: NGS enables the rapid characterization and identification of previously unknown and unfamiliar groups of viruses, contributing to understanding their genetic makeup and potential health implications. (2) Detection of unexpected viral pathogens: NGS can detect unexpected viral pathogens in clinical specimens, enhancing our capability for diagnosis and treatment of infections accurately. (3) Monitoring antiviral drug resistance: NGS allows for ultra-sensitive monitoring of resistance to antiviral drugs, beneficial in optimizing treatment regimens and the management of drug-resistant viral strains. (4) Exploration of viral diversity, evolution, and dissemination: NGS facilitates the study of viral diversity, evolution, and dissemination patterns, providing valuable insights into viral dynamics and transmission pathways. (5) Assessment of the human virome: NGS has been instrumental in assessing the human virome's composition and dynamics, shedding light on its role and significance in the health and management of diseases.

7.1 Introduction to NGS platforms

Almost all the outbreaks threatening public health in the past few decades were caused due to emergence of novel viruses like the H1N1 influenza pandemic, H7N9 avian influenza, and (SARS) Severe Acute Respiratory Syndrome, mostly from animal sources. Globalization, environmental changes, the rapidly growing human population occupying wildlife habitats, growth of the wet market are all major

doi:10.1088/978-0-7503-4987-1ch7

reasons for the spread of these novel pathogens causing endemic or pandemic situations. Consequently, novel pathogen identification can have an immense influence on human health and infectious diseases [1].

The infectious disease treatment development requires appropriate identification and characterization of the organism. There are mainly culture-dependent and culture-independent methods for investigating microbial infection etiology. However, some prior knowledge of the target organism must be detected by the techniques for identification of culture-independent methods (e.g., PCR) [2]. There are various PCR techniques such as the most common 16S rRNA (ribosomal RNA) gene sequence for detection of bacteria and the 28S-ITS gene sequence for fungi detection. These techniques have been scrutinized for their sensitivity. Hence, lack or delay in diagnosis has led to a lengthening of hospitalization duration, high morbidity, and mortality. The undiagnosed patients would require treatment with broad-spectrum therapy, which can lead to higher side effects and drug resistance [3]. The existing RNA viruses are variants constructed through evolution along with high mutation rates, and increased fitness in newly developed genotypes sometimes just in days of strong selective pressure [4].

Conventional detection techniques fail when there is no prior knowledge of the organism present. In particular, in certain infectious diseases like encephalitis, conventional methods fail in their identification of pathogens as much as in 70% of the cases [1]. Thus, new techniques have been explored for the detection of infectious disease which can lead to improvement in clinical outcomes for the patients. NGS technology possesses the ability to identify multiple organisms concurrently in one single sequencing run [2]. Just about all the infectious organisms (except prions), contain nucleic acid content—DNA or RNA—which makes them compliant to detection techniques based on nucleic acid. NGS can identify all the pathogenic organisms present in animal or human samples. Known for its deep and parallel sequencing capabilities, NGS has emerged as one of the most intriguing approaches for identifying newly emerging infectious pathogens in clinical samples. This technique involves sequencing of nucleic acids of the clinical sample into millions of sequences which leads to the detection of a targeted pathogen. The NGS library generates millions of copies of input nucleic acid in an unbiased manner even though it would be present in low quantity [1].

Because of the inception of Severe Acute Respiratory Syndrome Coronavirus 2 (SARS-CoV-2) in December 2019, research in NGS sequencing has grown considerably [3]. Various platforms for parallel sequencing genome sequencing have emerged, such as Illumina, Ion Torrent, PacBio, and Nanopore, and there are also various kits in the market that help in sequencing, like AmpliSeq, TrueSeq, Haloplex. Sanger's sequencing is first-generation sequencing, second-generation sequencing (SGS) includes 454 Roche, Ion Torrent, and Illumina while third-generation sequencing (TGS) includes PacBio, while Nanopore technology is the fourth-generation technique [5]. In this chapter, diverse NGS platforms along with their use in viral sequencing will be discussed.

7.2 Different platforms for sequencing and their principle and limitations

All the sequencing platforms have different ways of parallel sequencing. The several kinds of sequencing techniques, together with their benefits and drawbacks, are outlined in table 7.1.

7.2.1 Illumina

Illumina (San Diego, CA) uses the principle of 'sequence by synthesis'. In this type, billions of DNA clusters are generated on a flow cell (glass) by clonal amplification of sequenced DNA [6]. These clusters act as templates so that complementary strands are generated with fluorescently labeled reversible chain terminator nucleotides. Each nucleotide A, G, C, and T is labeled with a different fluorescent dye, which releases light in four different wavelength bands when excited by laser during each cycle of amplification. The level of accuracy achieved with the Illumina platform is very high [7] and produces the highest quality reads [8].

However, there are limitations to this platform, including prephrasing (generated due to remains of the nucleotide signal from the previous cycle merging with the next cycle), post-phasing (nucleotide incorporation missed due to incomplete withdrawal of the terminator), and cross-talk [6, 7]. There are various benchtop sequencers such as: MiniSeq, MiSeq series, iSeq 100, NextSeq 500 series, and NextSeq 1000 & 2000 series. The potential to achieve maximum reads per run increases with each platform which is 4, 25, 25, 400 million, and 1.1 billion, respectively. All the platforms have the potential for small WGS (whole-genome sequencing) of viruses and microbes, targeted gene sequencing (amplicon and gene panel based), miRNA, small RNA analysis, and targeted gene expression profiling. All the platforms except iSeq 100 can perform 16S metagenomic profiling. The NextSeq series platform also can perform metagenomics profiling (through shotgun as well as metatranscriptomics), methylation sequencing, transcriptome sequencing, single-cell profiling and also cell-free sequencing liquid biopsy analysis, exome, and large panel sequencing. All the platforms can read up to 2 × 150 bp except for MiSeq which has the potential to read 2 × 300 bp. The new-generation instrument can also amplify sequences in the paired-end manner (https://sapac.illumina.com/systems/sequencing-platforms.html).

7.2.2 Ion Torrent

Ion Life Technologies launched Ion Torrent PGM (Personal Genome Machine) in 2011, which is based on emulsion PCR in the same way as 454 GS Junior by Roche [8]. This is the second most prominently used NGS platform. It is a semiconductor-based, non-optical, revolutionary sequencing technology. The semiconductor chip contains millions of wells where DNA fragments get clonally amplified on beads. The amplification occurs by unmodified and unlabeled nucleotides, one by one, in a preset manner. The phosphodiester bonds break and release protons with each nucleotide addition, which generates changes in electric potential and pH and gets detected by

Table 7.1. Sequencing platforms.

Sequencing platform	Principle	Advantages	Disadvantages	Platforms	References
Illumina (SGS)	Sequencing by synthesis	Accuracy	Prephasing, post-phasing, cross-talk	iSeq 100, MiniSeq, MiSeq Series, NextSeq 500 Series and NextSeq 1000 & 2000 Series	[6, 7]
Ion Torrent PGM (SGS)	pH change detection	Lower cost	Homopolymer-associated indel errors	Ion GeneStudio S5 systems and Genexus systems	[7, 8]
PacBio (TGS)	Zero-mode waveguiding technology	High throughput, faster, long reads (50–60 kb or more), uniform coverage, single-molecule resolution	High error rate, less yield, high expense per base	RSII model and more recently, the Sequel™	[5, 9]
Nanopore (fourth-generation)	Pores formation by solid-state sensor technology and biological membrane systems	High throughput	A high error rate, however can be avoided by sequencing of large number of molecules	MinION, GridION, PromethION	[5]

semiconductor chips. The primary benefit of this technology is that it generates a read length of approximately 200 bp that can be used to fill gaps in assembly constructed by other technologies. Nevertheless, this length is much shorter than Roche-454 and PacBio but due to its lower cost, it can be preferable in many cases. However, it does not perform sequencing in a base-by-base manner like Illumina and hence can lead to single-nucleotide indels incorporation in the case of homopolymer stretches. Hence, unlike MiSeq Illumina, 454 GS Junior, and Ion Torrent sequencing instruments are shown to produce homopolymer indels (with an error rate of 0.38 and 1.5 errors per 100 bases, respectively) [7].

There are various NGS instruments of Ion Torrent—Ion GeneStudio S5 systems and Genexus systems. There are three systems available in the case of GeneStudio S5—Ion GeneStudio S5 system, Ion GeneStudio S5 Plus system, and Ion GeneStudio S5 Prime system with a maximum throughput of 15, 30 and 50 Gb, respectively. The range of 2–130 million reads is possible with the aid of five Ion S5 chips—Ion 510™ Chip (2–3 million reads), Ion 520™ Chip (4–6 million reads), Ion 530™ Chip (10–20 million reads), Ion 540™ Chip (60–80 million reads) and Ion 550™ Chip (100–130 million reads) (https://www.thermofisher.com/in/en/home/life-science/sequencing/next-generation-sequencing/ion-torrent-next-generation-sequencing-workflow/ion-torrent-next-generation-sequencing-run-sequence/ion-s5-ngs-targeted-sequencing.html).

7.2.3 PacBio

Pacific Bioscience (PacBio) is a TGS platform [5]. PacBio is also called 'SMRT (single-molecule real-time) sequencing'. It targets sequencing longer nucleotide sequences (DNA and RNA) up to 30–50 kb or longer and does not require pause between the reading steps (also called browse steps), contrary to the SGS platforms [5]. It is also faster than SGS. It provides a hundred times longer browse length than SGS. It can cover repeat sequences, high-GC sequences, and low-frequency mutations with high accuracy. However, there are chances of a higher error rate and it generates less yield. This technique has a low cost per base yet a high cost per run. The error rate could be 10%–15% and it is random. Therefore, after sequencing of ordination, the incorrect base can be identified directly. Hence it can be corrected by multiple sequencing and it can produce a consensus accuracy of more than 99.9% (Q50). It can perform sequencing with direct RNA as compared to SGS, where cDNA sequencing is required. It does not require PCR amplification. The data analysis is complex nevertheless it takes less than a day [9].

The PacBio works by binding engineered DNA polymerase to the DNA which is sequenced at the well's bottom (ZMW-zero-mode waveguide) in an SMRT flow cell. Each of the four nucleotides would be labeled using different phosphor-linked fluorophores, which help in distinguishing all four bases. ZMW is a tiny chamber, that directs light and the image is generated just below ZMW. Thus, the image occurs just in milliseconds after the nucleotide incorporation occurs, and after that, releasing the phosphate-linked fluorescent component and drifting it away from the bottom of ZMW and cannot be detected anymore. There are two platforms of

PacBio released—the new model of RSII and lately, the Sequel™ (https://www.pacb.com/technology/hifi-sequencing/sequel-system/) [9].

7.2.4 Nanopore

This is fourth-generation sequencing, built on the concept of DNA molecules being able to pass through holes, with each type of nucleotide being detected by their different currents. There are mainly two types of nanopores available: solid-state sensor technology and biological membrane. In the case of solid-state sensor technology, metal or metal alloy is used as a substrate for the nanopore formation. In the case of biological nanopores, lipid membrane-embedded transmembrane proteins are utilized. Two proteins: Mycobacterium smegmatis porin A (MspA) and alpha-hemolysin are mainly used to create pores and have been substantially studied. The motor proteins (e.g., highly processive DNA polymerase-phi29) are utilized to regulate the DNA passage rate across the pores. There are also other proteins such as exonuclease I or DNA helicase used for unwinding; then the DNA can move across the pores at the steady rate of tens of thousands of nucleotides. The recording of the characteristic electronic current produced by each passing nucleotide is recorded in real time. Hence, after passing of one DNA through the pore, it becomes free for the next DNA molecule. It is used for metagenomics and environmental samples, also in bacterial strain identification in the space station, as well as for haplotyping, viral genomics, and base modification identification. Similarly to PacBio, it can be used for epigenetic events and it is an RNA sequencing method and does not require PCR or cDNA sequencing. Hence, it can utilized for low-cost sequencing of RNA and DNA, genotyping, and environmental monitoring [5].

Though this method was initially put forth in the 1990s, ONT (Oxford Nanopore Technologies) has recently commercialized it, which has benchtop GridION (5 mimIONS in one module), portable MinION (512 nanopore flow cell channels) PromethION (48 flow cells, each containing 3000 nanopores; in development) (https://nanoporetech.com/products). They contain protein nanopores with electrically resistant polymer membranes, that generating changes in current when each nucleotide goes past the detector.

7.3 Novel virus discovery and the identification of unknown viral pathogens

Unknown viral pathogen detection can be a difficult and complex task, but technological advancement and methodological developments have made it easier to accomplish this. The globalization in the contemporary period has made it possible for viruses to travel from rural, undeveloped areas to every corner of the globe. Regardless of a person's nationality or ethnicity, viral infections have swiftly evolved to suit a variety of people [10]. The rapid evolution of viruses may be the cause of their widespread dissemination and rapid spread [11, 12]. As a result, managing viral illness emergencies by molecular identification of viral infections becomes extremely difficult due to the ongoing variation of the viral genome [13]. Worldwide, there are over 320 000 different types of mammalian viruses [14], and of those, only 200 are known to harbor human infections [15], according to some statistical models. A growing number of newly discovered viral diseases, such as SARS [16], Zika [17], or the more recent coronavirus 2019–CoV [18] outbreak, have been observed within the past few years. Before the widespread accessibility of molecular and serological diagnostics, pathogen detection was mostly accomplished through conventional microbiological techniques, such as cultivation on growth medium, cell cultures, and laboratory animals with subsequent microscopic examination, determination of pathogenic and antigenic characteristics, and metabolic profiling. Currently, a wide range of clinical procedures, such as Enzyme-Linked Immunosorbent Assay (ELISA), and FISH PCR with distinct variations are available for the detection of viruses. Depending on the amount of DNA/RNA templates from a disease in a sample, PCR allows us to precisely quantify pathogens in addition to detecting them [19]. Several methods can be employed to identify unknown viral pathogens.

7.3.1 Conventional techniques for identifying viral infections

The ELISA test has gained widespread usage because to its higher specificity and sensitivity, which are often reported at >90% [20, 21] with inexpensive sampling costs as well as the ease of processing samples and interpreting results. Because of these and other characteristics, ELISA has become a widely used tool for illness screening and prognosis but it has its limitations too. Since this test is primarily reliant upon antigen identification, heterologous antigen's cross-reactivity such as those unique to the influenza virus and the hepatitis C virus, might result in false-positive results [22]. ELISA only offers limited pathogen detection and an approximation of the viral burden; it is therefore unable to identify novel viruses [19].

Finding novel infections was made easier by the advancement of commercial Sanger sequencing software and molecular cloning techniques. Three steps comprise this approach's fundamental principle: (a) PCR amplification of a chosen region, (b) molecular cloning of the amplified fragments, and (c) the Sanger's method of sequencing for the results obtained from molecular cloning. Occasionally, nucleic acids from different viruses are distinguished via hybridization. In order to do this, a microarray is coated with complementary oligonucleotides that align with the conservative portions of the genomes of the chosen viral species, hence it necessitates at least a basic understanding of the target sequences. Because in this technique the sample had to contain a high concentration of viral nucleic acids and the amplification process was hampered by high quantities of host and microbiome DNA, the technique never gained traction in the diagnostics field [23].

Despite the abundant technologies available, real-time PCR is still among the most popular and potent tests accessible today, frequently used as a standard diagnostic procedure. A high degree of specificity is provided by real-time PCR, which can differentiate between infections that are closely related by looking for particular genetic markers. The detection and characterization of unknown pathogens is made possible by real-time PCR, which is an essential technique that greatly aids in the management and control of disease. Viral genera have been studied extensively through RT-PCR [24], for which an enormous number of primers have been developed [24–26]. These screening panels are highly sensitive and effective; however, they are not designed to detect novel strains or kinds with changed target sequences. Primer annealing errors may occur due to genetic similarities between known and unknown viruses, leading to false positives and taxonomic misidentification [20].

7.3.2 High throughput sequencing (HTS) for studying viral pathogens

The development of sophisticated techniques like NGS or HTS, has transformed biological and medical science research, including virology, by making it possible to genetically examine novel viruses without initially cultivating them. NGS is a potent and ground-breaking technique that quickly and extensively sequences molecules of DNA or RNA. HTS techniques sequence millions to billions of DNA fragments concurrently, in contrast to standard Sanger sequencing, which processes DNA one fragment at a time. Viral genome sequencing is already a crucial component of virological research [27] also helping medical professionals recognize complicated infections [28]. It has advanced the fields of evolutionary genomics and the study of molecular epidemiology over time [29, 30].

Direct analysis of genetic material obtained from environmental samples, known as metagenomics, proved to be an effective method for discovering viral infections that are currently unknown. Since all of the available nucleic acids are analyzed, it provides a way to look at the microbial population's taxonomic diversity in a biological or environmental sample. In metagenomics, viruses are identified by sequencing and analyzing nucleic acids (DNA or RNA) taken from clinical samples (blood, tissue, or body fluids) without knowing which pathogens are present beforehand [31]. This technique has further implications in transcriptomics and proteomics, which provide a deeper understanding of several features of infections, including drug resistance, processes of adaptation, and extensive interspecies communication networks [20]. Using shotgun sequencing, which has become widely used in clinical and environmental research and scientific investigations [32–34], metagenomics enables the identification and in-depth investigation of unidentified viral infections [35, 36]. In contrast to conventional methods [37], metagenomics eliminates the need for creating and manufacturing different primers for PCR reactions and their probes as well. This saves time, turning out to be vital during sudden viral outbreaks like the Ebola [38] or Zika [39] viruses when prompt, objective pathogen identification is essential to successfully containing the disease. When other diagnostic methods are insufficient to investigate cases of unknown clustered viral infections, such as in the case of the novel *Arenavirus*, unbiased HTS can also be helpful [40]. In RNA sequencing-based metagenomics, a better positive rate and the identification of more human viruses are the outcomes of RNA sequencing, which enables the detection of an essentially infinite number of infections concurrently. RNA sequencing can identify possible infections that may only be relevant in particular hosts or when discovered from specific sample types, as well as well-known respiratory viruses with clinical significance. Based on their genetic makeup, metagenomics can identify a wide range of infections, including unexpected or unknown viruses that conventional PCR panels could miss. By sequencing and analyzing the entire genetic material contained in the sample, metagenomics makes it possible to identify new viral strains or variations by comparing them to reference databases that are already in existence. Since metagenomics is not dependent on predetermined targets, it can be used to discover genetic variants or new infections without the need to redesign particular assays, which is frequently the case with traditional PCR panels. Because of the unbiased nature of metagenomics, it can be used to identify and track newly circulating viruses in populations, which is a useful tool for study and surveillance [41].

7.3.3 Novel viruses discovered via NGS

In a calf's diarrhoeal faeces, four distinct viruses were identified as, BoAstV, BCoV, BNoV and BKoV, while their dissemination and distribution were linked to the disease, according to metagenomics research. Furthermore, a degree of some co-infections was also found; co-infections or any particular combination of viruses increases the risk of calf diarrhea and necessitates a more thorough examination of both cases and controls [42].

Zhao *et al* 2022 [43] found 14 new viruses with the ability to distinguish colorectal cancer (CRC) patients from healthy controls with a substantial degree of accuracy. These viruses demonstrated potential as diagnostic biomarkers when they were either enriched or reduced in CRC patients. These fourteen viral genomes performed well in terms of diagnosis when merged into a biomarker panel. With the receiver operating characteristics represented by an area under the curve (AUC) of 0.87, the panel demonstrated distinction between patients with CRC and healthy controls within the training groups. Two distinct cohorts having varying ethnic backgrounds were used to further validate the biomarker panel's diagnostic performance. In both validation cohorts, the panel demonstrated strong CRC diagnostic performance, with AUCs of 0.85 and 0.73, respectively. The efficacy of the 14 viral indicators was evaluated about the fecal immunochemical test (FIT), a common screening test. FIT's AUC of 0.89 allowed it to discriminate between CRC patients and healthy controls; however, when the viral panel was added, the performance improved to an AUC of 0.95. These findings demonstrate the intriguing potential of the recently discovered viral genomes as useful diagnostic markers for CRC, providing encouraging opportunities for enhancing CRC screening and diagnosis methods.

7.4 Viral genome sequencing

NGS is frequently used to reconstruct whole viral genomes, even from unidentified or poorly described viruses. This can be done directly from clinical samples or from the preparations of culture-enriched viruses. The assay design can take many forms, such as overlapping amplicon sequencing and assembly, shotgun sequencing (random sequencing) done with complete amplicons of the genome, or shotgun metagenomic sequencing of random libraries [44]. NGS for viral genome sequencing is a potent technology that has transformed the field of virology by providing researchers with unparalleled data regarding viral evolution, transmission dynamics, and disease. The viral genome encodes every piece of data required for the virus to replicate and operate inside a host cell. The size, structure, and organization of viruses' genomes differ; some have segmented genomes, while others have linear or circular genomes.

7.4.1 Human virome characterization

The human microbiome's viral component is made up of several microbial communities that inhabit the body's different niches and is known as the human virome [45]. Molecular approaches have made it possible to identify several significant human viral infections, HHV8 (Human herpesvirus 8) [46], HCV (Hepatitis C virus) [47], and HEV (Hepatitis E virus) [48], that were not cultivable *in vitro*. NGS techniques have significantly changed the research investigation of the human virome, which makes it possible to quickly, objectively, and sensitively identify and characterize viruses. With the use of this method, full-length genomes by *de novo* pathways may be assembled out of the biological samples, allowing for the successful discovery of novel viruses far apart from those that are already known [49–51]. Studies have identified many DNA viruses present in high diversity on human skin through high-throughput sequencing, revealing the presence of viruses including resident and transitory viral populations. The effective and unbiased examination of viral genetic material at the skin surfaces has uncovered the presence of various families of viruses, including *Papillomaviridae*, *Polyomaviridae*, and *Circoviridae* [52, 53]. Human polyomaviruses and their possible connection to illness and cancer have been the subject of research. Research has brought to light the taxonomic and genetic diversity of hepatitis E virus, along with the quasispecies of the virus in individuals suffering from acute hepatitis E, especially those undergoing solid organ transplantation [54]. Human parechoviruses and a variety of enteric viruses are frequently found in stool samples from healthy people, including newborns, and human enterovirus infections are quite prevalent [55]. There is evidence to support the possibility of circovirus and cyclovirus cross-species transmission among farm animals. Human and chimpanzee feces are major sources of these viruses [56, 57]. These developments underscore the expanding comprehension of human virome, intricacy, and interindividual fluctuations along with possible influence over human well-being. A fascinating subgroup of viruses within the virome are those that may persist for an extended period in their host.

7.4.2 Detection of tumor viruses

The discovery of several viruses in human cancerous tissues has important clinical ramifications in oncology since viruses are known to be the cause of about 12% of all human malignancies [58]. With the development of paired-end (PE) reads and NGS technology, viruses in human cancerous tissue may now be found with previously unheard-of efficiency and precision. Several teams have used the enormous quantity of NGS data collected from human tissues to create computational methods for pathogen/virus discovery [59]. While identifying viruses inside human tissues is crucial for medical oncology, examining the locations of integration of viruses in chromosomes of host cells is also beneficial, considering that insertional mutagenesis occurs as a crucial stage in the progression of hepatocellular carcinoma (HCC) caused by the hepatitis B virus (HBV) [60].

Chen *et al* 2013 [61] created a novel algorithmic technique known as VirusSeq to use NGS data to find the sites of integration of known viruses inside the human genome. VirusSeq was assessed using RNA-Seq data from 239 HNSCC samples and 17 HCC samples. The results demonstrated that VirusSeq can reliably identify the integration sites of recognized viruses. VirusSeq is also capable of carrying out this task with whole-genome sequencing information that is derived from various human tissues. The primary constraint on the VirusSeq technique is its reliance on the known virus database responsible for the identification of potential viruses present in tissues of human carcinoma tissue. Novel viruses not included in the viral database will undoubtedly be missed by this. MCC (Merkel Cell Carcinoma) is an unusual, uncommon, and also severe kind of skin cancer among humans that usually impacts people who are elderly or have weakened immune systems; this characteristic has been linked to an infectious cause. After extracting the RNA from MCC samples, 454 pyrosequencing was used to examine it. Following the deletion of all digitized transcriptomes of sequences from human beings, a fusion transcript was discovered between a long T antigen sequence connected to murine polyomaviruses and a tyrosine phosphatase human receptor. Characterization and the entire sequencing of genome of this hitherto unidentified polyomavirus, named MCPyV (Merkel cell polyomavirus), began with this sequence. Only around 10% of the control tissues from various bodily sites, including the skin, had the virus, compared to 80% of MCC tissues. It was also shown that the clonal pattern of viral DNA integration into the tumor genome in MCPyV-positive MCCs strongly implied the virus's etiological participation in the pathophysiology of MCC [62].

Another area of viral oncology that benefited greatly from NGS technologies is the study of integration sites for retroviruses and retroviral vectors in the chromosomes of host cells. The malignant transformation could occur by using viral vectors for gene transfer which are integrated into the host genome because integrating the viral vector inside these genes may activate proto-oncogenes in hosts or inactivate tumor suppressor genes [62–64]. HIV [65] and retroviral integration sites, as well as HIV-based and retroviral vectors for gene therapy and cell reprogramming [66–70], have all been mapped using deep sequencing technology. The basis of deep sequencing techniques to identify retrovirus integration is 454 pyrosequencing of LM-PCR (linear amplification-mediated PCR) or ligation [69, 70] product sequences (LAM-PCR) [71]. Restriction enzymes are used by LAM-PCR as well as LM-PCR to break up DNA that contains proviruses. Subsequently, after digested DNA has been ligated with an appropriate linker, it is amplified by PCR using primers that anneal in the LTR as well as the linker sequence. The 454 high-throughput sequencing technique is then utilized to run a second PCR using nested primers containing linkers. For high-capacity sequencing, a restriction enzyme-free LAM-PCR technique was also created [72]. On the basis of MuA (bacterial transposase), a novel technique for locating integrated DNA locations was recently created.

Adaptors are inserted into genomic DNA using transposase so that 454 pyrosequencing can be used for PCR amplification and analysis. By recovering integration sites almost randomly, this technique could circumvent the bias brought on by restriction enzymes. It offered an indicator of clonal abundance in cells, which is essential in identifying the growth of cell clones which could signal the beginning of a malignant transformation [73].

7.4.3 Entire length sequencing of viral genomes

Sequencing the whole genomes of viruses is a challenging task since viral isolates contain tainting nucleic acids with contaminants from the host cells along with other agents, similar to viral metagenomics. Even among cases of very high viral load, the most thorough method of setting up a basic DNA library for shotgun sequencing or a cDNA library produced by randomly priming RNA produces a significant quantity of host-specific data rather than a thorough depiction of the viral sequences [40, 74, 75]. However, the read lengths might not be long enough to enable viral genomes to be assembled via *de novo* pathways; hence, longer read strategies—like 454 and Illumina technology—could be better [76].

Full genome sequencing of the human immunodeficiency virus (HIV) [77, 78], pandemic influenza viruses [51, 74, 79, 80] human herpesviruses [81, 82], and other viruses has been achieved using these methods. To get enough sequence coverage, very high throughput sequencing methods like the SOLiD platforms might be employed [76]. Marston *et al* 2013 [83] revealed the full genome sequences of previously known *Lyssaviruses* along with a unique novel *Lyssavirus* species using NGS. The technique comprised extracting RNA from cell monolayers, tissue culture supernatant, and diagnostic clinical tissue samples without the need for filtration, ultra-centrifugation, or viral enrichment procedures. By decreasing the rRNA and genomic DNA of host cells, this stage attempted to raise the proportion of RNA specific to viruses in the sample. The RNA samples were sequenced on the Roche 454 platform, which is known for its reliability and consistency in sequencing. *De novo* techniques were employed to assemble the acquired reads and provide consensus sequences covering the entire genome. The assembly procedure aided in the reconstruction of almost whole genomic sequences. Consensus sequences were compared to sequences of genomes of the identical *lyssavirus* species to verify the right sequences and distinguish between homopolymeric repeats and indels. Any feasible insertions or deletions were examined, and PCR products and, if necessary, Sanger sequencing was used to settle any differences. With a particular emphasis on the conserved genomic termini of *lyssaviruses*, the study used *Panlyssavirus* primers to generate PCR products for editing. With this stage, the accuracy and completeness of the derived genome sequences were guaranteed.

7.4.4 Exploration of variability in the viral genome and identification of viral quasispecies

The ability of viruses, especially RNA viruses, to quickly adapt to host immune selection pressure through evolution and mutation is remarkable. As a result, they produce a population known as quasispecies, which is made up of many different but closely related genomes. Precise identification of low-frequency variations may facilitate clinical decision-making in addition to offering priceless insights into molecular causes [84, 85]. Viral populations are diffuse and 'cloud-like,' which enables them to quickly adjust to evolving replicative circumstances thereby favoring already-existing variants that are more fit [86, 87]. As a result, a simple consensus sequence is insufficient to describe many significant viral features; instead, understanding the microvariants that exist within viral populations is necessary. These sequence variations might have a significant impact on viral virulence, immune response evasion, antiviral medication resistance, vaccine development, and production [88]. HIV quasispecies have been the subject of much research among RNA viruses because of their significance in the development of vaccines and their reaction to antiviral medication therapy [89]. Due to fast turnover rates, and an elevated viral load, with replication being facilitated by the error-prone, non-proofreading enzyme reverse transcriptase, HIV is very diverse within infected individuals. Recombination can transmit mutations between viral genomes, leading to notable alterations in virulence or antigenic shift, which is another factor that contributes to high diversity [90]. The analysis of the heavy and light chains of neutralizing antibodies comprising variable regions against HIV in blood drawn from people living with HIV-1 using 454 pyrosequencing methods is another exciting implementation of deep sequencing for HIV research. This analysis aims to comprehend the development of neutralizing antibodies in a broad way [91]. The genome of the human rhinovirus (HRV) was altered during lung transplantation in patients who had been infected with the same strain of the virus for over two years. The complete genome sequences of HRVs from samples taken at various stages of infection were analyzed and it was found that there was no phylogenetically discernible difference in the HRV populations in the lower and upper respiratory tracts during the infection, according to both conventional and Illumina ultra-deep sequencing, most probably due to ongoing mixing of viral populations. However, after several months of infection, particular modifications were observed in the VP2 immunogenic site 2 and the 5′UTR polypyrimidine tract of the HRV genome. These changes may account for the growth of the virus in lower airway environments. These are signs of possible adaptability to conditions with lower airways [92].

Compared to RNA viruses, DNA virus populations are thought to be the least complicated and varied. Data have been obtained through deep sequencing of DNA viral genomes, however, suggesting that infected people may have complicated genotype combinations of the virus and this positive selection might play a role in the diversification of various strains of viruses. There is also the situation with the HCMV (Human Cytomegalovirus), which can cause serious, sometimes fatal illness in immunocompromised persons and can leave latent infections in humans that last a lifetime. High intra-host variability among the HCMV genome was found in neonates having congenital HCMV infection using deep sequencing of amplified fragments derived from three variable HCMV genes [93] as well as long-range, overlapping amplified fragments covering the whole HCMV genome [94]. The genome diversity of HSV-1 (Herpes simplex virus 1) was also revealed by deep sequencing, which made it possible to identify virulence genes. The low-passage clinical isolate H129 and the laboratory strain F's genomic sequences were acquired using Illumina high-throughput sequencing, and they have been compared with the genomic sequence of an HSV-1 isolate that was more pathogenic (strain 17) [81]. HSV-1 H129, isolated from an encephalitic patient's brain, is the only known virus that can move across neural circuits in an anterograde manner [95]. Numerous variations in protein-coding between strains H129 and F and the genomic reference strain 17 were discovered, according to whole-genome sequencing. Some genes, such as the neurovirulence protein ICP34.5, were suggested to likely show accountability of strain H129's anterograde mutant phenotype, whereas a UL13 kinase's frameshift mutation may be the cause of strain F's decreased neurovirulence [81].

7.5 Monitoring antiviral drug resistance

Analysis for drug resistance should be done on specific haplotypes and mutations discovered during the initial NGS. This holds particular significance for viruses like HIV [96], HCV [97], influenza [98], and other viruses [99]. Drug resistance testing is particularly important for HIV because people with the virus must take their medication for the rest of their lives. Patients will have to transition to an alternative line of treatment if they become resistant to HIV drugs; however, this new treatment is possibly less researched and poses a greater danger to the health of patients. Furthermore, both the patient's proportion of mutations resistant to drugs as well as the outbreak's total number of drug-resistant individuals is continually rising [100]. This increases the difficulty of monitoring HIV medication resistance [101]. Drug resistance is usually detected by comparing the effectiveness of medications with genomic alterations [99]. It takes a non-linear approach to identify connections between drug resistance and mutations because different mutations typically have varying resistance powers and frequently act in concert [102, 103]. Depending on the outcomes of the first NGS data analysis, there are two key obstacles in drug resistance detection. They are related to the precision of haplotype and minority mutation detection. The first issue is that haplotypes with small drug-resistant mutations will be superior to other haplotypes that handle drug pressure if one exists. Consequently, drug-resistant haplotypes like these will eventually start to predominate [96, 104]. The second issue is that haplotypes, unlike mutations, are linked to drug resistance; yet, since haplotypes are more difficult to identify, analysis of their drug resistance can be greatly enhanced with much more accurate haplotyping instruments [105]. Since new medications that are effective against the hepatitis C virus (HCV) have recently been available, deep sequencing using NGS techniques is being employed more and more in clinical practice to identify HIV variants that are drug-resistant in low abundance and to identify small variations of the HCV [106]. The most reliable method for identifying mutations resistant to drugs among HIV-1 therapy targets, such as, integrase, protease, reverse transcriptase and the HIV env gene's V3 loop, is conventional direct sequencing of RT-PCR products, also known as 'population sequencing.' However, one of the main drawbacks of direct PCR sequencing is that it cannot identify drug-resistant variants that are found in fewer than 20%–25% of a patient's plasma sample's heterogeneous viral population [106–108].

Numerous investigations have demonstrated that subtle variations in drug resistance that were missed by sequencing based on populations are therapeutically significant because they frequently cause a novel antiretroviral treatment regimen to fail virally [107–109]. Multiple analyses utilizing 454 pyrosequencing for an in-depth examination of HIV reverse transcriptase and protease gene mutations showcased how précised this method is in identifying every drug-resistance mutation discovered through sequencing of the populations as well as its capacity to identify low-frequency mutations that are imperceptible through population sequencing [110–112]. Drug-resistant mutations in the integrase gene occur in response to integrase inhibitors. Before starting treatment, these types of mutations were found at extremely low levels by deep sequencing and may have been chosen by prior medication pressure [113, 114]. Utilizing 454 technology, deep sequencing has also been used to identify HBV resistance to nucleoside and nucleotide reverse-transcriptase inhibitors. Compared to traditional techniques based upon reverse hybridization and population sequencing, NGS technology proved to have enhanced sensitivity for discovering uncommon resistant mutations for HBV treatment [115, 116]. Furthermore, deep sequencing was used to identify the G-to-A hypermutation caused by the apolipoprotein B mRNA editing enzyme. This enzyme was previously thought to have existed in 0.6% of reverse-transcriptase genes [105]. Ultimately, HCV is being studied using the analysis of quasispecies and drug-resistant mutation information obtained from HIV with the introduction of new medications that target the HCV protease and polymerase. Moreover, deep sequencing technologies appear to be a viable tool for studying minority variations that are observed across the HCV quasispecies population both at baseline and when antiviral medication pressure was applied, offering fresh perspectives on the mechanisms underlying the acquisition of HCV resistance [117, 118].

7.6 Viral evolution and epidemiology of infections

NGS datasets offer a multitude of vital biological and epidemiological data that could be having a significant effect on public health and healthcare practices and initiatives. NGS technology allows for the assessment of viral populations within the host and complexity with unrivaled details. By analyzing NGS data, researchers can identify and characterize the diverse viral variants present within infected individuals, providing insights into the dynamics of viral populations. NGS datasets can be used to estimate an individual's infection age. Treatment choices and public health initiatives can benefit from knowledge of the infection's temporal progression [119]. NGS data can shed light on transmission network architectures and shed light on the spread of viruses among people. Controlling the spread of infectious diseases requires an understanding of transmission dynamics. NGS datasets make it possible to quickly gather and examine substantial amounts of sequencing data for monitoring purposes. Real-time monitoring can aid in the early detection of outbreaks and enable prompt public health actions [120–124]. Viral evolution and epidemiology of various viral infections are being studied using high throughput sequencing, tackling problems like viral superinfection, [125], tracking the emergence, development, and global dissemination of viral strains, such as HIV [90], or simulating how viruses evolve within their hosts and how immune escape mechanisms are weighed against the replication potential like that of HCV as well as HIV infections [118, 126, 127].

7.7 Concluding remarks

NGS datasets provide a thorough understanding of viral populations within hosts, enabling researchers to derive important biological and epidemiological data that can guide treatment choices, illness preventive tactics, and outbreak containment initiatives. Amongst the most fruitful usage of NGS is in diagnostic virology, where remarkable outcomes were obtained in the characterization and identification of various novel viruses, the revelation of unknown viral infections in patient specimens, the highly sensitive antiviral medication resistance monitoring, the exploration of diversity among various viral groups, their evolution, dissemination as well as assessment of human virome. Despite progress in discovering novel viruses and comprehending the intricacy of human viruses and virome, their exact makeup including their possible health effects on body surfaces and within tissues are still unknown. To fully understand how the virome contributes to disease and how it maintains health, more research is required. Future research should focus on understanding persistence mechanisms and evaluating the benefits and drawbacks of prolonged immune stimulation. Even though a lot of novel viruses have been discovered, it's still difficult to determine whether they cause disease. It will take further research on pathogenesis and clinical applications to determine the connections between particular viruses and human health effects.

Abbreviations

BCoV	bovine coronavirus
BoAstV	bovine astroviruses
CoV	coronavirus
CRC	colorectal cancer
FISH	fluorescence *in situ* hybridization
H1N1	hemagglutinin type 1 and neuraminidase type 1
HBV	hepatitis B virus
HCC	hepatocellular carcinoma
HCMV	human cytomegalovirus
HCV	hepatitis C virus
HEV	hepatitis E virus
HHV8	human herpesvirus 8
HIV	human immunodeficiency virus
HNSCC	head and neck squamous cell carcinoma
HRV	human rhinovirus
HSV1	herpes simplex virus 1
HTS	high throughput sequencing

ITS	internal transcribed spacer
LAM-PCR	linear amplification-mediated pcr
LM-PCR	ligation-mediated polymerase chain reaction
MCC	merkel cell carcinoma
MCPyV	merkel cell polyomavirus
MspA	mycobacterium smegmatis porin A
NGS	next generation sequencing
ONT	oxford nanopore technologies
PCR	polymerase chain reaction
PGM	personal genome machine
SARS	severe acute respiratory syndrome
SARS-CoV-2	severe acute respiratory syndrome coronavirus 2
SGS	second-generation sequencing
SMRT	singe molecule real time
TGS	third-generation sequencing
WGS	whole-genome sequencing
ZMW	zero-mode waveguide

References

[1] Chiu C Y 2013 Viral pathogen discovery *Curr. Opin. Microbiol.* **16** 468–78

[2] Gu W, Miller S and Chiu C Y 2019 Clinical metagenomic next-generation sequencing for pathogen detection *Annu. Rev. Pathol.: Mech. Dis* **14** 319–38

[3] Gu W, Deng X, Lee M, Sucu Y D, Arevalo S, Stryke D *et al* 2021 Rapid pathogen detection by metagenomic next-generation sequencing of infected body fluids *Nat. Med.* **27** 115–24

[4] Watson S J, Welkers M R A, Depledge D P, Coulter E, Breuer J M, de Jong M D *et al* 2013 Viral population analysis and minority-variant detection using short read next-generation sequencing *Philos. Trans. R. Soc B: Biol. Sci.* **368** 20120205

[5] Slatko B E, Gardner A F and Ausubel F M 2018 Overview of next-generation sequencing technologies *Curr. Protoc. Mol. Biol.* **122** e59

[6] Wang B, Wan L, Wang A and Li L M 2017 An adaptive decorrelation method removes Illumina DNA base-calling errors caused by crosstalk between adjacent clusters *Sci. Rep.* **7** 41348

[7] Singh R R 2020 Next-generation sequencing in high-sensitive detection of mutations in tumors: challenges, advances, and applications *J. Mol. Diagn* **22** 994–1007

[8] Loman N J, Misra R V, Dallman T J, Constantinidou C, Gharbia S E, Wain J and Pallen M J 2012 Performance comparison of benchtop high-throughput sequencing platforms *Nat. Biotechnol.* **30** 434–9

[9] Abde Aliy M, Bayeta S and Takale W 2022 Pacific bioscience sequence technology: Review *Int. J. Vet. Sci. Res.* **8** 27–33

[10] Haug C J, Kieny M P and Murgue B 2016 The Zika challenge *New Engl. J. Med.* **374** 1801–3

[11] Zhao Z, Li H, Wu X, Zhong Y, Zhang K, Zhang Y P, Boerwinkle E and Fu Y X 2004 Moderate mutation rate in the SARS coronavirus genome and its implications *BMC Evol. Biol.* **4** 1–9

[12] Donnelly C A, Fisher M C, Fraser C, Ghani A C, Riley S, Ferguson N M and Anderson R M 2004 Epidemiological and genetic analysis of severe acute respiratory syndrome *Lancet Infect. Dis* **4** 672–83

[13] Gardner S N, Kuczmarski T A, Vitalis E A and Slezak T R 2003 Limitations of TaqMan PCR for detecting divergent viral pathogens illustrated by hepatitis A, B, C, and E viruses and human immunodeficiency virus *J. Clin. Microbiol.* **41** 2417–27
[14] Anthony S J *et al* 2013 A strategy to estimate unknown viral diversity in mammals *MBio* **4** 10–128
[15] Woolhouse M, Scott F, Hudson Z, Howey R and Chase-Topping M 2012 Human viruses: discovery and emergence *Philos. Trans. R. Soc. B: Biol. Sci.* **367** 2864–71
[16] Vijayanand P, Wilkins E and Woodhead M 2004 Severe acute respiratory syndrome (SARS): a review *Clin. Med.* **4** 152
[17] Rather I A, Lone J B, Bajpai V K, Paek W K and Lim J 2017 Zika virus: an emerging worldwide threat *Front. Microbiol.* **8** 1417
[18] Hui D S *et al* 2020 The continuing 2019-nCoV epidemic threat of novel coronaviruses to global health—the latest 2019 novel coronavirus outbreak in Wuhan, China *Int. J. Infect. Dis.* **91** 264–6
[19] Kiselev D, Matsvay A, Abramov I, Dedkov V, Shipulin G and Khafizov K 2020 Current trends in diagnostics of viral infections of unknown etiology *Viruses* **12** 211
[20] Abdel-Hamid M, El-Daly M, El-Kafrawy S, Mikhail N, Strickland G T and Fix A D 2002 Comparison of second-and third-generation enzyme immunoassays for detecting antibodies to hepatitis C virus *J. Clin. Microbiol.* **40** 1656–9
[21] Döller G, Schuy W, Tjhen K Y, Stekeler B and Gerth H J 1992 Direct detection of influenza virus antigen in nasopharyngeal specimens by direct enzyme immunoassay in comparison with quantitating virus shedding *J. Clin. Microbiol.* **30** 866–9
[22] Kasprowicz V, Ward S M, Turner A, Grammatikos A, Nolan B E, Lewis-Ximenez L, Sharp C, Fleming W J, Sims V M and Walker S 2008 BD. Defining the directionality and quality of influenza virus–specific CD8+ T cell cross-reactivity in individuals infected with hepatitis C virus *J. Clin. Invest.* **118** 1143–53
[23] Cogswell F B, Bantar C E, Hughes T G, Gu Y and Philipp M T 1996 Host DNA can interfere with detection of Borrelia burgdorferi in skin biopsy specimens by PCR *J. Clin. Microbiol.* **34** 980–2
[24] VanDevanter D R, Warrener P, Bennett L, Schultz E R, Coulter S, Garber R L and Rose T M 1996 Detection and analysis of diverse herpes viral species by consensus primer PCR *J. Clin. Microbiol.* **34** 1666
[25] Weiss S *et al* 2012 Hantavirus in bat, sierra leone *Emerg. Infect. Dis* **18** 159
[26] Drosten C *et al* 2003 Identification of a novel coronavirus in patients with severe acute respiratory syndrome *New Engl. J. Med.* **348** 1967–76
[27] Radford A D, Chapman D, Dixon L, Chantrey J, Darby A C and Hall N 2012 Application of next-generation sequencing technologies in virology *J. Gen. Virol* **93** 1853
[28] Jerome H *et al* 2019 Metagenomic next-generation sequencing aids the diagnosis of viral infections in febrile returning travellers *J. Infect* **79** 383–8
[29] Riley L W and Blanton R E 2018 Advances in molecular epidemiology of infectious diseases: definitions, approaches, and scope of the field *Microbiol. Spectr* **6** 10–128
[30] Sukhum K V, Diorio-Toth L and Dantas G 2019 Genomic and metagenomic approaches for predictive surveillance of emerging pathogens and antibiotic resistance *Clin. Pharmacol. Ther.* **106** 512–24
[31] Cox-Foster D L *et al* 2007 A metagenomic survey of microbes in honey bee colony collapse disorder *Science* **318** 283–7

[32] Worthey E A *et al* 2011 Making a definitive diagnosis: successful clinical application of whole exome sequencing in a child with intractable inflammatory bowel disease *Genet. Med.* **13** 255–62
[33] Li C X, Shi M, Tian J H, Lin X D, Kang Y J, Chen L J, Qin X C, Xu J, Holmes E C and Zhang Y Z 2015 Unprecedented genomic diversity of RNA viruses in arthropods reveals the ancestry of negative-sense RNA viruses *eLife* **4** e05378
[34] Shi M *et al* 2016 Redefining the invertebrate RNA virosphere *Nature* **540** 539–43
[35] Venter J C *et al* 2004 Environmental genome shotgun sequencing of the Sargasso Sea *Science* **304** 66–74
[36] Mulcahy-O'Grady H and Workentine M L 2016 The challenge and potential of metagenomics in the clinic *Front. Immunol* **7** 29
[37] Thomson E *et al* 2016 Comparison of next-generation sequencing technologies for comprehensive assessment of full-length hepatitis C viral genomes *J. Clin. Microbiol.* **54** 2470–84
[38] Li T *et al* 2019 Metagenomic next-generation sequencing of the 2014 Ebola virus disease outbreak in the Democratic Republic of the Congo *J. Clin. Microbiol.* **57** 10–128
[39] Mlakar J *et al* 2016 Zika virus associated with microcephaly *New Engl. J. Med.* **374** 951–8
[40] Palacios G *et al* 2008 A new arenavirus in a cluster of fatal transplant-associated diseases *New Engl. J. Med.* **358** 991–8
[41] Graf E H, Simmon K E, Tardif K D, Hymas W, Flygare S, Eilbeck K, Yandell M and Schlaberg R 2016 Unbiased detection of respiratory viruses by use of RNA sequencing-based metagenomics: a systematic comparison to a commercial PCR panel *J. Clin. Microbiol.* **54** 1000–7
[42] Wu Q *et al* 2021 Next-generation sequencing reveals four novel viruses associated with calf diarrhea *Viruses* **13** 1907
[43] Zhao L *et al* 2022 Uncovering 1058 novel human enteric DNA viruses through deep long-read third-generation sequencing and their clinical impact *Gastroenterology* **163** 699–711
[44] Capobianchi M R, Giombini E and Rozera G 2013 Next-generation sequencing technology in clinical virology *Clin. Microbiol. Infect.* **19** 15–22
[45] Young G R, Eksmond U, Salcedo R, Alexopoulou L, Stoye J P and Kassiotis G 2012 Resurrection of endogenous retroviruses in antibody-deficient mice *Nature* **491** 774–8
[46] Chang Y, Cesarman E, Pessin M S, Lee F, Culpepper J, Knowles D M and Moore P S 1994 Identification of herpesvirus-like DNA sequences in AIDS-sssociated kaposi's sarcoma *Science* **266** 1865–9
[47] Houghton M 2009 Discovery of the hepatitis C virus *Liver Int.* **29** 82–8
[48] Gr R 1990 Isolation of a cDNA from the virus responsible for enterically transmitted non-A, non-B hepatitis *Science* **247** 1335–9
[49] Cheval J *et al* 2011 Evaluation of high-throughput sequencing for identifying known and unknown viruses in biological samples *J. Clin. Microbiol.* **49** 3268–75
[50] Wylie K M, Mihindukulasuriya K A, Sodergren E, Weinstock G M and Storch G A 2012 Sequence analysis of the human virome in febrile and afebrile children *PLoS One* **7** e27735
[51] Greninger A L *et al* 2010 A metagenomic analysis of pandemic influenza A (2009 H1N1) infection in patients from North America *PLoS One* **5** e13381
[52] Antonsson A, Erfurt C, Hazard K, Holmgren V, Simon M, Kataoka A, Hossain S, Håkangård C and Hansson B G 2003 Prevalence and type spectrum of human papillomaviruses in healthy skin samples collected in three continents *J. Gen. Virol.* **84** 1881–6

[53] Chen A C, McMillan N A and Antonsson A 2008 Human papillomavirus type spectrum in normal skin of individuals with or without a history of frequent sun exposure *J. Gen. Virol.* **89** 2891–7

[54] Dalianis T and Hirsch H H 2013 Human polyomaviruses in disease and cancer *Virology* **437** 63–72

[55] Kolehmainen P, Oikarinen S, Koskiniemi M, Simell O, Ilonen J, Knip M, Hyöty H and Tauriainen S 2012 Human parechoviruses are frequently detected in stool of healthy Finnish children *J. Clin. Virol* **54** 156–61

[56] Li L, Shan T, Soji O B, Alam M M, Kunz T H, Zaidi S Z and Delwart E 2011 Possible cross-species transmission of circoviruses and cycloviruses among farm animals *J. Gen. Virol* **92** 768

[57] Li L *et al* 2010 Multiple diverse circoviruses infect farm animals and are commonly found in human and chimpanzee feces *J. Virol* **84** 1674–82

[58] Zur Hausen H 2009 The search for infectious causes of human cancers: where and why *Virology* **392** 1-0

[59] Isakov O, Modai S and Shomron N 2011 Pathogen detection using short-RNA deep sequencing subtraction and assembly *Bioinformatics* **27** 2027–30

[60] Paterlini-Brechot P, Saigo K, Murakami Y, Chami M, Gozuacik D, Mugnier C, Lagorce D and Brechot C 2003 Hepatitis B virus-related insertional mutagenesis occurs frequently in human liver cancers and recurrently targets human telomerase gene *Oncogene* **22** 3911–6

[61] Chen Y, Yao H, Thompson E J, Tannir N M, Weinstein J N and Su X 2013 VirusSeq: software to identify viruses and their integration sites using next-generation sequencing of human cancer tissue *Bioinformatics* **29** 266–7

[62] Feng H, Shuda M, Chang Y and Moore P S 2008 Clonal integration of a polyomavirus in human Merkel cell carcinoma *Science* **319** 1096–100

[63] Howe S J *et al* 2008 Insertional mutagenesis combined with acquired somatic mutations causes leukemogenesis following gene therapy of SCID-X1 patients *J. Clin. Investig.* **118** 3143–50

[64] Bushman F, Lewinski M, Ciuffi A, Barr S, Leipzig J, Hannenhalli S and Hoffmann C 2005 Genome-wide analysis of retroviral DNA integration *Nat. Rev. Microbiol.* **3** 848–58

[65] Wang G P, Ciuffi A, Leipzig J, Berry C C and Bushman F D 2007 HIV integration site selection: analysis by massively parallel pyrosequencing reveals association with epigenetic modifications *Genome Res.* **17** 1186–94

[66] Varas F, Stadtfeld M, de Andres-Aguayo L, Maherali N, Di Tullio A, Pantano L, Notredame C, Hochedlinger K and Graf T 2009 Fibroblast-derived induced pluripotent stem cells show no common retroviral vector insertions *Stem Cells* **27** 300–6

[67] Winkler T, Cantilena A, Métais J Y, Xu X, Nguyen A D, Borate B, Antosiewicz-Bourget J E, Wolfsberg T G, Thomson J A and Dunbar C E 2010 No evidence for clonal selection due to lentiviral integration sites in human induced pluripotent stem cells *Stem Cells* **28** 687–94

[68] Kane N M *et al* 2010 Lentivirus-mediated reprogramming of somatic cells in the absence of transgenic transcription factors *Mol. Ther.* **18** 2139–45

[69] Cattoglio C *et al* 2010 High-definition mapping of retroviral integration sites identifies active regulatory elements in human multipotent hematopoietic progenitors *Blood, J. Am. Soc. Hematol.* **116** 5507–17

[70] Ciuffi A and Barr S D 2011 Identification of HIV integration sites in infected host genomic DNA *Methods* **53** 39–46

[71] Schmidt M, Schwarzwaelder K, Bartholomae C, Zaoui K, Ball C, Pilz I, Braun S, Glimm H and Von Kalle C 2007 High-resolution insertion-site analysis by linear amplification–mediated PCR (LAM-PCR) *Nat. Methods* **4** 1051–7
[72] Gabriel R *et al* 2009 Comprehensive genomic access to vector integration in clinical gene therapy *Nat. Med.* **15** 1431–6
[73] Brady T *et al* 2011 A method to sequence and quantify DNA integration for monitoring outcome in gene therapy *Nucleic Acids Res.* **39** e72
[74] Kuroda M *et al* 2010 Characterization of quasispecies of pandemic 2009 influenza A virus (A/H1N1/2009) by de novo sequencing using a next-generation DNA sequencer *PLoS One* **5** e10256
[75] Greninger A L, Runckel C, Chiu C Y, Haggerty T, Parsonnet J, Ganem D and DeRisi J L 2009 The complete genome of klassevirus–a novel picornavirus in pediatric stool *Virol. J.* **6** 1–9
[76] Legendre M, Santini S, Rico A, Abergel C and Claverie J M 2011 Breaking the 1000-gene barrier for Mimivirus using ultra-deep genome and transcriptome sequencing *Virol. J.* **8** 1–6
[77] Willerth S M, Pedro H A, Pachter L, Humeau L M, Arkin A P and Schaffer D V 2010 Development of a low bias method for characterizing viral populations using next generation sequencing technology *PLoS One* **5** e13564
[78] Bruselles A, Rozera G, Bartolini B, Prosperi M, Del Nonno F, Narciso P, Capobianchi M R and Abbate I 2009 Use of massive parallel pyrosequencing for near full-length characterization of a unique HIV Type 1 BF recombinant associated with a fatal primary infection *AIDS Res. Hum. Retrovir.* **25** 937–42
[79] Bartolini B *et al* 2011 Assembly and characterization of pandemic influenza A H1N1 genome in nasopharyngeal swabs using high-throughput pyrosequencing *Microbiologica-Q. J. Microbiol. Sci.* **34** 391
[80] Höper D, Hoffmann B and Beer M 2011 A comprehensive deep sequencing strategy for full-length genomes of influenza A *PLoS One* **6** e19075
[81] Szpara M L, Parsons L and Enquist L W 2010 Sequence variability in clinical and laboratory isolates of herpes simplex virus 1 reveals new mutations *J. Virol.* **84** 5303–13
[82] Kwok H, Tong A H, Lin C H, Lok S, Farrell P J, Kwong D L and Chiang A K 2012 Genomic sequencing and comparative analysis of Epstein–Barr virus genome isolated from primary nasopharyngeal carcinoma biopsy *PLoS One* **7** e36939
[83] Marston D A, McElhinney L M, Ellis R J, Horton D L, Wise E L, Leech S L, David D, de Lamballerie X and Fooks A R 2013 Next generation sequencing of viral RNA genomes *BMC Genomics* **14** 1–2
[84] Andino R and Domingo E 2015 Viral quasispecies *Virology* **479** 46–51
[85] Woo H J and Reifman J 2012 A quantitative quasispecies theory-based model of virus escape mutation under immune selection *Proc. Natl. Acad. Sci.* **109** 12980–5
[86] Novella I S, Domingo E and Holland J J 1995 Rapid viral quasispecies evolution: implications for vaccine and drug strategies *Mol. Med. Today* **1** 248–53
[87] Ruiz-Jarabo C M, Arias A, Baranowski E, Escarmís C and Domingo E 2000 Memory in viral quasispecies *J. Virol.* **74** 3543–7
[88] Barzon L, Lavezzo E, Militello V, Toppo S and Palù G 2011 Applications of next-generation sequencing technologies to diagnostic virology *Int. J. Mol. Sci.* **12** 7861–84
[89] Vrancken B, Lequime S, Theys K and Lemey P 2010 Covering all bases in HIV research: unveiling a hidden world of viral evolution *AIDS Rev.* **12** 89–102

[90] Tebit D M and Arts E J 2011 Tracking a century of global expansion and evolution of HIV to drive understanding and to combat disease *Lancet Infect. Dis.* **11** 45–56

[91] Wu X *et al* 2011 Focused evolution of HIV-1 neutralizing antibodies revealed by structures and deep sequencing *Science* **333** 1593–602

[92] Tapparel C, Cordey S, Junier T, Farinelli L, Van Belle S, Soccal P M, Aubert J D, Zdobnov E and Kaiser L 2011 Rhinovirus genome variation during chronic upper and lower respiratory tract infections *PLoS One* **6** e21163

[93] Görzer I, Guelly C, Trajanoski S and Puchhammer-Stöckl E 2010 Deep sequencing reveals highly complex dynamics of human cytomegalovirus genotypes in transplant patients over time *J. Virol.* **84** 7195–203

[94] Renzette N, Bhattacharjee B, Jensen J D, Gibson L and Kowalik T F 2011 Extensive genome-wide variability of human cytomegalovirus in congenitally infected infants *PLoS Pathog.* **7** e1001344

[95] Zemanick M C, Strick P L and Dix R D 1991 Direction of transneuronal transport of herpes simplex virus 1 in the primate motor system is strain-dependent *Proc. Natl. Acad. Sci.* **88** 8048–51

[96] Liu T F and Shafer R W 2006 Web resources for HIV type 1 genotypic-resistance test interpretation *Clin. Infect. Dis.* **42** 1608–18

[97] Lontok E *et al* 2015 Hepatitis C virus drug resistance–associated substitutions: state of the art summary *Hepatology* **62** 1623–32

[98] Pizzorno A, Abed Y and Boivin G 2011 Influenza drug resistance *Semin. Resp. Crit. Care Med.* **32** 409–22

[99] Irwin K K, Renzette N, Kowalik T F and Jensen J D 2016 Antiviral drug resistance as an adaptive process *Virus Evol.* **2** vew014

[100] Gibson K M, Steiner M C, Kassaye S, Maldarelli F, Grossman Z, Pérez-Losada M and Crandall K A 2019 A 28-year history of HIV-1 drug resistance and transmission in Washington, DC *Front. Microbiol.* **10** 369

[101] Assefa Y and Gilks c f 2017 Second-line antiretroviral therapy: so much to be done *Lancet HIV* **4** e424–5

[102] Flynn W F, Chang M W, Tan Z, Oliveira G, Yuan J, Okulicz J F, Torbett B E and Levy R M 2015 Deep sequencing of protease inhibitor resistant HIV patient isolates reveals patterns of correlated mutations in Gag and protease *PLoS Comput. Biol.* **11** e1004249

[103] Feder A F, Rhee S Y, Holmes S P, Shafer R W, Petrov D A and Pennings P S 2016 More effective drugs lead to harder selective sweeps in the evolution of drug resistance in HIV-1 *Elife* **5** e10670

[104] Johnson J A *et al* 2008 Minority HIV-1 drug resistance mutations are present in antiretroviral treatment–naïve populations and associate with reduced treatment efficacy *PLoS Med.* **5** e158

[105] Pawar S D, Freas C, Weber I T and Harrison R W 2018 Analysis of drug resistance in HIV protease *BMC Bioinf.* **19** 1–6

[106] Palmer S *et al* 2005 Multiple, linked human immunodeficiency virus type 1 drug resistance mutations in treatment-experienced patients are missed by standard genotype analysis *J. Clin. Microbiol.* **43** 406–13

[107] Jourdain G, Ngo-Giang-Huong N, Le Coeur S, Bowonwatanuwong C, Kantipong P, Leechanachai P, Ariyadej S, Leenasirimakul P, Hammer S and Lallemant M 2004

Intrapartum exposure to nevirapine and subsequent maternal responses to nevirapine-based antiretroviral therapy *New Engl. J. Med.* **351** 229–40

[108] Lecossier D, Shulman N S, Morand-Joubert L, Shafer R W, Joly V, Zolopa A R, Clavel F and Hance A J 2005 Detection of minority populations of HIV-1 expressing the K103N resistance mutation in patients failing nevirapine *JAIDS J. Acquir. Immune Defic. Syndr* **38** 37–42

[109] Palmer S, Boltz V, Martinson N, Maldarelli F, Gray G, McIntyre J, Mellors J, Morris L and Coffin J 2006 Persistence of nevirapine-resistant HIV-1 in women after single-dose nevirapine therapy for prevention of maternal-to-fetal HIV-1 transmission *Proc. Natl. Acad. Sci.* **103** 7094–9

[110] Wang C, Mitsuya Y, Gharizadeh B, Ronaghi M and Shafer R W 2007 Characterization of mutation spectra with ultra-deep pyrosequencing: application to HIV-1 drug resistance *Genome Res.* **17** 1195–201

[111] Hoffmann C, Minkah N, Leipzig J, Wang G, Arens M Q, Tebas P and Bushman F D 2007 DNA bar coding and pyrosequencing to identify rare HIV drug resistance mutations *Nucleic Acids Res.* **35** e91

[112] Simen B B *et al* 2009 Low-abundance drug-resistant viral variants in chronically HIV-infected, antiretroviral treatment–naive patients significantly impact treatment outcomes *J. Infect. Dis.* **199** 693–701

[113] Mukherjee R, Jensen S T, Male F, Bittinger K, Hodinka R L, Miller M D and Bushman F D 2011 Switching between raltegravir resistance pathways analyzed by deep sequencing *AIDS (London, England)* **25** 1951

[114] Codoñer F M *et al* 2010 Dynamic escape of pre-existing raltegravir-resistant HIV-1 from raltegravir selection pressure *Antivir. Res.* **88** 281–6

[115] Margeridon-Thermet S *et al* 2009 Ultra-deep pyrosequencing of hepatitis B virus quasispecies from nucleoside and nucleotide reverse-transcriptase inhibitor (NRTI)–treated patients and NRTI-naive patients *J. Infect. Dis.* **199** 1275–85

[116] Solmone M, Vincenti D, Prosperi M C, Bruselles A, Ippolito G and Capobianchi M 2009 Use of massively parallel ultradeep pyrosequencing to characterize the genetic diversity of hepatitis B virus in drug-resistant and drug-naive patients and to detect minor variants in reverse transcriptase and hepatitis BS antigen *J. Virol.* **83** 1718–26

[117] Verbinnen T, Van Marck H, Vandenbroucke I, Vijgen L, Claes M, Lin T I, Simmen K, Neyts J, Fanning G and Lenz O 2010 Tracking the evolution of multiple *in vitro* hepatitis C virus replicon variants under protease inhibitor selection pressure by 454 deep sequencing *J. Virol.* **84** 11124–33

[118] Delang L, Vliegen I, Froeyen M and Neyts J 2011 Comparative study of the genetic barriers and pathways towards resistance of selective inhibitors of hepatitis C virus replication *Antimicrob. Agents Chemother.* **55** 4103–13

[119] Knyazev S, Hughes L, Skums P and Zelikovsky A 2021 Epidemiological data analysis of viral quasispecies in the next-generation sequencing era *Brief. Bioinform.* **22** 96–108

[120] Beerenwinkel N *et al* 2005 Computational methods for the design of effective therapies against drug resistant HIV strains *Bioinformatics* **21** 3943–50

[121] Douek D C, Kwong P D and Nabel G J 2006 The rational design of an AIDS vaccine *Cell* **124** 677–81

[122] Gaschen B *et al* 2002 Diversity considerations in HIV-1 vaccine selection *Science* **296** 2354–60

[123] Holland J J, De La Torre J C and Steinhauer D A 1992 RNA virus populations as quasispecies *Genetic Diversity of RNA Viruses* (Springer) pp 1–20
[124] Rhee S Y, Liu T F, Holmes S P and Shafer R W 2007 HIV-1 subtype B protease and reverse transcriptase amino acid covariation *PLoS Comput. Biol.* **3** e87
[125] Redd A D *et al* 2011 Identification of HIV superinfection in seroconcordant couples in Rakai, Uganda, by use of next-generation deep sequencing *J. Clin. Microbiol.* **49** 2859–67
[126] Fischer W *et al* 2010 Transmission of single HIV-1 genomes and dynamics of early immune escape revealed by ultra-deep sequencing *PLoS One* **5** e12303
[127] Bull R A *et al* 2011 Sequential bottlenecks drive viral evolution in early acute hepatitis C virus infection *PLoS Pathog.* **7** e1002243

IOP Publishing

Viral Diseases
History and new developments in diagnostics and therapeutics
Arvind K Singh Chandel, Bhakti Tanna, Amisha Parmar, Gopal Patel and Neeraj S Thakur

Chapter 8

Nanotechnology in diagnostics

Yash Sharma, Kanak Chahar, Lopamudra Mishra, Lakshmi Kumari, Preeti Patel, Dilpreet Singh and Balak Das Kurmi

Nanotechnology is transforming the field of diagnostics by providing unprecedented precision and efficiency in disease detection. It has significantly enhanced the ability to detect pathogens, biomarkers, and even early-stage cancer cells with remarkable accuracy using nanoparticles (NPs), particularly gold and silver. This molecular-level interaction improves sensitivity while reducing the cost and complexity of diagnostic procedures. The advantages of nanotechnology in infection and cancer diagnostics, where timely and accurate detection is critical, are particularly noteworthy. It has facilitated the development of portable, point-of-care diagnostic tools that can deliver real-time results, thereby revolutionizing healthcare accessibility, especially in resource-limited settings. The promise of NPs to detect diseases at their earliest stages holds the potential for improving treatment outcomes and survival rates. However, while nanotechnology offers significant advantages, challenges remain, particularly regarding the safety and biocompatibility of NPs in clinical use. Despite these challenges, the future of diagnostics looks promising as advancements in nanotechnology pave the way for more personalized, efficient, and accessible healthcare solutions.

8.1 Introduction to nanotechnology and diagnosis

Although the creation or application of the smallest particles that are unseen to the human eye are not particularly novel inventions, the idea of nanotechnology has recently been at the forefront of scientific research. It has been discovered that an antique Roman glass cup contains colloidal NPs of silver and gold that are responsible for the phenomena that cause it to reflect various colours when lit. The flexibility and resistance of the fabled Damascene Sword have been attributed to nanometre-sized carbon particles that have been found to be present in it [1]. Nanotechnology is crucial in the life sciences, particularly as parts of functional biological units like deoxyribonucleic acid (DNA). For instance, ribosomes and RNA in live cells are primarily

doi:10.1088/978-0-7503-4987-1ch8

nanoscale in size. According to the United States Environmental Protection Agency, nanotechnology is the branch of science that uses nanoscale particles, studying its peculiar characteristics and employing these to achieve desired results in the fields of engineering, medicine, agriculture, or pharmaceuticals. Nanotechnology involves creating and using structures, devices, and systems that have novel properties and functions as a result of their small and/or intermediate size. An NP is any substance that has a size of less than one micron. Numerous helpful tools made possible by nanotechnology can be used to identify biomolecules and other analytes important for diagnosis [2]. Understanding NPs and their distinctive features may shed light on the peculiar reasons behind their use in various sectors, particularly in medical diagnosis.

Various medical textbooks have used different esplanations to describe medical diagnostics. However, capturing the main idea, the homepage of the website of the *Journal of Medical Diagnostic Methods* defines it as the discipline or practice of diagnosis which involves identifying and describing a disease state and its causal factors using signs and symptoms obtained from patient histories or from physical examinations of patients or their specimen with the aid of various diagnostic techniques. The main goal is to identify the medical condition that is being managed, treated, or endured. This is particularly true given that the first step in any attempt to cure or manage medical issue is to discover the underlying cause. Medical diagnosis has a lengthy history, going from the rudimentary organoleptic evaluation of body samples through the age of microscopy to the present-day usage of biosensors and body imaging. Therefore, incorporating nanotechnology to enhance diagnosis is not only a wise move, but also one that should be welcomed [3].

The new word 'nanodiagnostics' refers to the application of nanotechnology's ideas and approaches to diagnostics. The manipulation and evaluation of single molecules as well as the scaling down of platforms and systems to take use of the nanoscale features made possible by interactions between surfaces and biomolecules are all included, albeit they are not the only ones. In order to address the demand for clinical diagnostics, nanodiagnostics is a growing use of nanoscale technology. It involves identifying the pathophysiology of the ailment and the organisms that are responsible for it, as well as determining the disease status and any susceptibility to it. Nanoscale diagnostics made possible by nanotechnology has sparked a trend toward the usage of readily available, marketable handheld gadgets [2, 4]. As a rapidly growing area of molecular diagnostics, nanodiagnostics has had a significant impact on laboratory processes, offering fresh approaches for patient sample evaluation and the early detection of disease biomarkers with improved sensitivity and specificity. Since the majority of once-complex procedures are now integrated onto a single, straightforward device with the ability to be used for immediate diagnosis, diagnostic procedures have become less laborious but more sensitive thanks to the development and optimization of NP platforms for the detection of pathogens and cancer biomarkers [3].

8.2 Infection diagnosis

Noble metal NPs have been employed in proof-of-concept tests of a variety of biosensing technologies over the years for the selective and precise identification of

DNA/RNA sequences linked to infection and pathogens because of their optical and physicochemical features. These devices have been employed as fluorescence/chemiluminescence signal transduction substitutes or in conjunction with them. Due to their simplicity of synthesis and functionalization with DNA/RNA molecules, proteins, and other biomolecules, NPs are the best instrument for tagging biomolecular probes.

With proteins, DNA/RNA, and other biomolecules, NP-based systems have gradually included currently employed bioassays for detection of recognised biomarkers or nucleotide sequences, improving sensitivity and reducing costs. They can interact on the same scale as target biological molecules because of their nano-size scale, which presents a high ratio of surface area to volume. The detection of nucleic acids, proteins, pH changes, or tiny analytes utilizing colorimetric, fluorescence, mass spectrometry, electrochemical, and scattering techniques has been reported as a diagnostic strategy using NPs. Nanodiagnostic systems can conduct molecular tests more quickly, with greater sensitivity, greater flexibility, and at lower prices [5].

8.3 Gold and silver nanoparticles for molecular diagnostics

Methods for detecting biomolecules based on NPs made of noble metals, especially gold and silver, have received widespread use due to their distinctive physical and chemical characteristics [6]. They can be created as single inorganic compounds, alloys, or core shells, all of which have various sizes and shapes (such as spheres, rods, prisms, and stars) and carry various properties that can be used for biomolecule tagging and promoting biorecognition [7]. The high area to volume ratio of the nanosized particles facilitates functionalization with (bio)molecules.

Gold NPs (AuNPs) and silve NPs (AgNPs) exhibit remarkable visual characteristics, such as dazzling strong hues in solution, due to the localized surface plasmon resonance (LSPR). These properties are especially valuable for identifying pathogens and characterizing molecules [8]. The way that light interacts with the metal's surface electrons can be used to explain this occurrence. At the LSPR frequency, which falls within the visible region of the electromagnetic spectrum, there is a significant increase in electric field intensity, as well as in both scattering and absorption cross-sections. Due to surface plasmon amplification, optical cross-sections are significantly larger by at least five orders of magnitude than those of conventional dyes typically used for tagging biomolecules [9]. The surroundings, NP size, and shape all affect the LSPR band. Other intriguing characteristics of AuNPs and AgNPs are also used in molecular detection techniques, like the capacity to quench or amplify the fluorescence of a fluorophore nearby in a distance-dependent way. Fluorescence modulation is affected by factors such as the size of NPs, their coating, the wavelengths of both the incident and emitted light, and the inherent quantum yield of the fluorophore [10]. Nanosurfaces are also optimal for the enhancement of Raman spectrum, with increments of 105-times to 106-times the surface enhancement Raman spectroscopy (SERS) [11]. This allows for the use of organic dyes with defined Raman spectra to create specific fingerprints that are significantly amplified by NPs, facilitating the development of multi-label detection systems.

Other uses for AuNPs and AgNPs include metal conductivity, which takes advantage of the electrical signal amplification given by the NPs [12]. Several techniques of the production of AgNPs and AuNPs via chemical, physical, photochemical, and biological approaches have been documented.

Each approach has advantages and disadvantages based on cost, scalability, particle size, and size distribution [13, 14]. The reaction mechanism primarily involves the reduction of an Ag or Au salt, leading to the formation of neutral charged NPs. Subsequently, a capping agent 'restricts' the growth of NPs, stabilizing them in specific shapes and sizes. During synthesis, the capping agent can leave functional groups, such as carboxylic groups, available for further functionalization. Typically AuNPs and AgNPs are functionalized with biomolecules through thiol metal quasi-covalent bonds, having the strong affinity between the metal and sulfur found in biomolecules like proteins or easily introduced with oligonucleotides [14]. Direct bonding between amine groups and metals, or carboxyl groups of coating agents, is also used for functionalizing AuNPs with proteins, carbohydrates, and other polymers. This simple method makes AuNPs (and, to a lesser extent, AgNPs) particularly well-suited for easy and efficient biofunctionalization [13].

8.4 Biomarkers

A biomarker is a quantitative property that serves as an indicator for any biological state or condition. Infection biomarkers are usually molecules from the infecting agent—such as nucleic acids, proteins, cell walls, or metabolites—or host responses to infection, like antibodies, which can also be used as biomarkers [15]. Microbial pathogens are typically identified using traditional techniques like microscopy, cultivation on selective or differential media, or biochemical serological test, or molecular biology techniques. Traditional methods are often time-consuming and arduous, whereas molecular biological techniques are costly and impractical for clinical use. Furthermore, detecting biomarkers in biological fluid samples is problematic since most probes (for example, blood) contain components that disrupt biorecognition or affect the sensor's performance. For example, lateral flow cytometry and other colorimetric techniques are limited by sample properties like opacity or viscosity, which may affect the accuracy of the readout. A preliminary sample purification procedure is frequently used to overcome this problem [16]. While molecular diagnostic methods are often linked to disease diagnosis, it is important to recognize that they only detect the presence of the pathogen's molecular 'fingerprints'. Consequently, these assays do not offer direct information about the presence or metabolic activity of the microorganism in the tested samples.

Colorimetric, fluorescent, electrochemical, SERS, lateral flow, and other techniques may be used to identify noble metal NPs. Each has advantages and disadvantages. Colorimetric technologies are useful for rapid and simple screening, while SERS and fluorescence are useful for multiplex assays. Electrochemical systems offer high sensitivity, and lateral flow assays (LFAs) are advantageous for their portability [17].

8.5 Nanodiagnostics for nucleic acid

With whole-genome sequencing of pathogens, it is now possible to identify unique DNA fingerprints for various organisms and strains. The sequence variations found can be linked to specific characteristics [18]. Single nucleotide variants have been widely mapped and linked to phenotypic traits like antibiotic resistance and virulence [15]. Target sequences in clinical samples are typically present at low copy counts, making it challenging to identify nucleic acids directly without a step of amplification. This gene amplification stage, which takes around 2–3 h and requires specialized equipment, is often conducted via PCR or loop-mediated isothermal amplification (LAMP) [19]. For RNA, quantitative RT-PCR (qRT-PCR) [20] and nucleic acid sequence-based amplification are typically used [21].

8.6 Homogeneous colorimetric assays

The UV–vis spectrum behaviour of noble metal NPs is greatly influenced by size, shape, and interparticle spacing. As the distance between NPs decreases, the LSPR peak of AuNPs often undergoes a significant red shift, indicating that NPs aggregate in solution. This phenomenon forms the basis of many colorimetric detection methods. The aggregation of NPs can be induced by the hybridization of DNA crosslinkers, protein scaffolding, and/or increasing the ionic strength [22].

8.6.1 Unmodified nanoparticle

The distinct interactions of double-stranded DNA and single-stranded DNA onto the surface of AuNPs in relation to dsDNA sequences, forming inflexible non-adsorbent structures, ssDNA sequences non-specifically adsorb to the surface of the NPs, enhancing their stability. This enables the progress in the development of a detection method based on unmodified AuNP aggregation, in which ssDNA in contrast to the target is added to the AuNP solution, boosting its stability due to surface adsorption [23]. Following the addition of the target and salt, a DNA duplex is produced, exposing the NPs, which rapidly aggregate. This approach was used to identify hepatitis B virus (HBV), human immunodeficiency virus type 1 (HIV-I), Bacillus anthracis, and *Mycobacterium tuberculosis* with some changes [24]. A novel strategy combining unmodified AuNPs, rolling circle amplification, and thiol-modified primers; when amplification occurs, NPs attach to the thiol primers and do not aggregate when salt is added. It was possible to identify DNA with a limit of detection of 0.1 fM after isothermal amplification [25].

8.6.2 Cross-linking

Mirkin *et al* in 1996 explained selective DNA target recognition employing oligonucleotide functional AuNPs as gold nanoprobes in a cross-linking method, in which the target DNA functions as a linker between two distinct Au nanoprobes. The target's and the two probes' sequence complementarity causes NP aggregation and, as a result, a visual change from red to blue [26]. The very first approach developed for pathogen detection with a spot-and-read method for detection of mecA in methicillin-resistant *Staphylococcus aureus*{MRSA} directly from genomic DNA samples with a limit of detection (LOD) of 66 ng/VLL was based on this concept [27].

Following that, many cross-linking techniques for pathogen detection were published, with the crucial distinction between approaches, aside from target sequence and organism, being the requirement for preceding amplification of nucleic acid (i.e., PCR, LAMP, and NASBA). Some procedures claim to have an LOD that allows for direct nucleic acid detection. These include HIV-I, *Cryptosporidium parvum*, *M. tuberculosis* complex strains, and *Salmonella* sp. Identification. A cross-linking multiplex test for detecting Kaposi's sarcoma-associated herpesvirus (KSHV) and *Bartonella* was described. This experiment employed both Au and Ag nanoprobes, each of which detected a distinct target. Because gold and silver have different spectral characteristics, it is possible to distinguish between AgNPs and AuNPs aggregation in solution [28].

8.6.3 Non-cross-linking

Baptista *et al* published another colorimetric detection technique for nucleic acids based on AuNPs in 2006, when they reported the direct identification of *M. tuberculosis* genomic DNA from its clinical samples [29]. One advantage in the non-cross-linking approach is that it only requires one Au nanoprobe for molecular detection. Aggregation of Au nanoprobes is induced by elevating the ionic strength of the medium (i.e., salt addition), and colorimetric discrimination is possible due to the differential behaviour of Au nanoprobes in the presence (red due to Au-nanoprobe system stabilization) or absence (blue due to extensive aggregation) of a specific complementary target (figure 1.1(A)). Additional improvements were made to the protocol for single base changes (mutations) related with antibiotic resistance [30–32]. The non-cross-linking technique was recently implemented into a point-of-care (POC) platform and a mobile phone for image analysis, simplifying the detection procedure and decreasing equipment dependency [33].

8.7 Heterogeneous detection

8.7.1 Microarrays

Despite the fact that AgNPs have a larger attenuation coefficient and thus a higher spectrum signal, the bulk of colorimetric systems rely on AuNPs because they are more stable in solution and have higher functionalization efficiencies [34]. In some circumstances, AuNPs are employed for molecular detection and biofunctionalization before being stained with silver to create core–shell structures that combine the best features of both metals [35].

A silver staining procedure used in a microarray sandwich approach, in which certain nucleotides are placed to a platform and then target and probe hybridization is promoted. AuNPs are fixed to the matching areas of each target after a washing phase, and silver staining is conducted. It was possible to detect the *S. aureusmec* A gene (LOD = 100 fM) by studying the scattering [36].

Based on this strategy, Zhao *et al* [36] proposed using a microarray approach to detect influenza A virus. After PCR, they are able to detect and distinguish H5N1 from HINI and H3N2 strains with an LOD of 100 fM [37]. The similar technology for HPV detection was disclosed, aligned with an optical detection device and software for automated data analysis.

In contrast to field application, microarray-based techniques have the benefit of high throughput screening for a large number of samples for a few diseases or a small number of samples for a diverse range of pathogens. Microarray technologies, on the other hand, necessitate specialized equipment handled by dedicated technicians capable of handling high-density data and complicated analysis.

8.7.2 Lateral flow assay

POC testing can utilize LFAs as disposable platforms. Most of these devices use sandwich techniques, where a capture probe binds to the target analyte and a secondary probe detects the event on a suitable matrix, such as nitrocellulose, paper, or plastic [38, 39]. Regarding performance, LFAs operate in a straightforward manner: a liquid sample is applied to a sample pad, where it migrates to a conjugation pad and binds to the probe through capillary action. A second probe is immobilized and captures both the target and the first probe, forming a sandwich-like structure. This second probe is typically attached to the platform using streptavidin-coated microspheres, anti-streptavidin antibodies, and/or biotin-modified oligonucleotides that create streptavidin–biotin bonds [40]. To guarantee sample vector mobility, an adsorbent pad is always positioned on the platform's extremities. To prevent recognition or hybridization failure, a control line is utilized. LFAs are rapid, easy, and low-tech to perform; however, their primary drawback is sensitivity, which sometimes requires preceding amplification when dealing with nucleic acids [38].

8.7.3 Electrochemical assay

Electrochemical sensors are easy to use and manipulate, have excellent sensitivity and specificity, and may be easily transferred from laboratory settings to POC devices [41]. Electrochemical detection systems translate biomolecule identification into quantifiable changes in electrochemical parameters like redox kinetics, electrical impedance, or amperage [8]. An electrode, a capture probe, a reporting probe, and the target (such as DNA) are the usual components of an electrochemical DNA sensor. Capture probes can be immobilized on various nanomaterials, such as gold or magnetic NPs, although they are usually immobilized on the electrode surface (such as carbon or gold electrodes) and recognize the target DNA [42, 43]. The reporter probe generates an electrochemical signal in response to a reaction. The two probes work well together and hybridize in a sandwich fashion [44]. Recent advances in nanofabrication and microfluidics have made it possible to reduce the volume of samples and reagents, which has improved sensitivity and efficiency through miniaturization of sensors. Certain sensors, like the one detailed by Li *et al*, combine capture and reporting probes [45].

A reporter probe (an Au nanoprobe functionalized at the 5′ end) and a capture probe (a hairpin DNA attached on a glassy carbon electrode via the 3′ end) are used in this configuration to detect the presence of RNA from the hepatitis C virus (HCV). A shift in current/potential results from the hairpin's conformational shape changing as it gets closer to the AuNP and the electrode.

One benefit of using AuNPs in electrochemical sensors is the ability to functionalize enzymes to the surface using straightforward techniques. The nanoconjugates can be used to detect certain sequences or catalyze reactions that result in an electrochemical signal [41, 44]. An alkaline phosphatase and oligonucleotides are used to biofunctionalize the reporter Au nanoprobe, and the electrode surface is secured using a capture oligonucleotide probe. The substrate is para nitrophenol (p-NP), and the target is positioned between the reporter and capture probes. When the target is present, the enzyme hydrolyzes the substrate to produce para nitrophenyl phosphate (p-NPP), which is identified by differential pulse voltammetry (LOD of roughly 1.25 ng ml^{-1} of genomic DNA). Electrochemical detection of *V. cholerae* and *Salmonella enteritidis* was also achieved using magnetic NPs for target separation [46]. After magnetic separation, hydro chloric acid accelerates the dissolution of gold on a surface plasmon-coupled emission (SPCE) plate that tracks Au^{3+} ions. The authors reported detection limits of 5 and 100 ng ml^{-1}, respectively.

8.7.4 Fluorescence assay

Nano surface energy transferor NSET, is a phenomena that is commonly associated with fluorescence-coupled technologies on metal nanosurfaces [47]. NSET reflects fluorescence modulation near metal surfaces (governed by the LSPR of the NPs), just like the more common Forster resonance energy transfer (FRET) [48]. This is a distance-dependent interaction that takes place between 2 and 30 nm, double the range of FRET [49]. Typically, NSET-based nucleic acid detection systems consist of a fluorophore attached to an NP that strongly quenches its fluorescence; the presence of the target causes a conformational change that lengthens the fluorophore's bond with the NP, reducing the intensity of the quenching and enabling the detection of the fluorescence signal [50]. It has previously been established that colorimetric DNA detection can be achieved by using the difference in adsorption to AuNPs that ssDNA experiences compared to dsDNA. When a fluorophore is positioned close to the surface of NPs, it can modify the fluorescence that NPs release. This property has been used to develop straightforward sensing protocols that rely on the fluorophore-tagged oligonucleotide's differential adsorption onto the NP surface. When fluorescence is adsorbed to the surface, it is extinguished. Quenching efficiency is limited when a complementary target, such as dsDNA, is present because hybridization results in de-adsorption from the AuNPs' surface and a shift in the fluorophore's position [51].

Compared to colorimetric assays, fluorescence detection offers a major advantage because it enables the conjugation of many chromophores for different illnesses in multiplex assays, each with a distinct spectral signature. Additionally, a number of studies demonstrate a direct correlation between target concentration and signal strength, which enables the evaluation of infection load. The need for costly dye molecules and specialized detecting equipment is a major drawback [48].

8.7.5 Raman and SERS

It has been shown that the intersections between noble metal NP aggregates constitute SERS hotspots due to the overlap of LSPR fields [52]. A multiplex technique uses five distinct probes labeled with five different Raman dyes to detect five different viral agents, including the bacteria *B. anthracis* and the viruses hepatitis A (HVA), hepatitis B (HVB), HIV, Ebola, and varicella. In a sandwich test, the target hybridizes to an immobilized probe and a Raman-labelled Au nanoprobe, enabling sensitive SERS signal detection following silver deposition for signal intensification [53]. Wang *et al* proposed in 2013 another method for detecting infection situations that use the SERS-based methodology. The system functions as a beacon by using AgNPs functionalized with a dye-labelled oligonucleotide. The beacon is activated by the target's presence, which causes the SERS signal to decrease. The target is an RNA that has two radical S-adenosyl methionine domains (RSAD2), and the antiviral defense that results from these domains is known. In response to interferon stimulation or viral infection, such as human *cytomegalovirus*, influenza virus, HCV, dengue virus, alpha viruses, and retroviruses like HIV, RSAD2 has been found to be among the most highly upregulated genes. This technique may discriminate patients with symptomatic acute respiratory infections from healthy individuals with an accuracy of more than 95% [54].

SERS-based assays' primary benefits are without a doubt their sensitivity and multiplexing capabilities, but they also have some serious drawbacks, such as the need for specialized equipment and the difficulty of data processing.

8.7.6 Others

Other notable ways for detecting noble metal NPs have been published. These depend on combining detection techniques with the biobarcode test such as mass spectrometry, piezoelectric sensors, hyper-Rayleigh scattering, and sound detection [55].

The biobarcode test was used to identify nucleic acids, and numerous methods were followed for a variety of targets. Target separation is accomplished via DNA-functionalized magnetic NPs, and then bi-functionalized AuNPs hybridize to the target. These AuNPs are functionalized with a signature sequence and a specific sequence that recognizes the intended target in a 1:100 ratio. The thiol-Au links are broken after separation with magnetic NPs, requiring the characteristic sequences to be released and signal amplification to occur [56].

Yang *et al* [57] describe a method for detecting distinct signature sequences that employs MALDI TOF mass spectrometry. Using a multiplex assay with an LOD of 0.5 aM, they were able to identify DNA from HIV, HBV, HCV, and *Treponema pallidum* since each oligonucleotide has its own unique profile.

8.8 iPCR and other methods

Pathogen immunodetection has been described using gold spheres, rods, and AgNPs. These systems have used antibodies or aptamers to identify a variety of diseases using fluorescence, piezoelectric, SERS, and Rayleigh scattering assays [58]. Immune PCR (iPCR) was introduced in 1992 as a very sensitive approach for protein detection that combines antibodies and PCR. Antibodies conjugated with specific DNA sequences are utilized to target the antigen of interest, which is then amplified using PCR or LAMP [59]. Amplification of the DNA probe attached to the antibodies enables quantitative antigen determination. iPCR stands out as a very sensitive method for protein detection, distinguishing itself from other Au and AgNP methods by not relying on optical or electrochemical features; iPCR methods are sensitive because Au and AgNP are efficient transporters of biomolecules [60]. Amplification of the DNA probe attached to the antibodies enables quantitative antigen determination. iPCR stands out as a very sensitive method for protein detection, distinguishing itself from other Au and AgNP methods by not relying on optical or electrochemical features; iPCR methods are sensitive because Au and AgNP are efficient transporters of biomolecules [61]. This has been utilized to detect the nucleocapsid protein of the Hantaan virus. An ELISA plate covered with polyclonal antibodies and AuNPs containing a signature DNA and a monoclonal antibody against the target was utilized in this experiment. Heating released the characteristic sequence, which was then amplified using real-time PCR. Later, Perez *et al* separated respiratory syncytial virus using magnetic NPs rather than ELISA plates [62].

8.9 Nanotechnology in cancer diagnostics

Cancer mortality and incidence are rising all across the world. GLOBOCAN 2018 estimates that there will be more than 18.1 million new cases of cancer and 9.6 million deaths from the disease. [63, 64]. Early detection reduces cancer-related mortality significantly, for example, breast cancer patients with local metastases have a 5-year relative survival rate of over 90%, whereas those with distant metastases only have a 27% 5-year survival rate [65]. Imaging techniques and morphological study of tissues (histopathology) or cells (cytology) are currently used to aid in the early detection of cancer. The most commonly used imaging modalities, such as x-ray, MRI, computed tomography (CT), endoscope, and ultrasound, can identify cancer only when there is a visible alteration in the tissue. Thousands of cancer cells may have grown and perhaps metastasized by then. Furthermore, existing imaging technologies cannot distinguish between benign and malignant tumours [66]. Although nanotechnology has not yet been used in clinical trials for cancer diagnosis, it is already being used in a number of medical tests and screenings, such as the use of AuNPs in home pregnancy tests [67]. NPs are being used in cancer diagnostics to capture cancer biomarkers such as cancer-associated proteins, circulating tumour DNA, circulating tumour cells, and exosomes [68].

On the surfaces of NPs, different compounds such as aptamers, small molecules, peptides, and antibodies can be coated thickly. These compounds have the ability to

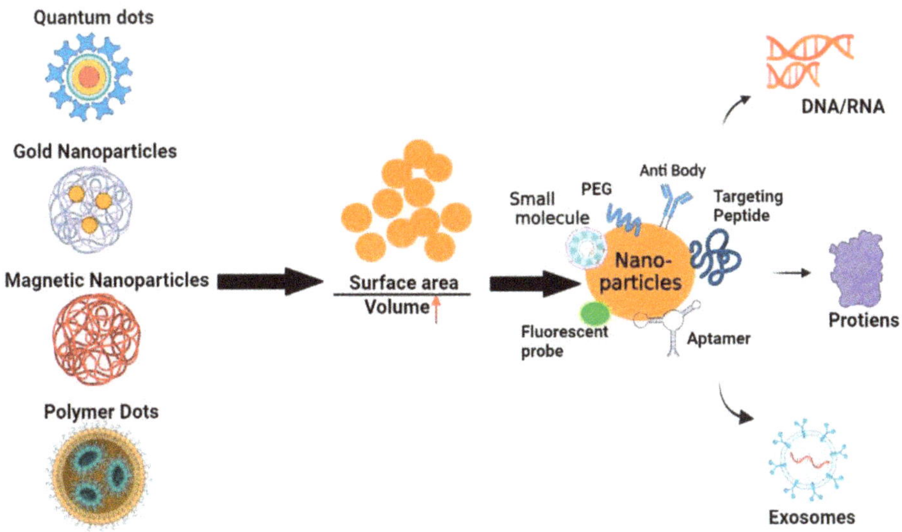

Figure 8.1. Improved cancer diagnosis and detection by nanotechnology. Reproduced from [87] CC BY 4.0.

attach to and recognize certain cancer molecules (figure 8.1). Experimen specificity and sensitivity can be enhanced by introducing cancer cells with several binding ligands to produce multivalent effects [69]. Real-time, simple, and affordable diagnostic methods based on nanotechnology are being developed as potential tools for cancer detection and diagnosis. [70].

8.9.1 Detection of circulating tumor cells

A cancer cell from the original tumor first invades the surrounding tissue during metastatic distribution. It then invades the blood and lymph systems' microvasculature (intravasation), survives and translocates through the bloodstream to microvessels in distant tissues, exits the bloodstream (extravasation), and survives in the microenvironment of distant tissues, which produces an appropriate foreign microenvironment for development [71]. People have reported using magnetic NPs (MNPs), AuNPs, quantum dots (QDs), nanowires, nanopillars, silicon nanopillars, carbon nanotubes, dendrimers, graphene oxide, and polymers for circulating tumor cells (CTC) detection (table 8.1) [72].

QDs have unique optical features that increase their utility in cancer cell identification. QDs are useful in the detection of low abundance compounds due to their high quantum yields. To improve QD electrical properties, hybridization of ZnO NDs with g-C_3N_4 QDs provides greater photoelectron transfer and separation efficiency. ZnO NDs and g-C_3N_4 QDs offer a wide range of applications because to their exceptional properties, and a photocatalyzed renewable self-powered cytosensing device based on ZnO NDs@g-C_3N_4 QDs was reported. The apparatus was utilized to detect CCRF-CEM cells (human acute lymphoblastic leukaemia cells) that express PTK7 by conjugating it to the membrane PTK7-specific aptamer Sgc8c.

Table 8.1. Nanotechnology for cancer cell detection.

Nanoparticle	Type of affinity probe	Specificity ligand	Type of cancer	References
Magnetic nanoparticle	Antibody	EpCAM	Colon/liver/lung/ breast	[73–75]
Quantum dots	Aptamer	PTK7	Leukaemia	[76]
Polymer dots	Antibody	EpCAM	Breast	[77]
Gold nanoparticles	Aptamer Antibody	Her2 Cd2/cd3	Breast Leukaemia	[78][79]
Carbon nanotubes	Antibody	EpCAM	Liver	[80]
Up-conversion nanoparticles	Antibody	Her2	Breast	[81]
Nanorod arrays	DNA aptamer	EpCAM	Breast	[82]
Nanoparticle coated silicon bead	Antibody	EpCAM/ CD146	Breast Colorectal	[83]
Nanofibers	Antibody	EpCAM	breast	[84]

According to the results, the appratus performs better in terms of detection range, detection limit, selectivity, and reproducibility. It only collected CCRF-CEM cells (500 cell/ml) and no other cell types like HL-60, K562, or HeLa cells. The scientists believe that the gadget has considerable potential as a platform for monitoring the course of leukaemia [76].

Non-toxic NPs with high quantum yields and photostability have been produced using polymer NPs derived from several conductive hydrophobic polymers. As a result, polymer dots (PDs) are perfect for CTC detection [77].

One method for functionalizing semiconducting PDs is via trapping of heterogeneous polymer chains in a single dot, aided by hydrophobic interactions during NP formation. A few amphiphilic polymers containing functional groups for future covalent conjugation of biomolecules, such as streptavidin and immunoglobulin G (IgG), display co-condensation with the majority of semiconducting polymers for NP surface alteration and functionalization. The PDs bioconjugate labelled cellular targets effectively and specifically, which includes a cell surface marker on human breast cancer cells, with no need for nonspecific binding detection. According to flow cytometry studies, the fluorescence of PD labelled MCF-7 cells was 25 times higher than that of QD labelled cells and 18 times higher than that of Alexa Fluor-labelled cells [85].

Up-conversion nanoparticles (UCNPs) are commonly used for fluorescent labelling because of their capacity to convert near-infrared (NIR) light to infrared (IR) light, resulting in fluorescence emission in the visible region of the spectrum with little background noise. Additionally, using NIR light as an excitation source protects normal tissues on the one hand while allowing deep tissue penetration on the other [86].

8.9.2 Detection using recognition of cell surface proteins

The primary method for detecting cancer cells is the binding of NP probes combine with moieties (protein, short peptides, antibodies, oligonucleotide aptamers) to surface markers on cancer cells as well as those entering cells and detecting genetic content. The first and most critical stage in the detection of cancer cells, such as CTCs, is capture or isolation. Despite the fact that physical features of the cell, such as size, deformability, and density, are occasionally exploited, capture is mostly dependent on the affinity of cell surface molecules on CTCs detected with materials such as antibodies or aptamers. Numerous studies have demonstrated that EpCAM is significantly expressed on CTCs from a variety of human malignancies, making it useful as a cell surface biomarker. As a result, anti-EpCAM compounds are frequently used in CTC screening. Epithelial-to-mesenchymal transition (EMT) of CTCs would result in ineffective positive sorting based on EpCAM expression. As a result, another option is to look for supplementary or replacement markers for EpCAM.

Various cell surface markers have been examined for the detection of CTCs, including vimentin, androgen receptor, glycan, major vault protein (MVP), and fibroblast activation protein (FAP). However, the majority of these markers are only seen in select cells, and several indicators are no longer present in CTCs that have undergone EMT. Supplementary mesenchymal CTCs are detected in the metastatic stages of cancer, therefore finding appropriate EMT markers to assess prognosis and metastasis in cancer patients is critical [87].

8.10 Nanotechnology for *in vivo* imaging

In addition to simplifying cancer diagnosis through the *ex vivo* identification of cancer cells and biomarkers in liquid biopsy samples, identifying malignant tissues within the body offers several benefits for cancer detection and treatment. A good NP probe for cancer detection should have a long circulation time, be selective to tumour tissue, and be non-toxic to neighbouring healthy tissue [88]. Related to the current research is a focus on NP probe accumulation in tumour tissue for cancer diagnosis in animal studies, primarily mouse designs.

NP probes can preferentially accumulate in tumour tissues by active or positive targeting, allowing for *in vivo* imaging and detection of cancer [89]. The key clinical application challenges are interactions between NPs and blood proteins, uptake and clearance by the reticuloendothelial system (RES), penetration into solid tumours, and optimal active (versus passive) targeting for cancer diagnostics. Fortunately, numerous advancements in these areas have been made.

8.10.1 Passive targeting

Passive targeting is defined as the preferential extravasation of 10- to 150-nm NPes from the circulation into tumour tissue. NPs can preferentially concentrate in tumour tissue because tight connections between endothelial cells in new blood vessels in tumours do not develop properly [90]. The enhanced permeability and retention (EPR) effect, which was discovered roughly 30 years ago by examining macromolecule transport into tumour tissues, is a type of passive NP entrance into the tumour microenvironment [91].

On the one hand, nanotechnology-based imaging is projected to improve the specificity and sensitivity of cancer diagnosis while reducing toxicity on the other. Using NPs and the EPR effect, they were able to create a new nano system for positron emission tomography (PET) imaging. A self-assembling amphiphilic dendrimer is used in the system to keep various PET reporting units at terminals. This dendrimer self-assembled into small homogeneous nano micelles that accumulated in tumours, allowing for efficient PET imaging. The nano system demonstrated improved imaging sensitivity and specificity due to dendrimer multivalence paired with passive tumour targeting mediated by EPR, with PET signal ratios increasing by roughly 14-fold when compared to the clinical gold standard 2-fluorodeoxyglucose ([18F] FDG) [92]. Furthermore, the dendrimer demonstrated an excellent safety profile and favourable pharmacokinetics for PET imaging. The researchers hope their findings will aid in the creation of dendrimer nano-systems for effective and promising cancer imaging.

8.10.2 Active targeting

Moreover, tumour visualizing using accumulating NPs through passive targeting using the EPR effect, researchers have conducted numerous studies on receptor recognition to actively target the surface of the cell tumour tissues. These technologies often enhance the number of NPs supplied to tumour tissue per unit time, hence improving the *in vivo* sensitivity tumour detecting techniques [89]. For early cancer diagnosis using high contrast imaging, active tumor targeting works better than passive targeting, which is dependent on the EPR effect. Green florescent protein and luciferase-transduced xenograft SKOV-3 ovarian cancer cells for *in vivo* imaging in a mouse model use a surface-enhanced resonance Raman scattering (SERRS) NP in conjunction with the folate receptor. No matter the size or location of the tumor, this technique—known as topically applied surface-enhanced resonance Raman ratiometric spectroscopy, or TAS3RS, was able to detect tumor lesions in a murine model of human ovarian adenocarcinoma by using an efficient ratiometric imaging approach with nontargeted SERRS-NP (nt-NP) and anti FR-SERRS-NP (FR-NP) multiplexing. During surgery, TAS3RS can identify little tumors that are left behind [93] (figure 8.2).

8.11 Clinical trials status of nanotechnology-based diagnostics

Although nanotechnology has been widely investigated in the laboratory for cancer diagnosis or detection, the ultimate purpose of these is clinical application investigations. Several forms of cancer diagnosis with nanotechnology techniques are now in clinical studies (table 8.2). MSKCC and Cornell University, for example, have produced hybrid silica NPs (C-dots) for PET imaging of patients with brain cancer or metastatic melanoma tumours. These NPs can be utilized to probe tumour cells when combined using cyclo-[Arg-Gly-Asp-Tyr] (cRGDY) peptides tagged with

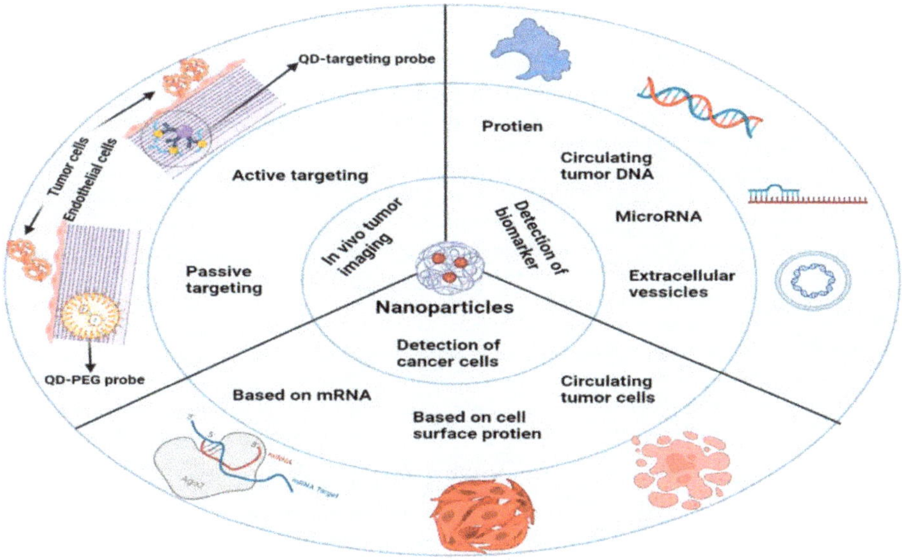

Figure 8.2. Diagrammatic representation of the uses of nanotechnology in cancer detection. Reproduced from [87] CC BY 4.0.

Table 8.2. List of clinical studies for applications using nanotechnology to diagnose cancer [87].

Title	Disease	Nanotechnology	Purpose	Phase
In colon cancer patients who have received neoadjuvant radiochemotherapy, carbon NPs are used as a lymph node tracer.	Cancer in rectal	Carbon NPs	Tracer of lymph node	Not relevant
Dynamic contrast-enhanced magnetic resonance imaging using ferrumoxytol and iron oxide NPs	Cancer: Head and Neck	NP iron oxide	Visualizing	Initial phase 1
Carbon nanoparticle application in laparoscopic colorectal surgery	Colorectal tumor	Carbon NP	Localization of tumors and mapping of lymph nodes	Not applicable
Mapping of sentinel lymph nodes in endometrial cancer	Neoplasm endomaterial	Carbon NP	Mapping of lymph nodes	Not relevant
Mapping of sentinel lymph nodes in cervical cancer	Uterine cervical neoplasm	Carbon NP	Mapping of lymph nodes	Not relevant

(Continued)

Table 8.2. (*Continued*)

Title	Disease	Nanotechnology	Purpose	Phase
Silica NPs with specific targeting for intraoperative real-time image-guided imaging of nodal metastases	Head and neck cancer Melanome cancer of the breast carcinoma of the colon	Fluorescent cRGDY-PEG-Cy5.5-C dots	Visualization/ Spatial	Phase 1/Phase 2
Using nanochip technology, patients with diffuse large B-cell lymphoma can be tracked along their course of treatment to identify relapses.	Lymphoma	NPs of lipoplex immunotethered	Observation and identification	Not relevant
Na-nose diagnosis of stomach lesions	Gastric cancer	Nano sensors	Diagnosis	
A microdosing research using 124I-labeled cRGDY silica nanomolecular particle tracer for PET imaging of patients with malignant brain tumors and melanoma	Brain tumors with malignancy and metastatic melanoma	124I-cRGDY-PEGdots	Place of Origin	Not relevant
Using 89Zr-cRGDY ultrasmall silica particle tracers for imaging patients with malignant brain tumors: a phase 1 microdosing study	Cancer of brain	89Zr-DFO-cRGDY-PEG-Cy5-C'dots	PET imaging	Phase 1

124I, which have the ability to bind to integrins only. Furthermore, cRGDY-PEG-Cy5.5-C dots, which are fluorescent cRGDY C-dots made for lymph node mapping and can be used to visualize malignant lymph nodes after surgery, were generated by another group of researchers, also from MSKCC. As research advances, it is expected that additional tools for cancer diagnosis based on nanotechnology will be introduced to clinics [87].

References

[1] Krukemeyer M *et al* 2015 History and possible uses of nanomedicine based on nanoparticles and nanotechnological progress *J. Nanomed. Nanotechnol.* **6** 336

[2] Baptista P V 2014 Nanodiagnostics: leaving the research lab to enter the clinics? *Diagnosis (Berl)* **1** 305–9

[3] Jackson T C, Patani B O and Jain Ekpa D E 2017 Nanotechnology in diagnosis: a review *Adv. Nanoparticles* **6** 93–102

[4] Jain K K 2003 Nanodiagnostics: application of nanotechnology in molecular diagnostics *Expert Rev. Mol. Diagn.* **3** 153–61

[5] Azzazy H M, Mansour M M and Kazmierczak S C 2006 Nanodiagnostics: a new frontier for clinical laboratory medicine *Clin. Chem.* **52** 1238–46
[6] Goluch E D *et al* 2006 A bio-barcode assay for on-chip attomolar-sensitivity protein detection *Lab Chip* **6** 1293–9
[7] Zhang Y *et al* 2012 Synthesis, properties, and optical applications of noble metal nanoparticle-biomolecule conjugates **57** 238–46
[8] Doria G *et al* 2012 Noble metal nanoparticles for biosensing applications *Sensors (Basel)* **12** 1657–87
[9] Dreaden E C *et al* 2012 The golden age: gold nanoparticles for biomedicine *Chem. Soc. Rev.* **41** 2740–79
[10] Kang K A *et al* 2011 Fluorescence manipulation by gold nanoparticles: from complete quenching to extensive enhancement *J. Nanobiotechnol.* **9** 16
[11] Le Ru E C *et al* 2007 Surface enhanced Raman scattering enhancement factors: a comprehensive study *J. Phys. Chem.* **111** 13794–803
[12] Jain P K *et al* 2006 Calculated absorption and scattering properties of gold nanoparticles of different size, shape, and composition: applications in biological imaging and biomedicine *J. Phys. Chem.* **B 110** 7238–48
[13] Tran Q H, Nguyen V Q and Le A-T 2013 Silver nanoparticles: synthesis, properties, toxicology, applications and perspectives *Adv. Nat. Sci: Nanosci. Nanotechnol.* **4** 033001
[14] Zhao P, Li N and Astruc D J 2013 State of the art in gold nanoparticle synthesis *Coord. Chem. Rev.* **257** 638–65
[15] Kaittanis C, Santra S and Perez J M 2010 Emerging nanotechnology-based strategies for the identification of microbial pathogenesis *Adv. Drug Deliv. Rev.* **62** 408–23
[16] Wei F, Lillehoj P B and Ho C M 2010 DNA diagnostics: nanotechnology-enhanced electrochemical detection of nucleic acids *Pediatr. Res.* **67** 458–68
[17] Rai M and Kon K 2015 *Nanotechnology in Diagnosis, Treatment and Prophylaxis of Infectious Diseases* (Amsterdam: Elsevier Science)
[18] Boyce J D, Cullen P A and Adler B 2004 Genomic-scale analysis of bacterial gene and protein expression in the host *Emerg. Infect. Dis.* **10** 1357–62
[19] Notomi T *et al* 2000 Loop-mediated isothermal amplification of DNA *Nucleic Acids Res.* **28** E63
[20] Freeman W M, Walker S J and Vrana K E 1999 Quantitative RT-PCR: pitfalls and potential *Biotechniques* **26** 112–22, 124–5
[21] Compton J 1991 Nucleic acid sequence-based amplification *Nature* **350** 91–2
[22] Baptista P V *et al* 2011 Nanoparticles in molecular diagnostics *Prog. Mol. Biol. Transl. Sci.* **104** 427–88
[23] Li H and Rothberg L 2004 Colorimetric detection of DNA sequences based on electrostatic interactions with unmodified gold nanoparticles *Proc. Natl Acad. Sci. USA* **101** 14036–9
[24] Hussain M M, Samir T M and Azzazy H M 2013 Unmodified gold nanoparticles for direct and rapid detection of *Mycobacterium tuberculosis* complex *Clin. Biochem.* **46** 633–7
[25] Fu Z, Zhou X and Xing D 2013 Sensitive colorimetric detection of Listeria monocytogenes based on isothermal gene amplification and unmodified gold nanoparticles *Methods* **64** 260–6
[26] Mirkin C A *et al* 1996 A DNA-based method for rationally assembling nanoparticles into macroscopic materials *Nature* **382** 607–9
[27] Storhoff J J *et al* 2004 Homogeneous detection of unamplified genomic DNA sequences based on colorimetric scatter of gold nanoparticle probes *Nat. Biotechnol.* **22** 883–7

[28] Mancuso M *et al* 2013 Multiplexed colorimetric detection of Kaposi's sarcoma associated herpesvirus and Bartonella DNA using gold and silver nanoparticles *Nanoscale* **5** 1678–86
[29] Baptista P V *et al* 2006 Gold-nanoparticle-probe-based assay for rapid and direct detection of *Mycobacterium tuberculosis* DNA in clinical samples *Clin. Chem.* **52** 1433–4
[30] Veigas B *et al* 2010 Au-nanoprobes for detection of SNPs associated with antibiotic resistance in *Mycobacterium tuberculosis Nanotechnology* **21** 415101
[31] Veigas B *et al* 2013 Isothermal DNA amplification coupled to Au-nanoprobes for detection of mutations associated to Rifampicin resistance in *Mycobacterium tuberculosis J. Nanobiotechnol.* **11** 38
[32] Pedrosa P *et al* 2014 Gold nanoprobes for multi loci assessment of multi-drug resistant tuberculosis *Tuberculosis (Edinb)* **94** 332–7
[33] Liandris E, Gazouli M, Andreadou M, Čomor M, Abazovic N, Sechi L A and Ikonomopoulos J 2009 Direct detection of unamplified DNA from pathogenic mycobacteria using DNA-derivatized gold nanoparticles *J. Microbiol. Mehods* **78** 260–4
[34] Love J C *et al* 2005 Self-assembled monolayers of thiolates on metals as a form of nanotechnology *Chem. Rev.* **105** 1103–69
[35] Agasti S S *et al* 2010 Nanoparticles for detection and diagnosis *Adv. Drug Deliv. Rev.* **62** 316–28
[36] Zhao J *et al* 2010 Multiplexed, rapid detection of H5N1 using a PCR-free nanoparticle-based genomic microarray assay *BMC Biotechnol.* **10** 74
[37] Li X Z *et al* 2013 Optical detection of nanoparticle-enhanced human papillomavirus genotyping microarrays *Biomed. Opt. Express* **4** 187–92
[38] Posthuma-Trumpie G A, Korf J and van Amerongen A 2009 Lateral flow (immuno)assay: its strengths, weaknesses, opportunities and threats. A literature survey *Anal. Bioanal. Chem.* **393** 569–82
[39] Anfossi L *et al* 2013 Lateral-flow immunoassays for mycotoxins and phycotoxins: a review *Anal. Bioanal. Chem.* **405** 467–80
[40] Hu J *et al* 2014 Advances in paper-based point-of-care diagnostics *Biosens. Bioelectron.* **54** 585–97
[41] Luo X and Davis J J 2013 Electrical biosensors and the label free detection of protein disease biomarkers *Chem. Soc. Rev.* **42** 5944–62
[42] Thiruppathiraja C *et al* 2011 Specific detection of *Mycobacterium* sp. genomic DNA using dual labeled gold nanoparticle based electrochemical biosensor *Anal. Biochem.* **417** 73–9
[43] Low K F, Karimah A and Yean C Y 2013 A thermostabilized magnetogenosensing assay for DNA sequence-specific detection and quantification of *Vibrio cholerae Biosens. Bioelectron.* **47** 38–44
[44] Wang Y *et al* 2008 Electrochemical sensors for clinic analysis *Sensors (Basel)* **8** 2043–81
[45] Li W *et al* 2012 Catalytic signal amplification of gold nanoparticles combining with conformation-switched hairpin DNA probe for hepatitis C virus quantification *Chem. Commun. (Camb.)* **48** 7877–9
[46] Vetrone S A, Huarng M C and Alocilja E C 2012 Detection of non-PCR amplified *S. enteritidis* genomic DNA from food matrices using a gold-nanoparticle DNA biosensor: a proof-of-concept study *Sensors (Basel)* **12** 10487–99
[47] Swierczewska M, Lee S and Chen X 2011 The design and application of fluorophore-gold nanoparticle activatable probes *Phys. Chem. Chem. Phys.* **13** 9929–41

[48] Griffin J *et al* 2009 Size- and distance-dependent nanoparticle surface-energy transfer (NSET) method for selective sensing of hepatitis C virus RNA *Chemistry* **15** 342–51
[49] Yun C S *et al* 2005 Nanometal surface energy transfer in optical rulers, breaking the FRET barrier *J. Am. Chem. Soc.* **127** 3115–9
[50] Rosa J *et al* 2012 Gold-nanobeacons for real-time monitoring of RNA synthesis *Biosens. Bioelectron.* **36** 161–7
[51] Darbha G K *et al* 2008 Miniaturized sensor for microbial pathogens DNA and chemical toxins *IEEE Sens. J.* **8** 693–700
[52] Park W H, Ahn S H and Kim Z H 2008 Surface-enhanced Raman scattering from a single nanoparticle-plane junction *Chem. Phys. Chem.* **9** 2491–4
[53] Cao Y C, Jin R and Mirkin C A 2002 Nanoparticles with Raman spectroscopic fingerprints for DNA and RNA detection *Science* **297** 1536–40
[54] Wang H N *et al* 2013 Surface-enhanced Raman scattering molecular sentinel nanoprobes for viral infection diagnostics *Anal. Chim. Acta* **786** 153–8
[55] Uludağ Y, Hammond R and Cooper M A 2010 A signal amplification assay for HSV type 1 viral DNA detection using nanoparticles and direct acoustic profiling *J. Nanobiotechnol.* **8** 1–12
[56] Nam J M, Park S J and Mirkin C A 2002 Bio-barcodes based on oligonucleotide-modified nanoparticles *J. Am. Chem. Soc.* **124** 3820–1
[57] Yang B *et al* 2010 Simultaneous detection of attomolar pathogen DNAs by Bio-MassCode mass spectrometry *Chem. Commun. (Camb)* **46** 8288–90
[58] Singh A K *et al* 2009 Gold nanorod based selective identification of *Escherichia coli* bacteria using two-photon rayleigh scattering spectroscopy *ACS Nano* **3** 1906–12
[59] Pourhassan-Moghaddam M *et al* 2013 Protein detection through different platforms of immuno-loop-mediated isothermal amplification *Nanoscale Res. Lett.* **8** 485
[60] Syed M A and Bokhari S H 2011 Gold nanoparticle based microbial detection and identification *J. Biomed. Nanotechnol.* **7** 229–37
[61] Chen L *et al* 2009 Gold nanoparticle enhanced immuno-PCR for ultrasensitive detection of Hantaan virus nucleocapsid protein *J. Immunol. Methods.* **346** 64–70
[62] Perez J W *et al* 2011 Detection of respiratory syncytial virus using nanoparticle amplified immuno-polymerase chain reaction *Anal. Biochem.* **410** 141–8
[63] Bray F *et al* 2018 Global cancer statistics 2018: GLOBOCAN estimates of incidence and mortality worldwide for 36 cancers in 185 countries *CA Cancer. J. Clin.* **68** 394–424
[64] The L 2018 GLOBOCAN 2018: counting the toll of cancer *Lancet* **392** 985
[65] Rezaianzadeh A *et al* 2017 The overall 5-year survival rate of breast cancer among Iranian women: A systematic review and meta-analysis of published studies *Breast Dis.* **37** 63–8
[66] Choi Y E, Kwak J W and Park J W 2010 Nanotechnology for early cancer detection *Sensors (Basel)* **10** 428–55
[67] Zhou W *et al* 2015 Gold nanoparticles for *in vitro* diagnostics *Chem. Rev.* **115** 10575–636
[68] Jia S *et al* 2017 Clinical and biological significance of circulating tumor cells, circulating tumor DNA, and exosomes as biomarkers in colorectal cancer *Oncotarget* **8** 55632–45
[69] Kumar B *et al* 2017 Mechanisms of tubulin binding ligands to target cancer cells: updates on their therapeutic potential and clinical trials *Curr. Cancer Drug Targets* **17** 357–75
[70] Chen X J *et al* 2018 Nanotechnology: a promising method for oral cancer detection and diagnosis *J. Nanobiotechnol.* **16** 52

[71] Chaffer C L and Weinberg R A 2011 A perspective on cancer cell metastasis *Science* **331** 1559–64
[72] Huang Q *et al* 2018 Nanotechnology-based strategies for early cancer diagnosis using circulating tumor cells as a liquid biopsy *Nanotheranostics* **2** 21–41
[73] Hong W *et al* 2016 Multifunctional magnetic nanowires: a novel breakthrough for ultrasensitive detection and isolation of rare cancer cells from non-metastatic early breast cancer patients using small volumes of blood *Biomaterials* **106** 78–86
[74] Wen C Y *et al* 2014 Quick-response magnetic nanospheres for rapid, efficient capture and sensitive detection of circulating tumor cells *ACS Nano* **8** 941–9
[75] Wu C H *et al* 2013 Versatile immunomagnetic nanocarrier platform for capturing cancer cells *ACS Nano* **7** 8816–23
[76] Pang X *et al* 2018 Construction of self-powered cytosensing device based on ZnO nanodisks@g-C(3)N(4) quantum dots and application in the detection of CCRF-CEM cells *Nano Energy* **46** 101–9
[77] Wu C *et al* 2010 Bioconjugation of ultrabright semiconducting polymer dots for specific cellular targeting *J. Am. Chem. Soc.* **132** 15410–7
[78] Zhu Y, Chandra P and Shim Y B 2013 Ultrasensitive and selective electrochemical diagnosis of breast cancer based on a hydrazine-Au nanoparticle-aptamer bioconjugate *Anal. Chem.* **85** 1058–64
[79] Zhang Y *et al* 2014 Immunomagnetic separation combined with inductively coupled plasma mass spectrometry for the detection of tumor cells using gold nanoparticle labeling *Anal. Chem.* **86** 8082–9
[80] Liu Y *et al* 2014 Construction of carbon nanotube based nanoarchitectures for selective impedimetric detection of cancer cells in whole blood *Analyst* **139** 5086–92
[81] Shen J *et al* 2014 Specific detection and simultaneously localized photothermal treatment of cancer cells using layer-by-layer assembled multifunctional nanoparticles *ACS Appl. Mater. Interfaces* **6** 6443–52
[82] Sun N *et al* 2016 A multiscale TiO2 nanorod array for ultrasensitive capture of circulating tumor cells *ACS Appl. Mater. Interfaces* **8** 12638–43
[83] Huang Q *et al* 2018 Gelatin nanoparticle-coated silicon beads for density-selective capture and release of heterogeneous circulating tumor cells with high purity *Theranostics* **8** 1624
[84] Wu X *et al* 2018 A micro-/nano-chip and quantum dots-based 3D cytosensor for quantitative analysis of circulating tumor cells *J. Nanobiotechnol.* **16** 1–9
[85] Wu C-S and Fan X J S L 2011 Development of a simple and sensitive quantum dot labeled magnetic immunoassay method for circulating tumor cell (MCF-7) detection *Sens. Lett.* **9** 546–51
[86] Li K *et al* 2019 Advances in the application of upconversion nanoparticles for detecting and treating cancers *Photodiagn. Photodyn. Ther.* **25** 177–92
[87] Zhang Y *et al* 2019 Nanotechnology in cancer diagnosis: progress, challenges and opportunities *J. Hematol. Oncol.* **12** 137
[88] Chinen A B *et al* 2015 Nanoparticle probes for the detection of cancer biomarkers, cells, and tissues by fluorescence *Chem. Rev.* **115** 10530–74
[89] Bertrand N *et al* 2014 Cancer nanotechnology: the impact of passive and active targeting in the era of modern cancer biology *Adv. Drug Deliv. Rev.* **66** 2–25
[90] Golombek S K *et al* 2018 Tumor targeting via EPR: Strategies to enhance patient responses *Adv. Drug Deliv. Rev.* **130** 17–38

[91] Matsumura Y and Maeda H 1986 A new concept for macromolecular therapeutics in cancer chemotherapy: mechanism of tumoritropic accumulation of proteins and the antitumor agent smancs *Cancer Res.* **46** 6387–92

[92] Garrigue P *et al* 2018 Self-assembling supramolecular dendrimer nanosystem for PET imaging of tumors *Proc. Natl Acad. Sci. USA* **115** 11454–9

[93] Oseledchyk A *et al* 2017 Folate-targeted surface-enhanced resonance raman scattering nanoprobe ratiometry for detection of microscopic ovarian cancer *ACS Nano* **11** 1488–97

Chapter 9

Antiviral agents: mechanisms of action and therapeutic insights

Bhingaradiya Nutan and Arvind K Singh Chandel

Because they specifically target different stages of the viral lifecycle, antiviral medicines are essential in the fight against viral infections. A thorough understanding of their mechanisms of action is essential to develop effective treatments for viral illnesses. This chapter thoroughly analyzes the various groups of antiviral drugs, clarifying their unique modes of action and their therapeutic implications. The topics cover a wide range, including immunological modulators, protease inhibitors, polymerase inhibitors, nucleoside analogs, and viral entry inhibitors. New antiviral tactics are also investigated, providing insight into fresh methods of fighting viral infections. In addition, the chapter highlights the opportunities and difficulties present in the ever-changing field of antiviral medication development, offering insightful information to researchers, physicians, and students in equal measure.

9.1 Introduction

Infectious diseases have been recognized since ancient times. Various microorganisms like bacteria, viruses, and fungi cause them. Viral infections are a common type of these diseases and stand as a dreadful challenge to global public health, presenting a vast spectrum of pathogens that can cause ailments ranging from mild inconveniences like the common cold to devastating pandemics that reshape societies [1]. In this complex landscape, delving into the depths of viral infections becomes not only an essential pursuit but a paramount one. This chapter serves as an extensive introduction to the multifaceted world of viral infections, offering an all-encompassing exploration of their structure, replication cycles, clinical manifestations, modes of transmission, immune responses, diagnostic approaches, treatment strategies, preventive measures, and the ever-evolving panorama of emerging viral threats.

doi:10.1088/978-0-7503-4987-1ch9

Viral infections are a subject of perpetual intrigue and study, continually enriched by scientific breakthroughs, epidemiological dynamics, and a deepening understanding of viral behavior. As we embark on this journey, we intend to lay a robust foundation for comprehending the complexities of viral infections. By providing a comprehensive overview, we aim to equip readers with a thorough grasp of the fundamental concepts and critical issues surrounding these enigmatic pathogens. Certainly, viral infections are a significant area of interest. Viruses cause viral infections, microscopic infectious agents composed of genetic material (DNA or RNA) surrounded by a protein coat [2]. These viruses can infect many living organisms, including humans, animals, plants, and bacteria. The structure of viruses is uncomplicated, comprising a protein coat, nucleic acid, viral enzymes, and occasionally a lipid envelope [3]. This simplicity contrasts with the intricate structures of fungi, helminths, and protozoa. Viruses, as obligate intracellular pathogens, rely on the host's cellular machinery for replication [4]. Drugs that can selectively target viruses are challenging due to the unique characteristics of viruses. Viruses are tiny agents that contain either DNA or RNA and can cause diseases in humans, animals, and plants. The ongoing battle between humans and viruses leads to different strategies being adopted by both sides.

The process of developing antiviral drugs includes several stages: identifying targets, screening potential compounds, generating and optimizing leads, conducting clinical studies, and finally, registering the drug. This process is vital because viral infections have caused millions of deaths throughout human history. The approval of the first antiviral drug, 'idoxuridine,' in June 1963 marked a significant milestone. Since then, many antiviral medications have been developed, helping millions worldwide.

Antiviral drugs, like antibiotics for bacteria, are a specific class of medications used to treat viral infections. However, unlike most antibiotics, antiviral drugs do not kill the viruses but inhibit their development [5]. Designing these drugs is difficult because viruses use the host's cells to replicate [6]. Therefore, finding drug targets that can interfere with the virus without damaging the host's cells is challenging. Moreover, the variation among viruses is the main difficulty in developing antiviral drugs and vaccines.

Computer-based drug discovery has become an essential tool in finding antiviral drugs. An example of this is nelfinavir, which was discovered in the 1990s to treat HIV infection [5]. Despite the utilization of modern tools and rigorous quality control measures, only a limited number of antiviral drugs receive approval for human use, often attributed to adverse side effects or the development of resistance to these drugs. The heightened awareness regarding viruses, their infection mechanisms, and the rapid evolution of novel strategies and techniques for antiviral interventions are expected to expedite the development of new antiviral drugs. The prevailing global situation indicates a continual rise in microbial threats at an accelerating pace, primarily driven by unprecedented climate change and globalization. This underscores the urgent need for proactive measures in the ongoing battle against emerging infectious diseases.

9.2 Importance of antiviral drugs

The importance of antiviral drugs in medicine and public health cannot be overstated. These drugs are designed to inhibit the replication and spread of viruses within the human body, and they play a vital role in managing and controlling viral infections. Here are several key reasons highlighting the importance of antiviral drugs (table 9.1).

Table 9.1. Importance of antiviral drugs in managing viral infections [6–8]. This table summarizes the critical roles of antiviral drugs in treating viral infections, reducing symptoms, preventing disease progression, managing outbreaks, preventing vertical transmission, and improving the quality of life for individuals affected by chronic viral infections.

Importance of antiviral drugs	Description
Treatment of viral infections:	Antiviral drugs are essential for treating a wide range of viral infections, including but not limited to HIV/AIDS, hepatitis B and C, influenza, herpes, and COVID-19. Without effective antiviral treatments, many of these infections could result in severe illness, complications, or even death [8].
Reducing symptoms:	Antiviral medications can alleviate symptoms associated with viral infections. For example, antiviral drugs for influenza can reduce the severity and duration of flu symptoms, helping patients recover more quickly [7].
Preventing disease progression:	In the case of chronic viral infections like HIV and hepatitis, antiviral drugs are crucial for preventing disease progression. They can slow down the replication of the virus, preserving the immune system and delaying the onset of complications [7, 8].
Managing outbreaks:	Antiviral drugs can be used in outbreak management and containment strategies. During epidemics or pandemics, such as the COVID-19 pandemic, antiviral medications can be administered to infected individuals to reduce viral transmission and ease the burden on healthcare systems [7].
Preventing vertical transmission:	Antiviral drugs can prevent the transmission of certain viruses from mother to child during pregnancy and childbirth. This is particularly important for preventing mother-to-child transmission of HIV and hepatitis B [6, 7].
Improving quality of life:	For individuals with chronic viral infections, antiviral therapy can significantly improve their quality of life by controlling the virus, reducing symptoms, and preventing complications.
Enhancing immune responses:	Some antiviral drugs boost the immune system's ability to fight off viral infections. They can enhance the body's natural defenses against viruses.

(*Continued*)

Table 9.1. (*Continued*)

Importance of antiviral drugs	Description
Pandemic preparedness:	Antiviral drugs are a vital component of preparedness plans for potential pandemics. They can be stockpiled and deployed as part of public health responses to emerging infectious diseases.
Reducing transmission:	Antiviral drugs can reduce viral shedding, making infected individuals less contagious to others. This is critical for preventing the spread of diseases in healthcare settings, households, and communities.
Combination therapies:	Antiviral drugs are often used in combination therapy, where multiple drugs with different mechanisms of action are employed. This approach can reduce the risk of drug resistance and enhance treatment effectiveness.
Research and development:	Antiviral drug research is ongoing, leading to the discovery of new drugs and therapies. This research contributes to understanding viruses and their interactions with the human body.
Vaccination complement:	While vaccines are essential for preventing viral infections, antiviral drugs provide treatment options for individuals who have already been infected. Vaccines and antiviral drugs form a comprehensive strategy for control of viral disease.

In summary, antiviral drugs are indispensable tools in the fight against viral infections. They save lives, improve patient outcomes, and are crucial for pandemic preparedness. Ongoing research and development in this field continue to expand our arsenal against viral diseases, highlighting their enduring importance in healthcare and public health.

9.3 Viral lifecycle and targets for antiviral drugs

9.3.1 Viral lifecycle

The viral lifecycle refers to the series of steps that a virus undergoes to infect host cells, replicate, and produce new viral particles. While the specific details of the lifecycle can vary depending on the type of virus, the general stages include [9]:

Attachment: The first step in the viral lifecycle involves the attachment of the virus to specific receptors on the surface of host cells. This attachment is mediated by viral surface proteins or other molecular structures that recognize and bind to complementary receptors on the host cell surface [10].

Entry: Once attached to the host cell, the virus enters the cell through various mechanisms, such as direct fusion with the host cell membrane, receptor-mediated endocytosis, or membrane penetration. This allows the viral genetic material (DNA or RNA) to gain access to the host cell's interior.

Uncoating: After entry, the virus undergoes uncoating, during which the viral capsid or envelope is disassembled, releasing the viral genetic material into the host cell cytoplasm. Uncoating can occur either immediately upon entry or after the virus has been transported to specific cellular compartments.

Replication and transcription: Once inside the host cell, the viral genetic material hijacks the host cell's machinery to replicate and transcribe viral RNA or DNA. This process may involve the production of viral proteins and the assembly of new viral genomes.

Translation and protein synthesis: The newly synthesized viral RNA or DNA directs the synthesis of viral proteins through the host cell's protein synthesis machinery. These viral proteins are essential for the assembly of new viral particles.

Assembly: As viral proteins and genetic material accumulate within the host cell, new viral particles are assembled at specific sites, such as the cell membrane or intracellular compartments. This process involves the packaging of viral genomes into capsids or envelopes, as well as the incorporation of viral envelope proteins.

Maturation: Once assembled, the newly formed viral particles undergo maturation, during which they acquire their final structural and functional characteristics. This may involve the cleavage of viral precursor proteins or other post-translational modifications.

Release: The final stage of the viral lifecycle involves the release of mature viral particles from the host cell. This can occur through various mechanisms, including budding from the host cell membrane, lysis of the host cell, or exocytosis. Released viral particles can then infect neighboring cells or spread to other hosts to initiate new rounds of infection.

Overall, the viral lifecycle represents a complex series of interactions between the virus and its host cell, with each stage presenting potential targets for antiviral intervention. Understanding the molecular mechanisms underlying the viral lifecycle is crucial for the development of effective antiviral therapies and vaccines to combat viral infections.

9.3.2 Targets for antiviral drugs

Antiviral drugs target specific components or processes involved in the viral lifecycle, aiming to inhibit viral replication, spread, and pathogenesis. Some common targets for antiviral drugs include the following.

9.3.2.1 Viral enzymes

Polymerases: Many antiviral drugs inhibit viral polymerases, enzymes responsible for replicating viral genomes (figure 9.1). Nucleoside/nucleotide analogs, such as acyclovir and tenofovir, mimic nucleotides and interfere with viral DNA or RNA synthesis [12, 13]. *Proteases:* Protease inhibitors block the activity of viral proteases, essential for processing viral polyproteins into functional proteins. Examples include lopinavir/ritonavir, used to treat HIV/AIDS [14]. *Neuraminidase*: Neuraminidase inhibitors, such as oseltamivir and zanamivir, prevent the release of newly formed viral particles from infected cells by inhibiting neuraminidase activity [15].

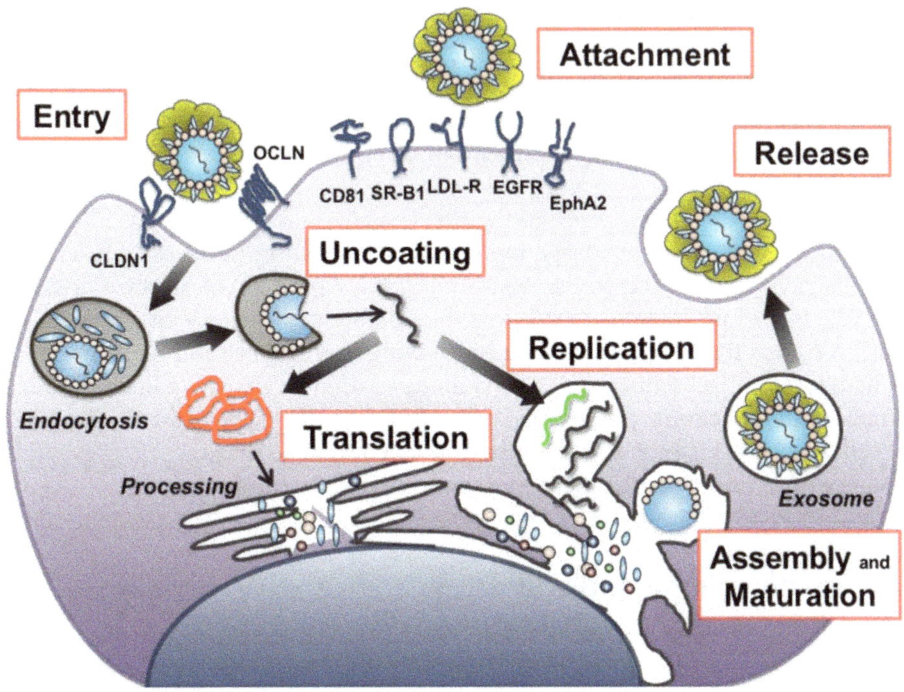

Figure 9.1. The virus replication cycle involves seven steps: attachment, entry, uncoating, translation, replication, assembly and maturation, and release. After attachment, the virus enters the cell through clathrin-mediated endocytosis. Uncoating occurs as the viral and cellular membranes fuse, releasing the RNA genome into the cytoplasm. Translation of the RNA produces a polyprotein precursor, which is then cleaved into individual proteins. Replication generates multiple copies of the viral genome via a replicative intermediate. Assembly and maturation occur in the endoplasmic reticulum, where viral progeny acquire their envelope proteins. Finally, virions are released from the cell, likely through exocytosis or cell-free transmission. Reprinted from [11], copyright (2016), with permission from Elsevier.

9.3.2.2 Viral fusion and entry

Fusion inhibitors: These drugs prevent the fusion of viral and host cell membranes, blocking viral entry into the host cell. Enfuvirtide is a fusion inhibitor used in the treatment of HIV/AIDS [16]. *Attachment Inhibitors*: Some antiviral drugs interfere with viral attachment to host cell receptors, preventing viral entry. Maraviroc, for example, blocks the interaction between HIV envelope glycoproteins and host cell receptors [17].

9.3.2.3 Host cell factors

CCR5 antagonists: CCR5 antagonists, such as maraviroc, block the CCR5 co-receptor on host cells, preventing HIV entry [18]. *Interferons*: Interferons modulate host immune responses to viral infections, inhibiting viral replication and promoting viral clearance [19].

9.3.2.4 Viral assembly and release

Maturation inhibitors: These drugs interfere with the maturation of viral particles, preventing their release from infected cells. Bevirimat, for instance, inhibits the maturation of HIV virions [20]. *Neuraminidase inhibitors*: Besides blocking viral release, neuraminidase inhibitors can also prevent viral entry, as mentioned earlier [21].

9.3.2.5 Viral proteins and processes

Reverse transcriptase: Drugs targeting viral reverse transcriptase, such as efavirenz and raltegravir, inhibit the conversion of viral RNA into DNA in retroviruses like HIV [22]. *Integrase:* Integrase inhibitors, like dolutegravir, block the integration of viral DNA into the host cell genome, preventing viral replication [23].

These targets represent critical points in the viral lifecycle where intervention can disrupt viral replication and spread. Combination therapy, utilizing drugs with different mechanisms of action, is often employed to enhance efficacy, prevent drug resistance, and improve treatment outcomes in viral infections.

9.4 Classification of antiviral drugs

9.4.1 Broad spectrum antivirals

These drugs are effective against a variety of viral pathogens (figure 9.2), offering a versatile approach to treating viral infections. Unlike specific antivirals, which target a particular virus or family of viruses, broad-spectrum antivirals can be useful when the causative agent is unknown or when multiple viruses are implicated in the infection. Examples of broad-spectrum antivirals include [24–27].

9.4.1.1 Ribavirin

Ribavirin is a nucleoside analog that effectively targets several RNA and DNA viruses, such as respiratory syncytial virus (RSV), hepatitis C virus (HCV), and some hemorrhagic fever viruses [27]. It works by inhibiting RNA synthesis, which interferes with viral replication, and it also has immunomodulatory properties. Ribavirin is used to treat various viral infections, including RSV, HCV, and specific viral hemorrhagic fevers like Lassa fever and Crimean–Congo hemorrhagic fever [28, 29]. Ribavirin interferes with viral replication by inhibiting RNA synthesis. It acts as a nucleoside analog, disrupting viral RNA replication. Additionally, it has immunomodulatory properties that enhance the host's immune response to viral infections [30]. Ribavirin is available in various formulations, including oral capsules, tablets, and inhalation solutions, depending on the indication [31, 32]. In combination with other antiviral drugs like interferons or direct-acting antivirals, ribavirin is used for the treatment of chronic hepatitis C infections [33]. It may also be administered via inhalation for severe cases of RSV infection, particularly in immunocompromised patients or those with underlying respiratory conditions [34]. Common side effects of ribavirin include hemolytic anemia, fatigue, nausea, and rash. It is contraindicated in pregnancy due to teratogenic effects [35].

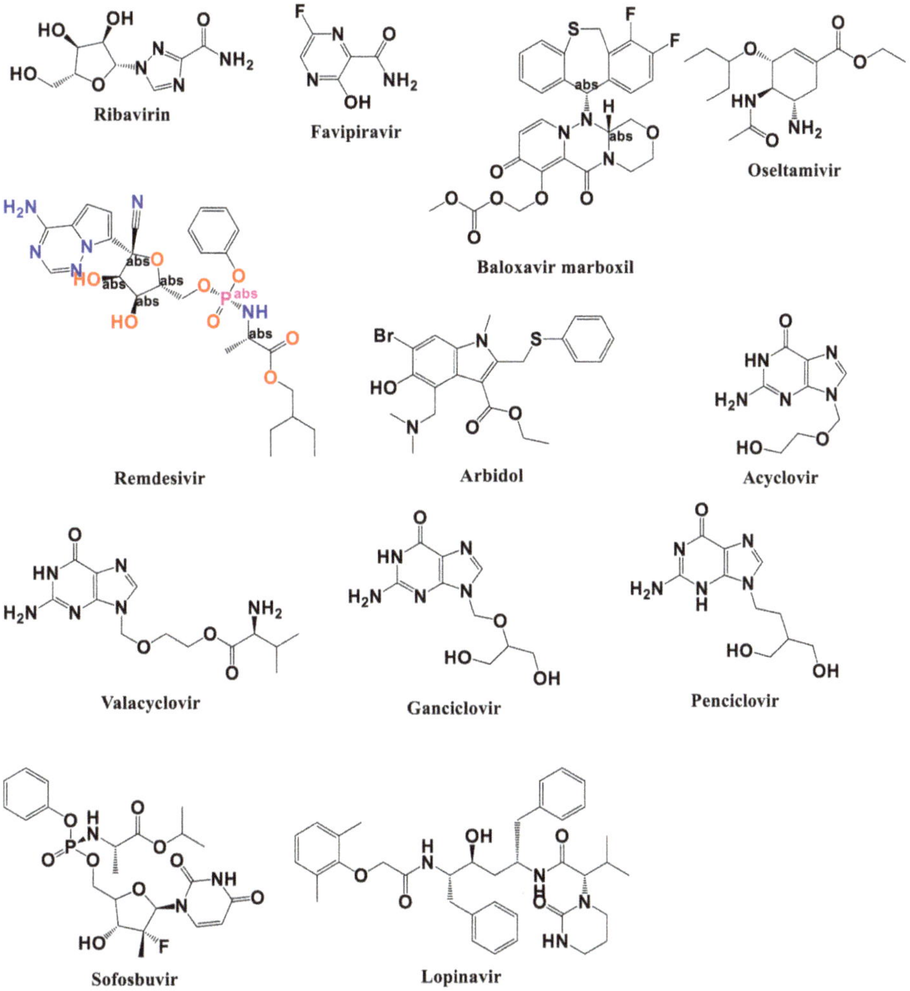

Figure 9.2. Chemical structures of antiviral drug molecules. (a), (d), (i), (j) and (l) Adapted from [40] with permission from the Royal Society of Chemistry. (b) adapted from [6], copyright (2016) with permission from Elsevier.

9.4.1.2 Favipiravir

Favipiravir is an RNA polymerase inhibitor that has demonstrated activity against a broad spectrum of RNA viruses, including influenza viruses, Ebola virus, and certain coronaviruses [36]. It works by blocking viral RNA replication. Favipiravir is primarily indicated for the treatment of influenza virus infections. Favipiravir is a nucleoside analog that inhibits viral RNA polymerase, specifically the RNA-dependent RNA polymerase (RdRp). By mimicking the structure of viral RNA nucleotides, favipiravir is incorporated into the viral RNA chain during replication, leading to premature chain termination and inhibition of viral RNA synthesis [37]. Favipiravir is typically administered orally in tablet form. It is available in different dosages depending on the indication and country-specific guidelines. In clinical practice, favipiravir is used for the treatment of influenza virus infections, particularly in cases of seasonal influenza or influenza outbreaks [38]. It has also been explored for the treatment of emerging viral diseases, such as Ebola virus disease and COVID-19. Common side effects of favipiravir include gastrointestinal symptoms (e.g., nausea, vomiting, diarrhea), elevated serum uric acid levels (hyperuricemia), and potential teratogenic effects, particularly if used during pregnancy [39].

9.4.1.3 Remdesivir

Originally developed to treat Ebola virus disease, remdesivir is a nucleotide analog inhibitor of viral RNA polymerases. It has shown efficacy against a range of RNA viruses, including coronaviruses like SARS-CoV-2, the virus responsible for COVID-19 [41, 42]. Remdesivir, also known by its chemical name GS-5734, is a prodrug of an adenosine nucleotide analog. Its chemical structure consists of a nucleoside analog with a modified sugar moiety, a 1′-cyano group, and a phosphoramidate prodrug moiety attached to the 5′ position of the sugar [43]. This modification allows for increased stability and enhanced cellular uptake compared to the parent nucleoside. Remdesivir works by inhibiting viral RNA polymerases, enzymes essential for viral replication. As a nucleotide analog, Remdesivir is incorporated into viral RNA during replication, leading to premature termination of RNA synthesis and inhibition of viral replication [37, 44]. Its broad-spectrum activity stems from its ability to target the replication machinery of various RNA viruses, including coronaviruses, filoviruses (e.g., Ebola virus), and paramyxoviruses. Remdesivir gained emergency use authorization (EUA) from regulatory agencies for the treatment of COVID-19 in hospitalized patients [45]. Clinical trials have shown that Remdesivir can shorten the time to recovery in some patients with severe COVID-19, although its impact on mortality remains a subject of debate. It is typically administered intravenously and is recommended for use in hospitalized patients with severe COVID-19 who require supplemental oxygen or mechanical ventilation. Common side effects of Remdesivir include nausea, vomiting, and elevated liver enzymes [46]. Rare but serious adverse effects, such as hypersensitivity reactions and acute kidney injury, have also been reported. As with any medication, the benefits and risks of Remdesivir should be carefully weighed before use. Remdesivir was developed through collaboration between Gilead Sciences and various research institutions. It was initially explored as a potential treatment for Ebola virus disease and later repurposed for other viral infections, including COVID-19. Clinical trials evaluating its efficacy and safety in COVID-19 patients have been conducted worldwide, contributing to the growing body of evidence supporting its use in the management of severe COVID-19 [45, 46]. Overall, Remdesivir represents an important addition to the armamentarium of antiviral drugs, offering a potential treatment option for severe COVID-19 and other viral infections. Its development and clinical use underscore the importance of continued research and collaboration in combating emerging infectious diseases.

9.4.1.4 Baloxavir marboxil

Baloxavir marboxil is a cap-dependent endonuclease inhibitor approved for the treatment of acute uncomplicated influenza in certain populations. It targets the cap-snatching mechanism of viral RNA transcription, inhibiting viral replication. Baloxavir marboxil is indicated for the treatment of acute uncomplicated influenza in patients 12 years of age and older who have been symptomatic for no more than 48 h. It is effective against both influenza A and B viruses. Baloxavir marboxil inhibits viral replication by targeting the cap-dependent endonuclease enzyme within the influenza virus. This enzyme is crucial for viral RNA transcription, and inhibition of its activity disrupts viral replication and spread. Baloxavir marboxil is administered orally as a single-dose tablet. The drug is used for the treatment of influenza infections, particularly in cases where rapid symptom relief is desired. It is effective against both seasonal influenza strains and certain strains with resistance to other antiviral medications, such as adamantanes and neuraminidase inhibitors. Common side effects of baloxavir marboxil include diarrhea, bronchitis, headache, and nausea. It may also cause abnormal laboratory test results, including elevated liver enzymes. Resistance to baloxavir marboxil can develop with prolonged use, particularly due to mutations in the viral endonuclease target. Therefore, the drug is recommended for use only in the early stages of influenza infection and should be used judiciously to minimize the risk of resistance.

9.4.1.5 Arbidol (umifenovir)

Arbidol is a broad-spectrum antiviral agent with activity against enveloped and non-enveloped viruses, including influenza viruses, HCV, and some coronaviruses. It interferes with viral entry by inhibiting viral fusion with host cell membranes. Arbidol is indicated for the treatment and prevention of acute respiratory viral infections caused by influenza viruses, including seasonal influenza and potentially pandemic strains. It is also used for the prophylaxis of influenza in high-risk populations and as an adjunctive therapy for viral pneumonia caused by influenza and other respiratory viruses. The exact mechanism of action of arbidol is not fully understood. However, it is believed to exert its antiviral effects through multiple mechanisms, including inhibiting viral fusion with host cell membranes, interfering with viral entry and replication, and modulating host immune responses to viral infections. Arbidol is typically administered orally in tablet or capsule form. The dosing regimen may vary depending on the indication and severity of the viral infection. Arbidol is commonly used for the treatment and prevention of influenza virus infections, particularly in regions where influenza outbreaks are prevalent. It may also be used as a prophylactic measure during influenza seasons or in high-risk populations, such as healthcare workers or individuals with underlying health conditions. Common side effects of arbidol include gastrointestinal symptoms (e.g., nausea, vomiting, diarrhea), headache, dizziness, and allergic reactions. It is generally well-tolerated, but adverse effects may occur in some individuals. Arbidol has been shown to be generally safe and effective for the treatment and prevention of influenza virus infections in clinical studies. However, more research is needed to fully understand its efficacy in different populations and against various viral strains.

9.4.1.6 Interferons

Interferons are a group of cytokines that possess broad-spectrum antiviral activity. They stimulate the immune system to produce antiviral proteins, inhibit viral replication, and modulate immune responses. Interferon-alpha, beta, and gamma are commonly used clinically for various viral infections. There are three main types of interferons: alpha, beta, and gamma. Each type has distinct functions and is produced by different cell types. Interferons have various therapeutic uses, including the treatment of viral infections (such as hepatitis B and C, human papillomavirus), certain cancers (such as melanoma and leukemia), autoimmune diseases (such as multiple sclerosis and rheumatoid arthritis), and as immunomodulatory agents. Interferons exert their effects by binding to specific cell surface receptors, leading to the activation of various signaling pathways within the cell. This activation triggers the expression of hundreds of interferon-stimulated genes (ISGs), which have antiviral, antiproliferative, and immunomodulatory effects. Interferons are typically administered via injection (subcutaneous or intramuscular) due to poor oral bioavailability. They are available as recombinant proteins or pegylated formulations (PEGylated interferons), which have an extended half-life in the body.

Types and examples:

- *Interferon-alpha:* Used primarily for the treatment of viral hepatitis (hepatitis B and C), certain cancers (such as hairy cell leukemia and Kaposi's sarcoma), and some autoimmune diseases.
- *Interferon-beta:* Used for the treatment of multiple sclerosis (MS) to reduce the frequency and severity of relapses.
- *Interferon-gamma:* Used in the treatment of chronic granulomatous disease (CGD) and osteopetrosis, and is being investigated for other conditions.

Common side effects of interferon therapy include flu-like symptoms (such as fever, chills, fatigue), injection site reactions, hematologic abnormalities (such as leukopenia and thrombocytopenia), and neuropsychiatric effects (such as depression and anxiety). Despite their therapeutic benefits, interferon therapy can be associated with significant side effects and limited efficacy in some patients. Additionally, the development of resistance to interferon therapy can occur in certain viral infections. Interferons play a vital role in innate immunity and have diverse therapeutic applications in the treatment of viral infections, cancers, and autoimmune diseases. However, their use requires careful consideration of potential side effects and individual patient characteristics. These broad-spectrum antiviral drugs offer a valuable therapeutic option for managing viral infections, especially in cases where the specific viral pathogen is unidentified or where multiple viruses may be involved in the disease process.

9.5 Specific antiviral

9.5.1 Oseltamivir (Tamiflu)

Oseltamivir is a specific antiviral medication used to treat and prevent influenza A and influenza B viruses. It inhibits the neuraminidase enzyme, which is essential for the release of new viral particles from infected cells, thereby reducing viral spread. It is typically administered orally as capsules or suspension. Used for the treatment of influenza infections, especially within 48 h of symptom onset, to reduce the duration and severity of symptoms and to prevent complications. Common side effects include nausea, vomiting, headache, and neuropsychiatric effects.

9.5.2 Acyclovir

Acyclovir is used to treat infections caused by herpes simplex virus (HSV) and varicella-zoster virus (VZV). Acyclovir is a nucleoside analog that inhibits viral DNA synthesis by acting as a substrate for viral DNA polymerase, leading to chain termination. Available in various formulations including oral, topical, and intravenous. Used for the treatment of genital herpes, cold sores, shingles, and chickenpox. Common side effects include nausea, vomiting, diarrhea, and headache. Intravenous administration may cause nephrotoxicity. Acyclovir, acting as the precursor to 2′-deoxyguanosine, works to combat viral infections through a series of steps that humanize its approach. The process begins with the activation of acyclovir into its active form, acyclovir triphosphate, by viral enzymes such as thymidine kinase from HSV-infected cells or phosphotransferase from cytomegalovirus. Following activation, acyclovir triphosphate enters a covert mission within the infected cell, disrupting viral DNA synthesis by outcompeting a crucial building block—2′-deoxyguanosine triphosphate. This strategic interference leads to the termination of viral DNA chain elongation, preventing further replication. Importantly, this integration of acyclovir into the viral DNA is irreversible, akin to locking a door that cannot be opened. The humanized aspect of acyclovir's action lies in its selective nature. While it efficiently targets viral DNA replication, its impact on uninfected cells is minimal, reducing the risk of side effects. Furthermore, the majority of acyclovir is excreted unchanged in urine, underscoring its efficiency in specifically addressing viral infections.

In terms of dosage, acyclovir's effectiveness is evidenced by its ability to achieve therapeutic plasma concentrations with relatively low doses, making it a practical option for treating infections caused by HSV and VZV. However, the dosing regimen for varicella-zoster infection is tailored to its shorter plasma half-life, requiring more frequent administration. Acyclovir emerges as a humanized ally in the battle against viral infections, showcasing a strategic and selective approach that minimizes collateral damage to uninfected cells. Its efficacy in treating specific viral strains further positions it as a valuable weapon in the medical arsenal.

9.5.3 Valacyclovir

Valacyclovir is an oral medication that quickly turns into acyclovir once ingested. This is made possible through the action of valacyclovir hydrolase in the digestive tract and liver. The transformation happens immediately after ingestion, resulting in enhanced bioavailability that is three-to-several-times higher than that of acyclovir alone. Valacyclovir is a highly effective treatment for infections caused by the HSV and VZV. It can also be used to prevent cytomegalovirus. As a prodrug, it is easily absorbed by the body and is a practical and powerful option for antiviral therapy.

9.5.4 Ganciclovir

Ganciclovir is a newer antiviral medication that differs from acyclovir in its chemical structure. Specifically, it has a hydroxymethyl group in position 3′ of a non-cyclic side chain, which allows it to serve as a building block for DNA chain terminators. Despite similarities in absorption and mechanism of action with acyclovir, ganciclovir's unique structure gives it additional capabilities. When cells are infected with cytomegalovirus, ganciclovir is transformed into ganciclovir monophosphate by viral-encoded phosphotransferase. This conversion is more efficient than that of acyclovir, leading to a more prolonged presence of intracellular ganciclovir triphosphate, which can last up to 12 h (compared to 1–2 h for acyclovir). This unique characteristic contributes to ganciclovir's superior efficacy in treating cytomegalovirus infections. When ganciclovir is administered intravenously, it can achieve peak plasma concentrations of more than 3 μM, which is an effective level to inhibit most strains of cytomegalovirus. This makes intravenous ganciclovir highly effective for both preventing and treating cytomegalovirus infections. Although oral ganciclovir has also been useful for preventing cytomegalovirus, its bioavailability is limited (8%–9%). In antiviral therapy, valacyclovir and ganciclovir are both important. Valacyclovir is effective against herpesviruses due to its high bioavailability, and ganciclovir is a potent weapon against cytomegalovirus due to its unique properties.

9.5.5 Penciclovir

Penciclovir, an antiviral medication, is commonly used to combat infections triggered by HSV. It stands out in several ways: Penciclovir is a drug that inhibits the activity of viral DNA polymerase, which is a crucial enzyme for the replication of the HSV. It's commonly used as a topical cream, and is directly applied to the affected skin or mucous membranes. This makes it effective for conditions like cold sores (herpes labialis) around the mouth. The drug becomes active within infected cells when viral thymidine kinase triggers its transformation into its active form, penciclovir triphosphate. Penciclovir triphosphate works by disrupting the synthesis of viral DNA. It does this by acting as a faulty substrate for viral DNA polymerase, which prevents further replication. Penciclovir is very selective, and only activates in cells infected by the HSV. This is thanks to viral thymidine kinase. The drug is effective for other localized HSV infections, not just cold sores. Side effects are generally mild, with occasional local skin reactions at the application site. In some studies, penciclovir has demonstrated a longer intracellular half-life than acyclovir. This means it may require less frequent dosing. However, treatment decisions involving penciclovir should be made in consultation with healthcare professionals. This is to take into account the specific condition and medical history of the individual.

9.5.6 Sofosbuvir

Sofosbuvir is used in combination with other medications to treat chronic HCV infections. It is a nucleotide analog inhibitor of the HCV NS5B RNA-dependent RNA polymerase, which is essential for viral RNA synthesis. Administered orally as tablets. Used as part of combination therapy for the treatment of chronic HCV infections, often with other direct-acting antiviral agents. Common side effects include fatigue, headache, nausea, and insomnia.

9.5.7 Lopinavir/ritonavir

Lopinavir/ritonavir is used in combination with other medications to treat HIV-1 infection. Lopinavir inhibits the HIV-1 protease enzyme, which is essential for the maturation of infectious viral particles, while ritonavir is a pharmacokinetic enhancer that increases lopinavir's plasma concentration. It can be administered orally as tablets or oral solution, and is used as part of combination antiretroviral therapy (cART) for the treatment of HIV-1 infection. Common side effects include gastrointestinal disturbances, elevated liver enzymes, and lipid abnormalities. These examples demonstrate specific antiviral drugs tailored to target particular viral infections, thereby providing effective treatment options with fewer off-target effects compared to broad-spectrum antivirals.

9.6 Mode of action of antiviral drugs

9.6.1 Inhibition of viral entry

Blockade of viral attachment: Maraviroc is a CCR5 antagonist used in the treatment of HIV/AIDS. It blocks the interaction between the HIV envelope glycoprotein gp120 and the CCR5 co-receptor on host CD4+ T cells, preventing viral attachment and entry into the cells.

Inhibition of membrane fusion: Enfuvirtide is an HIV fusion inhibitor that prevents viral entry by binding to the viral protein gp41, inhibiting the conformational changes necessary for viral membrane fusion with the host cell membrane, preventing the fusion of the viral and cellular membranes and subsequent entry of the virus into the host cell.

9.6.2 Inhibition of viral replication and transcription

Nucleoside/nucleotide analogs and their incorporation: Acyclovir is a nucleoside analog used in the treatment of HSV and VZV infections. It is phosphorylated by viral thymidine kinase and incorporated into viral DNA, leading to chain termination and inhibition of viral DNA synthesis.

Polymerase inhibitors and their mechanisms: Sofosbuvir is a nucleotide analog inhibitor of the HCV NS5B RNA-dependent RNA polymerase. It is metabolized intracellularly to the active triphosphate form, which competes with natural nucleotides, causing premature chain termination during viral RNA synthesis. Remdesivir is a broad-spectrum antiviral medication with activity against multiple

RNA viruses, including Ebola virus and SARS-CoV-2. It acts as a nucleotide analog inhibitor of viral RNA-dependent RNA polymerases, interfering with viral RNA synthesis.

9.6.3 Disruption of viral protein synthesis

Protease inhibitors and their role: Lopinavir is a protease inhibitor used in combination therapy for HIV/AIDS. It inhibits the viral protease enzyme, preventing the cleavage of viral polyproteins into functional components necessary for viral maturation and infectivity. Ritonavir is a protease inhibitor used in the treatment of HIV/AIDS. It inhibits the activity of the HIV-1 protease enzyme, preventing the cleavage of viral polyproteins into functional components necessary for viral replication.

9.6.4 Inhibition of viral assembly and release

Mechanisms of action for assembly inhibitors: Oseltamivir is a neuraminidase inhibitor used in the treatment and prevention of influenza A and B viruses. By inhibiting the neuraminidase enzyme, it prevents the release of newly formed viral particles from infected cells, reducing viral spread.

9.6.5 Stimulation of the immune response

Immunomodulators and their effects: Interferon-alpha is a type of immunomodulator used in the treatment of chronic viral hepatitis B and C infections. It stimulates the host immune response, enhancing antiviral activity, and inhibiting viral replication.

9.6.6 RNA interference (RNAi) as a therapeutic approach

siRNA and miRNA-based strategies: Patisiran is an RNA interference (RNAi) therapeutic used in the treatment of hereditary transthyretin-mediated amyloidosis (ATTR). It utilizes small interfering RNAs (siRNAs) to target and degrade specific mRNA molecules encoding the transthyretin protein, reducing the production of abnormal protein aggregates.

9.7 Resistance mechanisms

9.7.1 Emergence of antiviral resistance

Antiviral resistance refers to the ability of viruses to evade the effects of antiviral drugs, rendering them less effective or ineffective in controlling viral infections.

Resistance can emerge due to various factors, including viral mutations, selective pressure from antiviral therapy, and improper use of antiviral drugs.

9.7.2 Mechanisms of resistance development

Mutation of target viral genes: Viral mutations can lead to changes in the target viral genes that are essential for antiviral drug efficacy. These mutations may result in structural alterations of viral proteins targeted by the drug, reducing or abolishing drug binding and inhibitory effects. For example, mutations in the viral polymerase gene can confer resistance to nucleoside or nucleotide analogs by altering the enzyme's active site, preventing drug incorporation or enhancing drug excision.

Altered drug metabolism: Some viruses may develop resistance through alterations in drug metabolism pathways, leading to reduced activation or increased inactivation of antiviral drugs. For instance, viruses may upregulate drug-metabolizing enzymes or efflux transporters, leading to enhanced drug clearance and decreased intracellular drug concentrations.

Reduced drug uptake: Resistance can also arise from reduced uptake of antiviral drugs into infected cells, thereby limiting their intracellular concentrations and inhibitory effects on viral replication. This may occur due to mutations or alterations in cell surface receptors or transporters involved in drug uptake.

9.8 Strategies to mitigate resistance:

Combination therapy: Using multiple antiviral drugs with different mechanisms of action can reduce the likelihood of resistance emergence by targeting multiple steps in the viral replication cycle simultaneously.

Drug cycling or rotation: Alternating between different antiviral drugs or treatment regimens over time can help prevent the development of resistance by reducing the selective pressure exerted by a single drug.

Monitoring and surveillance: Regular monitoring of viral load and drug susceptibility can help detect the emergence of resistance early, allowing for timely adjustments to treatment strategies.

Development of new drugs: Continued research and development of novel antiviral drugs with distinct mechanisms of action can provide alternative treatment options and overcome resistance.

These strategies aim to minimize the emergence and spread of antiviral resistance, ensuring the continued efficacy of antiviral therapy in controlling viral infections.

9.9 Clinical applications

9.9.1 Common antiviral drugs and their clinical use

- Antiviral drugs are used to treat a variety of viral infections and can be categorized based on their mechanism of action and target virus.
- Common antiviral drugs include nucleoside/nucleotide analogs (e.g., acyclovir, tenofovir), protease inhibitors (e.g., lopinavir/ritonavir), polymerase inhibitors (e.g., sofosbuvir, remdesivir), neuraminidase inhibitors (e.g., oseltamivir), and interferons (e.g., interferon-alpha).
- These drugs are used for the treatment of viral infections such as influenza, HIV/AIDS, hepatitis B and C, HSV, VZV, and RSV, among others.

A. **Treatment of specific viral infections:**
    - Antiviral drugs are tailored to target specific viruses based on their mechanism of action and efficacy against particular viral pathogens.

- For example, oseltamivir and zanamivir are used for the treatment of influenza virus infections, while acyclovir and valacyclovir are effective against herpes simplex and VZV infections.
- Sofosbuvir and ledipasvir are used in combination therapy for the treatment of chronic HCV infections, while tenofovir and emtricitabine are used for the treatment of HIV/AIDS.

B. **Prophylactic use of antiviral drugs:**

- Antiviral drugs are also used prophylactically to prevent viral infections in certain high-risk populations or settings.
- For example, oseltamivir and zanamivir may be used prophylactically during influenza outbreaks or in individuals at high risk of complications from influenza.
- Antiretroviral drugs such as tenofovir/emtricitabine (Truvada) are used as pre-exposure prophylaxis (PrEP) to prevent HIV transmission in individuals at risk of HIV infection.

9.10 Challenges and limitations in clinical practice

Antiviral drug resistance: The emergence of antiviral resistance poses a significant challenge in clinical practice, limiting the efficacy of available treatments and necessitating the development of new drugs and treatment strategies.

Adverse effects: Antiviral drugs can cause various adverse effects, including gastrointestinal disturbances, hepatotoxicity, nephrotoxicity, and hematologic abnormalities, which may limit their tolerability and adherence to treatment.

Limited efficacy: Some viral infections, such as chronic hepatitis B and HIV/AIDS, may require lifelong treatment with antiviral drugs, and achieving a cure may not always be feasible.

Cost and accessibility: Access to antiviral drugs may be limited by factors such as cost, availability, and healthcare infrastructure, particularly in resource-limited settings.

Despite these challenges, antiviral drugs play a crucial role in the management and prevention of viral infections, improving patient outcomes and reducing the burden of viral diseases worldwide. Continued research and development efforts are needed to address existing limitations and optimize the clinical use of antiviral therapy.

9.11 Future directions

A. **Emerging antiviral therapies:**

- The field of antiviral therapy continues to evolve with the development of novel therapeutic agents targeting various stages of the viral lifecycle.
- Emerging antiviral therapies include new classes of drugs such as host-targeted antivirals, viral entry inhibitors, and immune modulators that

aim to enhance the body's natural defense mechanisms against viral infections.
- Additionally, advancements in antiviral drug discovery, including high-throughput screening, computational modeling, and structure-based drug design, are driving the identification of new drug candidates with potent antiviral activity.

B. **Advancements in drug delivery and personalized medicine:**
- Drug delivery technologies are advancing rapidly, enabling targeted and controlled release of antiviral drugs to specific tissues or cell types affected by viral infections.
- Personalized medicine approaches, such as pharmacogenomics and biomarker-based therapy selection, are being increasingly employed to optimize antiviral treatment regimens and improve patient outcomes.
- Nanotechnology-based drug delivery systems, gene editing techniques, and RNA interference (RNAi) technologies hold promise for the development of precision antiviral therapies tailored to individual patient characteristics and viral susceptibility profiles.

C. **Potential for novel antiviral targets:**
- Ongoing research efforts are focused on identifying novel targets for antiviral therapy, including viral and host factors essential for viral replication, pathogenesis, and immune evasion.
- Host-directed therapies that target host cell factors involved in viral entry, replication, and immune responses are gaining attention as potential antiviral strategies with broad-spectrum activity and reduced risk of resistance.
- Advancements in understanding virus–host interactions, viral evolution, and immune evasion mechanisms are informing the development of innovative antiviral approaches, including immunotherapies, therapeutic vaccines, and RNA-based therapies targeting viral RNA or host factors essential for viral replication.

Overall, future directions in antiviral therapy are focused on the development of innovative therapeutic approaches that target specific viral pathogens, enhance host immune responses, and minimize the emergence of drug resistance. These advancements hold promise for improving the treatment and prevention of viral infections and addressing unmet medical needs in the field of infectious diseases.

9.12 Conclusion

Antiviral drugs play a crucial role in the treatment and prevention of viral infections by targeting specific stages of the viral lifecycle or modulating host immune responses. Common antiviral drug classes include nucleoside/nucleotide analogs, protease inhibitors, polymerase inhibitors, neuraminidase inhibitors, and interferons, each with distinct mechanisms of action and clinical applications. Resistance to antiviral drugs poses a significant challenge in clinical practice and can arise due to mutations in viral target genes, altered drug metabolism, or reduced drug uptake. Strategies to mitigate resistance include combination therapy, drug cycling, monitoring and surveillance, and the development of new drugs with alternative mechanisms of action.

Ongoing research in antiviral drug development is essential for addressing emerging viral threats, combating drug resistance, and improving treatment outcomes for viral infections. Advancements in drug discovery, delivery technologies, and personalized medicine hold promise for the development of more effective and targeted antiviral therapies. Collaborative efforts between academia, industry, and government agencies are critical for accelerating the pace of antiviral drug development and translating scientific discoveries into clinical applications.

The future of antiviral therapy is promising, with ongoing research efforts focused on identifying novel drug targets, optimizing drug delivery systems, and advancing personalized medicine approaches. With the continued emergence of new viral pathogens and the threat of viral pandemics, there is a growing need for innovative antiviral therapies capable of addressing evolving viral challenges. By harnessing the power of interdisciplinary research, innovation, and global collaboration, the field of antiviral therapy is poised to make significant strides in improving public health and combating viral diseases in the years to come.

In conclusion, antiviral therapy remains a cornerstone of modern medicine, offering effective treatment and prevention options for a wide range of viral infections. Continued investment in research and development is essential for driving innovation, overcoming challenges, and realizing the full potential of antiviral therapy in improving patient outcomes and reducing the global burden of viral diseases.

Abbreviations

AIDS	Acquired immunodeficiency syndrome
cART	Combination antiretroviral therapy
CCR5	C-C chemokine receptor type 5
CGD	Chronic granulomatous disease
COVID-19	Coronavirus disease 2019
DNA	Deoxyribonucleic acid
EUA	Emergency use authorization
HCV	Hepatitis C virus
HIV	Human immunodeficiency virus
HSV	Herpes simplex virus
PrEP	Pre-exposure prophylaxis
RdRp	RNA-dependent RNA polymerase
RNA	Ribonucleic acid
RNAi	RNA interference
RSV	Respiratory syncytial virus
SARS-CoV-2	Severe acute respiratory syndrome-related coronavirus
siRNAs	Small interfering RNAs
VZV	Varicella-zoster virus

References

[1] Casanova J-L and Abel L 2013 The genetic theory of infectious diseases: a brief history and selected illustrations *Annu. Rev. Genomics Hum. Genet.* **14** 215–43

[2] Payne S 2022 *Viruses: From Understanding to Investigation* (Amsterdam: Elsevier)

[3] Milgroom M G 2023 *Viruses, Biology of Infectious Disease : From Molecules to Ecosystems* (Berlin: Springer) pp 35–54

[4] Schmid-Hempel P 2021 *Evolutionary Parasitology: The Integrated Study of Infections, Immunology, Ecology, and Genetics* (Oxford: Oxford University Press)

[5] Gini G 2023 The impact of artificial intelligence methods on drug design *Cheminformatics, QSAR and Machine Learning Applications for Novel Drug Development* (Amsterdam: Elsevier) pp 89–137

[6] Adamson C S, Chibale K, Goss R J M, Jaspars M, Newman D J and Dorrington R A 2021 Antiviral drug discovery: preparing for the next pandemic *Chem. Soc. Rev.* **50** 3647–55

[7] Dolgin E 2021 The race for antiviral drugs to beat COVID-and the next pandemic *Nature* **592** 340–3

[8] Salave S, Rana D, Bodar A, Khunt D, Prajapati B and Patel J 2023 Viral infections: current treatment options *Viral Drug Delivery. Systems: Advances in Treatment of Infectious Diseases* (Berlin: Springer) pp 65–89

[9] Jones J E, Le Sage V and Lakdawala S S 2021 Viral and host heterogeneity and their effects on the viral life cycle *Nat. Rev. Microbiol.* **19** 272–82

[10] Chakraborty A, Ko C, Henning C, Lucko A, Harris J M, Chen F, Zhuang X, Wettengel J M, Roessler S and Protzer U 2020 Synchronised infection identifies early rate-limiting steps in the hepatitis B virus life cycle *Cell. Microbiol.* **22** e13250

[11] Dustin L B, Bartolini B, Capobianchi M R and Pistello M 2016 Hepatitis C virus: life cycle in cells, infection and host response, and analysis of molecular markers influencing the outcome of infection and response to therapy *Clin. Microbiol. Infect.* **22** 826–32

[12] Dronina J, Bubniene U S and Ramanavicius A 2021 The application of DNA polymerases and Cas9 as representative of DNA-modifying enzymes group in DNA sensor design *Biosens. Bioelectron.* **175** 112867

[13] Te Velthuis A J W, Grimes J M and Fodor E 2021 Structural insights into RNA polymerases of negative-sense RNA viruses *Nat. Rev. Microbiol.* **19** 303–18

[14] Zephyr J, Yilmaz N K and Schiffer C A 2021 *Viral proteases: structure, mechanism and inhibition, Enzyme* (Amsterdam: Elsevier) pp 301–33

[15] Lin X, Liu X-Y, Zhang B, Qin A-Q, Hui K-M, Shi K, Liu Y, Gabriel D and Li X J 2022 A rapid influenza diagnostic test based on detection of viral neuraminidase activity *Sci. Rep.* **12** 505

[16] Pattnaik G P and Chakraborty H 2020 Entry inhibitors: efficient means to block viral infection *J. Membr. Biol.* **253** 425–44

[17] Jóźwik I K, Passos D O and Lyumkis D 2020 Structural biology of HIV integrase strand transfer inhibitors *Trends Pharmacol. Sci.* **41** 611–26

[18] Qi B, Fang Q, Liu S, Hou W, Li J, Huang Y and Shi J 2020 Advances of CCR5 antagonists: from small molecules to macromolecules *Eur. J. Med. Chem.* **208** 112819

[19] Rojas J M, Alejo A, Martín V and Sevilla N 2021 Viral pathogen-induced mechanisms to antagonize mammalian interferon (IFN) signaling pathway *Cell. Mol. Life Sci.* **78** 1423–44

[20] Mallery D L, Kleinpeter A B, Renner N, Faysal K M R, Novikova M, Kiss L, Wilson M S C, Ahsan B, Ke Z and Briggs J A G 2021 A stable immature lattice packages IP6 for HIV capsid maturation *Sci. Adv.* **7** eabe4716

[21] Mtambo S E, Amoako D G, Somboro A M, Agoni C, Lawal M M, Gumede N S, Khan R B and Kumalo H M 2021 Influenza viruses: harnessing the crucial role of the M2 ion-channel and neuraminidase toward inhibitor design *Molecules* **26** 880

[22] Selyutina A, Persaud M, Lee K, KewalRamani V and Diaz-Griffero F 2020 Nuclear import of the HIV-1 core precedes reverse transcription and uncoating *Cell. Rep.* **32** 108201

[23] Maertens G N, Engelman A N and Cherepanov P 2022 Structure and function of retroviral integrase *Nat. Rev. Microbiol.* **20** 20–34

[24] Andersen P I, Ianevski A, Lysvand H, Vitkauskiene A, Oksenych V, Bjørås M, Telling K, Lutsar I, Dumpis U and Irie Y 2020 Discovery and development of safe-in-man broad-spectrum antiviral agents *Int. J. Infect. Dis.* **93** 268–76

[25] Ekins S, Lane T R and Madrid P B 2020 Tilorone: a broad-spectrum antiviral invented in the USA and commercialized in Russia and beyond *Pharm. Res.* **37** 1–8

[26] Xu J, Shi P-Y, Li H and Zhou J 2020 Broad spectrum antiviral agent niclosamide and its therapeutic potential *ACS Infect. Dis.* **6** 909–15

[27] Cho N J and Glenn J S 2020 Materials science approaches in the development of broad-spectrum antiviral therapies *Nat. Mater.* **19** 813–6

[28] Bugert J J, Hucke F, Zanetta P, Bassetto M and Brancale A 2020 Antivirals in medical biodefense *Virus Genes* **56** 150–67

[29] Huchting J 2020 Targeting viral genome synthesis as broad-spectrum approach against RNA virus infections *Antivir. Chem. Chemother.* **28** 2040206620976786

[30] Mahajan S, Choudhary S, Kumar P and Tomar S 2021 Antiviral strategies targeting host factors and mechanisms obliging+ ssRNA viral pathogens *Bioorg. Med. Chem.* **46** 116356

[31] Barlow A, Landolf K M, Barlow B, Yeung S Y A, Heavner J J, Claassen C W and Heavner M S 2020 Review of emerging pharmacotherapy for the treatment of coronavirus disease 2019 *Pharmacother. J. Hum. Pharmacol. Drug Ther.* **40** 416–37

[32] Yang T, Oliyai R and Kent K M 2022 The making of the one pill—developing single tablet regimens for HIV and for HCV *Antivir. Ther.* **27** 13596535211067606

[33] Alarfaj S J, Alzahrani A, Alotaibi A, Almutairi M, Hakami M, Alhomaid N, Alharthi N, Korayem G B and Alghamdi A 2022 The effectiveness and safety of direct-acting antivirals for hepatitis C virus treatment: a single-center experience in Saudi Arabia *Saudi Pharm. J.* **30** 1448–53

[34] Tejada S, Martinez-Reviejo R, Karakoc H N, Peña-López Y, Manuel O and Rello J 2022 Ribavirin for treatment of subjects with respiratory syncytial virus-related infection: a systematic review and meta-analysis *Adv. Ther.* **39** 4037–51

[35] Priyadharsini R 2021 Antiviral drugs *Introduction to Basics of Pharmacology and Toxicology, Volume 2: Essentials of Systemic Pharmacology—From Principles to Practice* (Springer) pp 927–57

[36] Shiraki K and Daikoku T 2020 Favipiravir, an anti-influenza drug against life-threatening RNA virus infections *Pharmacol. Ther.* **209** 107512

[37] Khan S, Attar F, Bloukh S H, Sharifi M, Nabi F, Bai Q, Khan R H and Falahati M 2021 A review on the interaction of nucleoside analogues with SARS-CoV-2 RNA dependent RNA polymerase *Int. J. Biol. Macromol.* **181** 605–11

[38] Du Y and Chen X 2020 Favipiravir: pharmacokinetics and concerns about clinical trials for 2019-nCoV infection *Clin. Pharmacol. Ther.* **108** 242–7

[39] Hassanipour S, Arab-Zozani M, Amani B, Heidarzad F, Fathalipour M and Martinez-de-Hoyo R 2021 The efficacy and safety of Favipiravir in treatment of COVID-19: a systematic review and meta-analysis of clinical trials *Sci. Rep.* **11** 11022

[40] Bassetto M, Massarotti A, Coluccia A and Brancale A 2016 Structural biology in antiviral drug discovery *Curr. Opin. Pharmacol.* **30** 116–30

[41] Wang J, Reiss K, Shi Y, Lolis E, Lisi G P and Batista V S 2021 Mechanism of inhibition of the reproduction of SARS-CoV-2 and Ebola viruses by remdesivir *Biochemistry* **60** 1869–75

[42] Nili A, Farbod A, Neishabouri A, Mozafarihashjin M, Tavakolpour S and Mahmoudi H 2020 Remdesivir: a beacon of hope from Ebola virus disease to COVID-19 *Rev. Med. Virol.* **30** 1–13

[43] Cannalire R, Cerchia C, Beccari A R, Di Leva F S and Summa V 2020 Targeting SARS-CoV-2 proteases and polymerase for COVID-19 treatment: state of the art and future opportunities *J. Med. Chem.* **65** 2716–46

[44] Johnson K A and Dangerfield T 2021 Mechanisms of inhibition of viral RNA replication by nucleotide analogs *Enzym* **49** 39–62

[45] Tran A and Witek T J Jr. 2021 , The emergency use authorization of pharmaceuticals: history and utility during the COVID-19 pandemic *Pharmaceut. Med.* **35** 203–13

[46] Rizk J G, Forthal D N, Kalantar-Zadeh K, Mehra M R, Lavie C J, Rizk Y, Pfeiffer J P and Lewin J C 2021 Expanded Access programs, compassionate drug use, and emergency use authorizations during the COVID-19 pandemic *Drug Discov. Today* **26** 593–603

IOP Publishing

Viral Diseases
History and new developments in diagnostics and therapeutics
Arvind K Singh Chandel, Bhakti Tanna, Amisha Parmar, Gopal Patel and Neeraj S Thakur

Chapter 10

Ethnopharmacological approaches for COVID-19 therapy

Niyati Gupta and Bhakti Tanna

Ethnopharmacology is a fascinating field that explores the traditional medicinal knowledge of various cultures and communities. It often involves the study of plants and their bioactive compounds for potential therapeutic applications. With regards to COVID-19, researchers have been particularly interested in exploring medicinal plants and natural products that may have antiviral properties or could modulate the immune response to the virus. One area of interest in COVID-19 research is the virus's interaction with the angiotensin-converting enzyme 2 (ACE2) receptor, which is crucial for viral entrance into host cells. Some studies have focused on natural products that may inhibit this interaction, potentially blocking viral entry and replication. While research in this area is ongoing, certain medicinal plants and their constituents have shown promising results in laboratory studies. However, it is essential to approach these findings with caution, as laboratory studies do not always translate directly to clinical efficacy in humans. Further research, including clinical trials, is needed to evaluate the effectiveness and safety of these natural products for preventing or treating COVID-19. Moreover, while medicinal plants and natural products can offer potential therapeutic benefits, they should not be considered a substitute for standard medical care or public health measures such as vaccination and physical distancing.

10.1 Introduction

The emergence of human civilization and culture materialized around 12,000 years ago. According to social anthropologists and botanists, a small human community started the cultivation of plants on the banks of rivers Tigris and Euphrates, presently located in Iraq. It was revolutionary as for the first time in the history of Earth, food was being produced by domestication and cultivation. Oats, wheat, barley, and sesamum were possibly the first plants to be cultivated. The cultivators

doi:10.1088/978-0-7503-4987-1ch10

could be termed as the first ethnobotanists. By trial and error, the cultivation of edible plants and even the plants that could be used to treat diseases were being cultivated perfectly. The term ethnopharmacology was first coined in 1967 in San Francisco at an international symposium while discussing traditional psychoactive drugs. With time many scientists tried to define the term but could not do it justice. Ethno—(meaning 'culture' or 'people'), pharmacology (meaning 'drug') as a trans-disciplinary exploration covers the social and biological sciences [1].

Studying ethnopharmacology has some major advantages. It uses the knowledge of ancient people, because if the drug plant has been used by native cultures over a long duration, it must have a rationale. Drug discovery is a lengthy and expensive affair. Discovery of a new drug takes 12–15 years and can cost as much as $231 million. In addition to that, out of 10 000 synthesized molecules, an average of only one drug will receive US FDA (United States Food and Drug Administration) approval for the marketing. Thus, a plant with ancient utilization for a disease has a higher chance of containing active compound than the thousand synthetic drugs produced. Another benefit of using medicinal plants for treatment purposes is to get scientific validation for their advantageous and disadvantageous effects, which would eventually help these treatments get accepted in other developed countries. This can be economically valuable, as WHO (World Health Organization) had given an estimation that 80% of the population live in developing countries of which 80% do use medicinal plants for their primary ailments [2].

Medicinal plants have provided raw materials for one-third of our current antimicrobial agents over the centuries, and many of the allopathic medicines have their origins in traditional medicine. It is stated in the literature that 80% of currently used drugs have been obtained from natural resources such as medicinal plants, microorganisms etc [3]. Many of the laboratory scientists may not even be aware of the fact that many reagents used by them are actually obtained from natural resources and the development is due to the knowledge of ancient times. Such an example is the galantamine drug, used for treatment of Alzheimer's disease; many chemotherapeutic drugs such as taxols, vincristine, camptothecan etc are obtained from natural sources [4]. Ethnopharmacology, is the interconnection of many disciplines, such as botany, pharmacology, culture, health, economics etc. The use of active ingredients from the medicinal plants to cure common ailments is the traditional approach of ethno-pharmacology [5]. Recently, the outbreak of COVID-19 and its variants forced the research community to work on its treatments and vaccines at a fast pace [6]. The introduction of coronavirus in 2020 made people aware about their immunity and personal hygiene [7]. Hence plant-based alternative therapeutic choices have grabbed everyone's attention [6]. Thus, in this chapter various medicinal plants that have been studied for the treatment of coronavirus infection are included.

10.2 Use of molecular docking in unravelling potential of medicinal plants for the interventions of COVID-19

Molecular docking helps to target specific proteins responsible for infection and their binding to various molecules to unravel their potential as therapy. It can be used to evaluate proteins' ligand complex formation and their structural stability, which helps in predicting the drug target binding ability and finding the compounds which possess higher biological potency [8]. Since 2020, there has been many studies targeting natural products to evaluate their potential in the treatment of the global pandemic. However, these types of *in silico* studies have to be established by *in vivo* studies [58].

In a study conducted by Güler *et al* [9] they investigated various flavonoid compounds present in the ethanolic extract of *Anatolian propolis* and then evaluated them against ACE-II receptor inhibitor potential using molecular docking. They downloaded the ACE-II protein crystal structure online from data bank website (http://www.rcsb.org/pdb). Flavonoid compounds were obtained from PubChem and Hyperchem software was used to draw them and then geometric optimization was used for conformational search. Docking simulations were done using the Lamarckian genetic algorithm and Autodock 4.2 and were used for possible docking modes between the enzyme and selected compounds. They found that ethanolic extract (specifically rutin) has shown to be a good competitive inhibitor for the ACE-II enzyme and hence can be explored for COVID-19 treatment. Another study involving *Nigella sativa* L. also known as black cumin has been suggested for ingestion for COVID-19 interventions in societies commonly [10]. The molecular docking study for its compounds was done against the dimensional structure of the virus obtained from Protein Data Bank and chemical compounds were obtained from PubChem and were tested against various chemicals being tested clinically such as chloroquine. They found that Nigellidine gave scores close to chloroquine and even better scores than hydroxychloroquine. Another compound α-Hederin gave a better score than favipiravir and even chloroquine and hydroxychloroquine. Thus, proving their potential.

One more study by Shah *et al* [11], involving *Cressa cretica* active constituent 3, 5-Dicaffeoylquinic acid and Quercetin showed effectiveness as compared to standard Remdesivir with good docking score and hydrogen bond and hydrophobic relationship noted with the active site of M^{pro}, the protease crystal structure of COVID-19. *C. cretica* plant mirrors the best parts of Sanjeevani, which is one the least understood and most desired herbs in Indian culture and is the subject of much dispute. Three plants—*C. cretica*, *Dendrobium plicatile*, and *Selaginella bryopteris* are the main categories of Sanjeevani, amongst which *C. cretica* is widely used for asthma, diabetes, stomachic, etc in traditional medicines and it is the most commonly available holophytic herb. *In silico* study targeting curcumin and its derivatives targeting ACE2, IL (interleukin)-1β, IL-6 TNF α (tumor necrosis factor-alpha), and PAR-1 (protease-activated receptor) host receptor, shows that it helps in the treatment of the early response to viral infection and also its cure. Specifically, after DFT (density functional theory) and MDS (molecular dynamics simulation), hydrazinocurcumin showed the highest activity against ACE2 and PAR-1 target proteins [12].

Thus, this *in silico* docking analysis, can be used to search for the most useful treatments in much less time than the conventional techniques which can take years. The screening process becomes less time-consuming, which can save plenty of time and resources. Many studies are exploring various traditionally used herbs in the interventions of COVID-19 by *in silico* analysis. In this chapter, a few of them are mentioned in table 10.1 given below.

Table 10.1. *In silico* studies to unravel natural products effective in COVID-19 treatment.

Medicinal plant	Natural product	Method	Target	References
Anatolian propolis	Flavonoid—specifically Rutin	Molecular docking (*in silico* analysis)	ACE-II enzyme	[9]
Nigella sativa L.	Nigellidine, α-Hederin; dithymoquinone (DTQ)	Molecular docking (*in silico* analysis)	$_{3cl}$pro$_{/M}$pro COVID-19; 3clpro/Mpro SARS-coronavirus three dimensional structures; increased potential of binding at SARS-CoV-2: ACE2 interface	[10]
Cressa cretica	3,5-Dicaffeoylquinic acid and Quercetin	Molecular docking (*in silico* analysis)	M^{pro} receptor of COVID-19	[11]
Bupleurum chinense DC. Cyathula officinalis Kuan	Quercetin	Molecular docking (*in silico* analysis—Network pharmacol)	Binds to ACE2, impairs the interaction between S protein and ACE2	[8]
Hippophae rhamnoides L.	Isorhamnetin	CMC, Molecular docking	Binds to S protein and ACE2, inhibites SARS-CoV-2 spike pseudotyped virus entering $ACE2^{h}$cell	[8]
Pueraria lobata(Willd.) Ohwi	Puerarin	Network pharmacology, Molecular docking	Binds to ACE2 and S protein, impairs the interaction between S protein and ACE2	[8]
Carthamus tinctorius L.	Rutin	Molecular docking (*in silico* analysis)	Binds to S protein and ACE2	[8]
Glycyrrhiza uralensis Fisch	Euchrenone, Glycyrrhizic acid	Network pharmacology, Molecular docking	Binds to ACE2, M^{pro} and RdRp	[8]
Honey and propolis (bees glue)	*p*-coumaric acid, ellagic acid, kaempferol, and quercetin	AutoDock Vina software	M^{pro}, RdRp	[13]
Mangosteen; Javanese turmeric	Javanese turmeric; Javanese turmeric	Molecular docking (*in silico* analysis)	M^{pro}	[14]
Red wine, Chinese hawthorn, and blackberry	Antiviral phytocompounds	ADME and Lipinski rules (*In silico* analysis)	$3CL^{pro}$ and (ACE2)	[15]
Ophiocoma dentata	Steroid compounds	Molecular docking, ADMET analysis, and *in silico* toxicity studies as well as *in vitro* analysis	M^{pro}, nsp and RdRp	[16]
Sargassum spinuligerum	Phlorotannins	Molecular docking (*in silico* analysis)	M^{pro}	[17]
Marine sponge (*Lissodendoryx* sp.)	Eribulin, a macrocyclic ketone analogue of the marine compound halichondrin B	Autodock Vina and MDS	RdRp	[18]
Sesamum indicum L.	Hydroxymatairesinol	Molecular docking (*in silico* analysis)	M^{pro}	[19]

RdRp: RNA-dependent RNA polymerase.
M^{pro}: Main protease.
ADME: absorption, distribution, metabolism and excretion.
$3CL^{pro}$: hydrolytic enzyme.
ACE2: angiotensin-converting enzyme 2.
NSP: nonstructural protein.

10.3 Natural products from medicinal plants and their mechanisms for COVID-19 intervention

Many natural products have been shown to aid in the prevention of contagious infection through COVID-19, with the use of medicinal plants, coupled with a reduction in its severity by alleviating the effects of SARS-CoV-2 infection similar to the release of inflammatory cytokines leading to acute respiratory distress syndrome, multiorgan dysfunction, and dysregulation of cytokine storm and immunity [20].

Herbal medicine adjuncts in treating the symptoms of COVID-19 infection along with modern medicine [21]. During the COVID-19 outbreak, widely known herbal medicines with antiviral properties were being administered as an extra supportive treatment to suppress SARS-CoV-2, since standard treatments were not effective enough. Therefore, they are effective in reducing and managing the risk of COVID-19 infection.

Elevations in inflammatory indicators, including erythrocyte sedimentation rate (ESR), C-reactive protein (CRP), and interleukin-6 (IL-6), have been linked to worsened outcomes and illness severity; these findings are most likely connected to cytokine storm [22]. In addition to direct antiviral effects, herbal drugs have been shown to have anti-inflammatory properties that contribute significantly to COVID-19 treatment. A single botanical plant may contain a diverse spectrum of chemical substances that would be responsible for its antiviral, anti-inflammatory, immunomodulatory, and other activities. This gives it versatility based on strong efficacy evidence. Some herbal medicines used to treat COVID-19 are summarized below.

Based on the method of management, different approaches were being utilized for the treatment. Cases of headache, symptoms of fever, mild infection, sweat, red tongue tip, dry cough, floating pulse, thirst, and sore throat, were treated with Yinqiao san and Sangju yin, which is a combination of various natural herbs [23]. In severe cases of infections with high-grade fever, chest stiffness, sweating, dry cough, fatigue, nausea, breathing difficulty, bloating, yellow coating, and red or dark red tongue, preventive and supportive management of COVID-19 infection was achieved through reducing the immune system by utilizing *Thymus vulgaris*, *Glycyrrhiza glabra*, *Althea officinalis*, *ginseng* and *Allium sativum* [24]. Previous research has revealed that consuming echinacea supplements may be associated with decreased levels of the pro-inflammatory cytokines TNF, IL-6, and IL-8 and higher levels of the anti-inflammatory cytokine IL-10 [25].

Interestingly, curcumin has been proven *in silico* studies to limit SARS-CoV-2 entry into cells and viral multiplication, while a recent experimental study suggests that bromelain may also block viral entry into cells.

Some natural products such as *amygdalinum*, *Gymnanthemum*, *N. sativa*, *Azadirachta indica*, *G. glabra*, *Eurycoma longifolia*, *ginseng*, *A. officinalis*, *A. sativum*, *T. vulgaris* can be used as adjuvant therapy and are beneficial in the prevention and treatment of COVID-19 by strengthening the immune system.

10.3.1 *Gymnanthemum amygdalinum*

This has immune-boosting properties when used in conjunction with vaccinations. This plant has traditionally been utilized to relieve fever, headaches, cough, and diarrhea.

Aqueous extracts from *Gymnanthemum amygdalina* have been shown in studies to enhance human immune system activity, as seen by an increase in CD4+ T-cells and leukocytes. These findings suggest the plant's potential use as a supplemental treatment in human immunodeficiency virus (HIV) antiretroviral regimens. Additionally, it can control the amounts of substances and cytokines that promote inflammation [26].

10.3.2 *Azadirachta indica* (neem)

Fever has been the primary clinical symptom of COVID-19, for the treatment of which, neem has proven valuable outcomes. Traditionally, neem leaf decoction has been used to treat fever caused by COVID-19 infection. Additionally, it reports immunoregulatory and anti-inflammatory benefits to strengthen immune response [27] Moreover, neem leaf extracts including its metabolic components, such as flavonoids and polysaccharides, are known to exhibit direct antiviral efficacy against different kinds of viruses via animal experiments and *in silico* docking research [28]. More specifically, molecular docking research for SARS-CoV-2 has demonstrated an inhibitory effect by binding onto the SARS-CoV-2 envelope, membrane, and glycoproteins owing to the presence of medicinal constituents such as nimbolin, nimocin, and cycloartenol [29].

10.3.3 *Nigella sativa* (black cumin)

By tradition, black cumin is reported to have a wide range of indications including upper respiratory conditions or diseases such as asthma due to its significant anti-inflammatory and anti-hypersensitivity effects which aid in relieving asthma symptoms.

Plant extracts of *N. sativa* seeds reduce the amount of viral, alpha-fetoprotein, establishing the antiviral property. According to some reports, it also enhances the liver function parameters in hepatitis C patients [30]. In an animal study, black cumin seed oil reduces viral counts to an unknown amount by exhibiting antiviral and immunomodulatory effects on the cytomegalovirus. It also augments the immune response by increasing CD3 and CD4 levels and release of interferon-gamma (IFN-γ) from Natural Killer (NK) T-cells and macrophages [31].

10.3.4 *Allium sativum* and *Allium cepa*

Onion (*Allium cepa*) and garlic (*A. sativum*) have usually been used for the initial treatment of COVID-19 infection. Garlic can inhibit the SARS-CoV-2, as perceived by *in silico* studies. It acts by the formation of hydrogen bonds between amino acids with the binding site of the primary structural protease of SARS-CoV-2 along with the bioactive components of the protease that produce the virus. It also leads to a significant upregulation of the T helper cells, cytotoxic T-cells, and NK cells, as well as downregulation of the levels of leptin, leptin receptor, IL-6, proliferator-activated receptor gamma (PPAR-γ), and TNF-α [32]. Because of its ability to modulate cytokine secretion, immunoglobulin production, phagocytosis, and macrophage activation, it is an effective option for the management of COVID-19 infection.

Onion is also a good candidate for the management of COVID-19 disease due to the presence of its anti-inflammatory, antithrombotic, antihypertensive, antimicrobial, antimutagenic, prebiotic activities, anticarcinogenic, immunomodulatory, antithrombotic, anti-inflammatory, antidiabetic, and antioxidant, and antiviral effect [32].

10.3.5 Glycyrrhiza glabra

Glycyrrhizin effectively inhibits the replication of SARS-cov-2 (FFM-1 and FFM-2). It is discovered to be non-cytotoxic to the host cells while simultaneously inhibiting the virus's cytopathic effect. It inhibits virus replication and, penetration and adsorption of the virus into the host cells [33]. It also produces nitrous oxide synthase, signifying the release of nitrous oxide which it generates for the inhibition of virus replication. The action against SARS-CoV-2 can be significantly enhanced through modification of the glutamate receptor structures, especially by producing amino-acid conjugates and amide derivatives, but it can be at the cost of elevated cytotoxicity.

Other additional potential medicinal plants that are being used to treat and prevent the COVID-19 infection are listed in table 10.2.

10.4 Traditional Chinese medicine (TCM) for the treatment of COVID-19

Chinese medicine has been used in China since ancient times. The knowledge of Chinese herbalists has helped gather tremendous knowledge that has been beneficial in fighting various diseases for thousands of years and has also helped during the outbreak of COVID-19. It is a well-known fact that TCM has various biological properties such as antiviral, anti-inflammatory, immunoregulation properties, etc and thus it has also shown significant potential in the medication of COVID-19 [34].

Many herbal formulations in TCM have been tested for the treatment of COVID-19 and have shown high activity against it. One of the tested TCMs was Jinhua Qinggan granule (JHQGG), which is a mixture of herbal drugs that was first developed for treating H1N1 influenza and has also shown high activity in the treatment of COVID-19 patients [35]. This formulation appeared to decrease critical biomarkers of COVID-19, such as LI-6 (interleukins-6) and NLS (neutrophil/lymphocyte ratio) and hence it manifested its potential for its use in mild to severe patients. The formulations such as XBJ (Xuebijing injection), QFPD (QingfeiPaidu Decoction), and HXZQ (Huoxiang Zhengqi Powder) exhibited activity by regulation of PI3K (phosphatidylinositol-3 kinase)-Akt (total protein kinase B) pathway which plays a critical role in virus spread and replication [34, 36]. Amongst these, QFPD is a general prescription drug for the treatment; it has also shown inhibition of inflammation and has also exhibited recovery in clinical trials. QFPD is combination of 22 different herbal compounds such as Fried *Glycyrrhiza uralensis, Cinnamomun cassia*, *Gypsum Fibrosum*, ginger-processed Pinelliaternata, Ginger, *Polyporus umbellatus*, *Asari Radix* et Rhizoma, *Ephedrae Herba*, Dioscorea opposite Rhizoma, *Armeniacae Semen Amarum*, *Poria cocos*, *Atractylodes macrocephala*, *Aster tararicus*, *Bupleuri Radix*, *Scutellaria baicalensis Geor*, *Belamcandae Rhizoma*, tangerine peel, Alismaorientalein, *Aurantii Fructus Immaturus*, *Farfarae Flos* and

Table 10.2. Natural products and their mechanism involved in the treatment of COVID-19 [20].

Natural source	Compound	Biological role	Activity against COVID-19
Nigella sativa	Thymoquinone	Antioxidant immune-regulatory, anti-inflammatory, and antioxidant benefits	Prevent the SARS-CoV-2 entry; inhibits viral replication
Apples, raspberries, onions, red grapes, cherries, citrus fruits, and green leafy vegetables	Quercetin	Antioxidant, anti-inflammatory, anti-cancerous, antiviral, anti-bacterial, and immunomodulatory	Inhibition of 3CL protease activity and viral entry inside the host cell
Blueberries, kiwis, coffee, cherries, apples, And tea	Caffeic acid	Antioxidant, anti-inflammatory, anti-bacterial and antiviral	Inhibit the virus attachment to the host cell; Binds 3CL protease inhibits the viral replication
Mimusopscaffra, Ilex paraguarieni, and Glechoma hederacea	Ursolic acid	Anti-inflammatory, anti-bacterial effects, antioxidant, anti-cancer, and antidiabetic	Potently block the M^{Pro}enzyme
Raspberries, strawberries, pomegranate, persimmon, grapes, blackcurrants, plums, mango, guava, walnuts, almonds, longan seeds, green tea, and *Momordica charantia*	Ellagic acid	Antioxidant and anti-proliferative, Inhibit fibrosis, oxidative stress, and inflammation in the diabetic liver	Inhibits the MPro and RdRp ; Prevent viral attachment and internalization to the host cell
Vanilla bean *Thymus vulgaris*, ocimum, origanum, *Monarda genera*, members of verbenaceae, scrophulariaceae, ranunculaceae, and apiaceae families	Vanillin Thymol	Anti-clastogenic, antimicrobial agent, antioxidant Antioxidant, local anesthetic, anti-carcinogenesis, anti-nociceptive, cicatrizing, antiseptic, as well as a potential as a growth enhancer and immunomodulator	M^{Pro} inhibition Inhibit the viral spike protein; prevent the SARS-CoV-2 entry, potent disinfectants.
Rosemary, perilla, sage, mint, and basil	Rosmarinic acid	Antispasmodic, analgesic, anti-rheumatic, diuretic, and antiepileptic agent food flavoring agent,	Inhibition of viral entry, replication

Agastache rugosa [34, 37]. It is a combination of HXZQ that has been shown to prevent and treat COVID-19, as well as improve patient symptoms. There are various other TCMs with well-established mechanisms for preventing the disease such as Lianhua Qingwen Prescription (LHQW), Jinhua Qinggan Granules (JHQG), Shengjiang powder (SJS), Huashibaidu prescription (HSBD), Maxing

Shigan Decoction (MXSG), Reduning Injection (RDN), Shengmai injection (SMI), Yiqi Fumai Lyophilized Injection (YQFM), Tanreqing Injection (TRQ), Shufeng Jiedu Capsules(SFJD) that have proven to possess various pathways through which they can inhibit the infection and help in disease treatment [34]. Amongst these formulations, LH capsule has been shown to increase patient's rate of recovery (91.5% versus 82.4%) even when compared to Western medicines during prospective, randomized controlled trials; as well as in CT (computed tomography) (83.8% versus 64.1%); and in clinical recovery rates (78.9% versus 66.2%) [38]. TCM combined with Western medicine, exhibited potential improvement in COVID-19 prognosis [39]. Apart from these compositions, various natural products have been shown to help in overcoming the disease like genkwanin and derivative of quercetin from pogostemonis herb; β-sitosterol, aloe-emodin, rhein, catechins from rhubarb; other natural products such as glycyrrhizin, nicotinamide quercetin, (-)-epigallocatechin gallate; combination of curcumin, vitamin C and glycyrrhizin [34].

Natural products from TCM have been tested and have shown different mechanisms through which they inhibit the SARS-CoV-2 infection at varying stages. ACE2 enzyme inhibition was observed in forsythoside A (*Forsythiae fructus* (Lianqiao) fruit), rhein (*Rheum palmatum* (Yaoyong Dahuang)), quercetin (*Ginkgo biloba* (Yingxing)), neochlorogenic acid (*Lonicera japonica* (Jingyinhua)), ephedrine (*Ephedrae Herba* (Mahuang)) using enzyme inhibition assay. Antiviral effects were exerted on the infected Vero cell line by digitoxin (*Digitalis purpurea* (Yangdihuang)), tetrandrine (*Stephania tetrandra* (Fengfangji)), glycyrrhizin (*G. uralensis* (Gancao)), resveratrol (*Polygonum cuspidatum* (Huzhang)), pterostilbene (*Pterocarpus santalinus* (Zitan)), cepharanthine (*Stephania japonica* (Qianjinteng)), ginsenoside Rb1 (*Panax ginseng* (Renshen)). Hesperidin from *Citrus aurantium* (Suancheng) has shown block spike-ACE2 interaction using target-based virtual ligand screening. Sequence alignment and homology modeling indicated the spike's crucial targets to be 3Clpro (3C-like protease), PLpro (papain-like protease) which has been targeted by baicalein and scutellarein (*Scutellaria baicalensis* (Huangqin)), shikonin (*Lithospermum erythrorhizon (*Zicao)), theaflavin (black tea), tanshinone IIA, Dihydrotanshinone I, crytotanshinone & dihydrotanshinone I (*Salvia miltiorrhiza* (Danshen)), sinigrin and hesperetin (*Isatis indigotica* root (Banlangen)), luteolin (Jinyinhua), etc [40].

In a retrospective study, the mortality rate was decreased by up to 82.2% in patients treated with TCM to those treated with non-TCM [41]. In a cohort study, Hanshiyi formula (HSYF) TCM and control were given to patients and the patients moving from progressed to severe stage were observed to be 0% and 6.5%, respectively, in a statistically significant manner [42]. Thus, the successful utilization of TCM is due not only to its inhibition of viruses but also to blocking infection, reducing inflammatory response, regulating immune response, and boosting body repair mechanisms. Thus, TCM contemplates the ideology of 'preventive treatment of disease' [43].

10.5 Pre-clinical and clinical trials

The development of potential anti-COVID-19 natural products and herbal medicines is of great importance, as plant-based therapeutics have shown promising efficacy against various viruses by strengthening the immune system. These promising medicines can only be marketed in countries around the world when pre-clinical and clinical trials are successful.

Screening of natural products for *in vitro* and *in vivo* activity has mainly been concerned with preventing viral reproduction, as determined by the PCR evaluation of viral RNA and determination of IC50 value reported. The prevention of the cytopathic effect on infected cells and of inflammatory markers like interleukins are among the other most often researched methods [44]. For evaluation of SARS-CoV-2 replication, Vero E6 cell lines are being used predominantly. In particular, targets vis. papain-like protease, protease, NSP-14, NSP-15, RNA-dependent RNA polymerase, TMPRSS2, and spike protein are being studied *in vitro*.

In a pre-clinical study for the determination of the effects of parthenolide in COVID-19 patients, parthenolide showed significant inhibition of pro-inflammatory pathways, especially the LPS and NF-kB pathways. As per the obtained results, parthenolide significantly reduced IL-1, IL-2, IL-6, IL-8, and TNF-α production pathways, developed in a number of human cell line models both *in vivo* and *in vitro* (monocytes, macrophages, neutrophils) [45, 46].

A study found that *Adhatoda Vesica* extract reduced airway inflammation, TGF-β1, IL-6, and HIF-1α levels, and enhanced mouse survival rates in pulmonary fibrosis and sepsis models. It also inhibited siRNA-induced inflammation and blood coagulation abnormalities in mice. The lung transcriptome showed decreased expression of hypoxia, inflammation, TGF-β1, and angiogenesis genes, but adaptive immunity-related genes increased [47].

After pre-clinical studies, involving the assessment of potential treatments or interventions in laboratory and animal settings, the next step in the process of developing new medical treatments is typically clinical research considering human subjects to assess safety, efficacy, and potential adverse effects of the natural product.

Clinical research to assess the safety and effectiveness of ZingiVir as an add-on medication in COVID-19 patients, showed a remarkable recovery in COVID-19 patients. Also, the use of herbal medicines like ashwagandha, tulsi, amruth (giloy), and turmeric as add-on treatment in COVID-19 patients has shown better recovery in terms of indications and symptoms of COVID-19 patients. Refer to the table 10.3 below for other significant clinical trials.

10.6 Conclusion

It is not possible to track down all the medicinal plants that are being used for ethnopharmacology purposes. However, in this chapter, we have tried to cover a major share of those used or tested for SARS-CoV-2 treatment. There are numerous studies involving molecular docking that represent a potential natural product's action on a molecule. Using this knowledge, the product can be screened and evaluated by *in vitro* and *in vivo* analysis. Thereafter, clinical research needs to be conducted to confirm their role. Therefore, in our chapter, we have tried to cover plants, their natural products, their potential mechanisms towards SARS-CoV-2 as

Treatment details	Study title	Type of trial (design of study)	Remarks	References
ZingiVir-H	Clinical research on safety and efficacy of ZingiVir-H as an add-on therapy in COVID-19 patients.	Interventional (Other)	Zingivir-H consumption with the standard of care in COVID-19 confirmed patients showed a remarkable recovery compared to that of a placebo	[48]
Herbal formulation—aayudh advance)	To study the effectiveness of herbal formulation aayudh advance as a supplementary treatment for the coronavirus 2019 (COVID-19) infected patients	Interventional, randomized, parallel-group, active-controlled	Aayush advance 'when given concomitantly with standard of care, was found to be 100% safe, devoid of any drug-drug interaction, effective as virucidal to reduce viral load, and increased the recovery rate when compared to standard of care alone when tested in mild symptomatic COVID-19 patients	[49]
Kabasura, kudineer	Effectiveness of siddha medicine, kabasura, kudineer and vitamin c–zinc supplementation in the management of mild COVID-19 patients	Interventional, randomized, parallel group	The role of vitamin C with zinc supplementation in the management of COVID-19 is still not clear. Therefore, study will compare the effect of kabasura kudineer and vitamin C with zinc supplementation in terms of negative conversion of SARS-COV 2 infection	[50]
Ayurveda rasayana along with conventional guidelines for healthcare workers	Role of chyawanprash in the prevention of COVID-19 in healthcare workers	Interventional, randomized, parallel-group	No adverse effect was found in the study	[51]

(Continued)

Table 10.3. (*Continued*)

Treatment details	Study title	Type of trial (design of study)	Remarks	References
Ayurveda protocol	Effect of ayurvedic intervention in COVID-19 positive cases	Interventional, single-arm trial, completed	Ayurveda treatment protocol includes sanshamani, nagaradi kwath, amalaki churna, and golden milk to improve the strength of the patient	[49]
Purified aqueous extract of cocculus hirsutus (AQCH)	A study to evaluate the effect and safety of a phytopharmaceutical drug in treatment of coronavirus infection	Interventional, randomized, parallel-group	Clinical improvement was observed in COVID patients in terms of disease severity	[52]
Chayapanprash (an ayurvedic herbal preparation)	Ayurvedic intervention (chyawanprash) in the prevention of COVID-19 pandemic among healthcare personnel	Interventional, single arm	This remedy was found to be a possible safe prophylactic remedy for COVID-19	[53]
Amrta karuna syrup	Clinical trial on immunity and antiviral for quarantine patients of COVID-19	Interventional, randomized, parallel-group, active-controlled	The formulation was found to be immunomodulatory	[54]
Virulina along with standard treatment tocol	A clinical trial to know the effect of Virulina® for treatment of COVID positive patients	Interventional, randomized, parallel-group, placebo controlled	The formulation was found to boost the immunity of the patients and help ease the symptoms	[55]
Astha-15 capsule	A clinical trial to evaluate the safety and efficacy of polyherbal capsule Astha-15 used as an add-on therapy with standard care of therapy as an immunity booster in the suspected and COVID-19 diagnosed patients	Interventional, randomized, parallel-group, placebo	A better recovery rate was observed	[54]

Immunity kit	Use of herbal medicine like tulsi, amruth (giloy), turmeric, ashwagandha as add on treatment in COVID-19 patients	Interventional, single arm	Upon using the ayurvedic formulation as add on treatment, the recovery was better in terms of signs and symptoms of COVID-19 patients	[54]
Arogya Kashayam -20	Intervention of ayurvedic medicine (arogya kashayam) in COVID-19 positive cases (asymptomatic and mild symptomatic)	Interventional, randomized, parallel group, active-controlled	The unani regimen was found to be effective against the mild symptoms of COVID-19	[56]
Khameera marwareed Tiryaq-e —Arba Unani joshanda/decoction behidana (Cydonia oblonga) 3 gm, unnab (Zizyphus jujube) 5 in number, sapistan (Cordia myxa) 9 in numbers	A study on unani regimen for the prevention of high/moderate risk population of COVID-19	Interventional non-randomized, multiple arm	Improvement was found in the immune status of COVID patients	[57]
Tab. Bresol and tab. Septilin	Role of herbal immunomodulators in mild COVID-19 confirmed cases	Interventional, randomized, parallel-group, active-controlled	Use of herbal immunomodulators as an add-on treatment improved the recovery rate of COVID-19 patients	[58]
Add–on personalized Ayurveda intervention to ICMR guideline on COVID-19	The COVID-19 study with Ayurveda add-on to ICMR guideline	Interventional, randomized, parallel-group	The efficacy of treatment was measured in terms of average stay of patients in the hospital to become COVID negative	[59]

(*Continued*)

Table 10.3. (*Continued*)

Treatment details	Study title	Type of trial (design of study)	Remarks	References
1.Kabasura kudineer 2. Shakti drops 3. Turmeric plus tablets	Kabasura kudineer, shakti drops and turmeric plus in the management of COVID-19	Interventional (Others)	A better recovery rate was observed in terms of signs and symptoms of stages 1 and 2 of COVID-19 cases on the addition of ayurvedic medicines, thereby improving the quality of life of stage 1 and 2 COVID-19 patients	[60]
1.Dashamula kwatha and pathyadi kwatha with trikatu churna 2. Sansamani vati 3. AYUSH 64 4. Yastimadhu Ghanavati	Effect of ayurveda medicine in COVID-19 mild symptoms	Interventional randomized, parallel-group, active-controlled	No adverse reaction was observed and improvement in signs and symptoms	[58]
Cap. IP	Safety and efficacy of ayurvedic capsule in mild to moderate COVID-19 infection	Interventional, randomized, parallel group	Improvement was observed in respiratory symptoms of COVID patients	[61]

well as the status of clinical trials if conducted. We have also focused on TCM as it has been in use for centuries. There are many natural and medicinal products in use that have shown beneficial effects.

Abbreviations

ACE2	Angiotensin-converting enzyme 2
ADME	Absorption, distribution, metabolism and excretion
CRP	C-reactive protein
ESR	Erythrocyte sedimentation rate
IL	Interleukin
MDS	Molecular dynamics simulation
NLS	Neutrophil/lymphocyte ratio
nsp	Nonstructural protein
RdRp	RNA-dependent RNA polymerase
TCM	Traditional Chinese medicine
TGF	Transforming growth factor
TNF	Tumor necrosis factor
USFDA	United States Food and Drug Administration
WHO	World Health Organization

References

[1] Pushpangadan P, George V, Ijinu T P and Rajasekharan S 2016 *Ethnobotany, Ethnobiology, Ethnopharmacology, Bioprospecting of Traditional Knowledge and Evolution of Benefit Sharing. Indian Ethnobotany: Emerging Trends* (Jodhpur: The Scientific Publisher) pp 1–23

[2] Farnsworth N R 1993 Ethnopharmacology and future drug development: the North American experience *J. Ethnopharmacol.* **38** 137–43

[3] Gahamanyi N, Munyaneza E, Dukuzimana E, Tuyiringire N, Pan C H and Komba E V 2021 Ethnobotany, ethnopharmacology, and phytochemistry of medicinal plants used for treating human diarrheal cases in Rwanda: a review *Antibiotics* **10** 1231

[4] Heinrich M and Bremner P 2006 Ethnobotany and ethnopharmacy-their role for anti-cancer drug development *Curr. Drug Targets* **7** 239–45

[5] Ortega F 2009 Medicinal plants in the evolution of therapeutics—a case of applied ethnopharmacology *Ethnopharmacology. sl: Encyclopedia of Life Support Systems* (UNESCO-EOLSS) pp 160–82

[6] Lim X Y, Teh B P and Tan T Y 2021 Medicinal plants in COVID-19: potential and limitations *Front. Pharmacol.* **12** 611408

[7] Mukhopadhyay S and Palbag S 2021 Ethnopharmacology and pharmacology of ayurvedic plant Ativisha *J. Ayurvedic Herb. Med.* **7** 46–8

[8] Liu H M, Liu X M, Yuan X Y, Xu C, Wang F, Lin J Z, Xu R C and Zhang D K 2021 Screening S protein–ACE2 blockers from natural products: strategies and advances in the discovery of potential inhibitors of COVID-19 *Eur. J. Med. Chem.* **226** 113857

[9] Güler H I, Şal F A, Can Z, Kara Y, Yildiz O, Beldüz A O, Canakci S and Kolayli S 2021 Targeting CoV-2 spike RBD and ACE-2 interaction with flavonoids of *Anatolian propolis* by *in silico* and *in vitro* studies in terms of possible COVID-19 therapeutics *Turk. J. Biol.* **45** 530–48

[10] Bouchentouf S and Missoum N Identification of compounds from *Nigella sativa* as new potential inhibitors of 2019 Novel Coronavirus (COVID-19): Molecular docking study https://chemrxiv.org/engage/chemrxiv/article-details/60c7495c469df4070af43bbf
[11] Shah S, Chaple D, Arora S, Yende S, Mehta C and Nayak U 2022 Prospecting for *Cressa cretica* to treat COVID-19 via *in silico* molecular docking models of the SARS-CoV-2 *J. Biomol. Struct. Dyn.* **40** 5643–52
[12] Noor H, Ikram A, Rathinavel T, Kumarasamy S, Nasir Iqbal M and Bashir Z 2022 Immunomodulatory and anti-cytokine therapeutic potential of curcumin and its derivatives for treating COVID-19–a computational modeling *J. Biomol. Struct. Dyn.* **40** 5769–84
[13] Shaldam M A, Yahya G, Mohamed N H, Abdel-Daim M M and Al Naggar Y 2021 *In silico* screening of potent bioactive compounds from honeybee products against COVID-19 target enzymes *Environ. Sci. Pollut. Res.* **28** 40507–14
[14] Sumaryada T and Pramudita C A 2021 Molecular docking evaluation of some Indonesian's popular herbals for a possible COVID-19 treatment *Biointerface Res. Appl. Chem.* **11** 9827–35
[15] Xu J, Gao L, Liang H and Chen S D 2021 *In silico* screening of potential anti–COVID-19 bioactive natural constituents from food sources by molecular docking *Nutrition* **82** 111049
[16] Abd El Hafez M S, AbdEl-Wahab M G, Seadawy M G, El-Hosseny M F, Beskales O, Saber Ali Abdel-Hamid A, El Demellawy M A and Ghareeb D A 2022 Characterization, in-silico, and in-vitro study of a new steroid derivative from *Ophiocoma dentata* as a potential treatment for COVID-19 *Sci. Rep.* **12** 5846
[17] Geahchan S, Ehrlich H and Rahman M A 2021 The anti-viral applications of marine resources for COVID-19 treatment: an overview *Marine Drugs* **19** 409
[18] Piplani S, Singh P K, Winkler D A and Petrovsky N 2021 Computationally repurposed drugs and natural products against RNA dependent RNA polymerase as potential COVID-19 therapies *Mol. Biomed.* **2** 28
[19] Allam A E, Amen Y, Ashour A, Assaf H K, Hassan H A, Abdel-Rahman I M, Sayed A M and Shimizu K 2021 *In silico* study of natural compounds from sesame against COVID-19 by targeting M pro, PL pro and RdRp *RSC Adv.* **11** 22398–408
[20] Demeke C A, Woldeyohanins A E and Kifle Z D 2021 Herbal medicine use for the management of COVID-19: a review article *Metab. Open* **12** 100141
[21] Ang L, Song E, Lee H W and Lee M S 2020 Herbal medicine for the treatment of coronavirus disease 2019 (COVID-19): a systematic review and meta-analysis of randomized controlled trials *J. Clin. Med.* **9** 1583
[22] Zeng F, Huang Y, Guo Y, Yin M, Chen X, Xiao L and Deng G 2020 Association of inflammatory markers with the severity of COVID-19: a meta-analysis *Int. J. Infect. Dis.* **96** 467–74
[23] Liu L S, Lei N, Lin Q, Wang W L, Yan H W and Duan X H 2015 The effects and mechanism of Yinqiao Powder on upper respiratory tract infection *Int. J. Biotechnol. Wellness Indus.* **4** 57
[24] Wang J, Zhu X, Sun Y, Zhang X and Zhang W 2020 Efficacy and safety of traditional Chinese medicine combined with routine western medicine for the asymptomatic novel coronavirus disease (COVID-19): a Bayesian network meta-analysis protocol *Medicine* **99** e21927
[25] Aucoin M *et al* 2021 A systematic review on the effects of Echinacea supplementation on cytokine levels: is there a role in COVID-19? *Metab. Open* **11** 100115

[26] Grubben G J and Denton O A 2004 *Plant Resources of Tropical Africa 2. Vegetables* (Earthprint Ltd)

[27] Paterson R *et al* 2020 The emerging spectrum of COVID-19 neurology: clinical, radiological and laboratory findings *Brain* **143** 3104–20

[28] Lage G A, Medeiros F D, Furtado W D, Takahashi J A, Filho J D and Pimenta L P 2014 The first report on flavonoid isolation from *Annona crassiflora* Mart *Nat. Prod. Res.* **28** 808–11

[29] Borkotoky S and Banerjee M 2021 A computational prediction of SARS-CoV-2 structural protein inhibitors from *Azadirachta indica* (Neem) *J. Biomol. Struct. Dyn.* **39** 4111–21

[30] Abdel-Moneim A, Morsy B M, Mahmoud A M, Abo-Seif M A and Zanaty M I 2013 Beneficial therapeutic effects of *Nigella sativa* and/or *Zingiber officinale* in HCV patients in Egypt *EXCLI J.* **12** 943

[31] Salem A M, Bamosa A O, Qutub H O, Gupta R K, Badar A, Elnour A and Afzal M N 2017 Effect of *Nigella sativa* supplementation on lung function and inflammatory mediators in partly controlled asthma: a randomized controlled trial *Ann. Saudi Med.* **37** 64–71

[32] Khubber S, Hashemifesharaki R, Mohammadi M and Gharibzahedi S M 2020 Garlic (*Allium sativum* L.): a potential unique therapeutic food rich in organosulfur and flavonoid compounds to fight with COVID-19 *Nutr. J.* **19** 1–3

[33] Cinatl J, Morgenstern B, Bauer G, Chandra P, Rabenau H and Doerr H 2003 Glycyrrhizin, an active component of liquorice roots, and replication of SARS-associated coronavirus *Lancet* **361** 2045–6

[34] Yu-Jie D A, Shi-Yao W, Shuai-Shuai G O, Jin-Cheng L I, Fang L I and Jun-Ping K O 2020 Recent advances of traditional Chinese medicine on the prevention and treatment of COVID-19 *Chin. J. Nat. Med.* **18** 881–9

[35] Kageyama Y, Aida K, Kawauchi K, Morimoto M, Ebisui T, Akiyama T and Nakamura T 2022 Jinhua Qinggan granule, a Chinese herbal medicine against COVID-19, induces rapid changes in the neutrophil/lymphocyte ratio and plasma levels of IL-6 and IFN-γ: an open-label, single-arm pilot study *World Acad. Sci. J.* **4** 1–8

[36] Du H T, Wang P, Ma Q Y, Li N, Ding J, Sun T F, Wang C G, Wang D D, Zhang H M and Zhang L M 2020 Preliminary study on the effective components and mechanism of Huoxiang Zhengqi Decoction in inhibiting the replication of novel coronavirus *Mod. Tradit. Chin. Med. Mater. Med.-World Sci. Technol.* **22** 645–51

[37] Peng X J, Yang X J, Xu G, Chen Y B, Yang C H, Gong W L, Han D and Liu F 2020 Investigating clinical efficacy and mechanism of qingfei paidu decoction for treatment of COVID-19 based on integrative pharmacology *Chin. J. Exp. Tradit. Med. For.* **24** 6–13

[38] Hu K *et al* 2021 Efficacy and safety of Lianhuaqingwen capsules, a repurposed Chinese herb, in patients with coronavirus disease 2019: a multicenter, prospective, randomized controlled trial *Phytomedicine* **85** 153242

[39] Xiao M *et al* 2020 Efficacy of Huoxiang Zhengqi dropping pills and Lianhua Qingwen granules in treatment of COVID-19: a randomized controlled trial *Pharmacol. Res.* **161** 105126

[40] Lyu M *et al* 2021 Traditional Chinese medicine in COVID-19 *Acta Pharm. Sin.* B **11** 3337–63

[41] Chen G *et al* 2020 Chinese herbal medicine reduces mortality in patients with severe and critical Coronavirus disease 2019: a retrospective cohort study *Front. Med.* **14** 752–9

[42] Tian J *et al* 2020 Hanshiyi Formula, a medicine for SARS-CoV2 infection in China, reduced the proportion of mild and moderate COVID-19 patients turning to severe status: a cohort study *Pharmacol. Res.* **161** 105127

[43] Ren J L, Zhang A H and Wang X J 2020 Traditional Chinese medicine for COVID-19 treatment *Pharmacol. Res.* **155** 104743

[44] Mousavi S, Zare S, Mirzaei M and Feizi A 2022 Novel drug design for treatment of COVID-19: a systematic review of preclinical studies *Can. J. Infect. Dis. Med. Microbiol.* **2022** 2044282

[45] Magni P, Ruscica M, Dozio E, Rizzi E, Beretta G and Facino R M 2012 Parthenolide inhibits the LPS-induced secretion of IL-6 and TNF-α and NF-κB nuclear translocation in BV-2 microglia *Phytotherapy Res.* **26** 1405–9

[46] Wang M and Li Q 2015 Parthenolide could become a promising and stable drug with anti-inflammatory effects *Nat. Prod. Res.* **29** 1092–101

[47] Gheware A *et al* 2021 Adhatoda Vasica attenuates inflammatory and hypoxic responses in preclinical mouse models: potential for repurposing in COVID-19-like conditions *Respir. Res.* **22** 1–5

[48] Sasidharan S, Hareendran Nair J, Srinivasakumar K P, Paul J, Madhu Kumar R, Rajendran K, Saibannavar A A and Nirali S 2022 An efficacy and safety report based on randomized controlled single-blinded multi-centre clinical trial of ZingiVir-H, a novel herbo-mineral formulation designed as an add-on therapy in adult patients with mild to moderate COVID-19 *PLoS One* **17** e0276773

[49] Singh R S *et al* 2021 Promising traditional Indian medicinal plants for the management of novel Coronavirus disease: a systematic review *Phytother. Res.* **35** 4456–84

[50] Jabaris S L and Kudineer V K 2021 A Siddha medicine against COVID-19 infection: scope and future perspective *Int. J. Complement Alt. Med.* **14** 173–4

[51] Gupta A *et al* 2021 Chyawanprash for the prevention of COVID-19 infection among healthcare workers: a randomized controlled trial *medRxiv* https://doi.org/10.1101/2021.02.17.21251899

[52] Joglekar S *et al* 2022 Efficacy and safety of a phytopharmaceutical drug derived from cocculus hirsutus in adults with moderate COVID-19: a phase 2, open-label, multicenter, randomized controlled trial *Infect. Dis. Ther.* **11** 807–26

[53] Jindal N, Rajput S, Yadav B, Mundada P, Singhal R, Varshney S, Srikanth R K and Dhiman K S 2021 Chyawanprash as add on to the standard of care in preventing COVID-19 infection among apparently healthy health care workers–a single arm, longitudinal study *AAM* **10** 204–19

[54] Rao M V, Juneja A, Maulik M, Adhikari T, Sharma S, Gupta J, Panchal Y and Yadav N 2021 Emerging trends from COVID-19 research registered in the Clinical Trials Registry-India *Indian J. Med. Res.* **153** 26

[55] Sewda D *et al* 2023 A double-blind, placebo-controlled, randomized clinical trial to evaluate the efficacy and safety of Virulina® along with standard treatment as per hospital protocol for the treatment of novel coronavirus (COVID-19) *J. Drug Del. Therapeut.* **13** 91–7

[56] Shukla U and Ujjaliya N 2023 Evaluation of addon effectiveness of Arogya kashayam-20 in mild-to-moderate COVID-19 cases – A randomized controlled study *AYUHOM* **10** 28–32

[57] Nikhat S and Fazil M 2023 Critical review and mechanistic insights into the health-protective and immunomodulatory activity of Tiryāq (Theriac) from the purview of Unani medicine *Brain Behav. Immun. Integrat.* **4** 100021

[58] Ali A A, Bugarcic A, Naumovski N and Ghildyal R 2022 Ayurvedic formulations: potential COVID-19 therapeutics? *Phytomed. Plus* **2** 100286

[59] García-Martínez B I, Ruiz-Ramos M, Pedraza-Chaverri J, Santiago-Osorio E and Mendoza-Núñez V M 2022 Influence of age and dose on the effect of resveratrol for glycemic control in type 2 diabetes mellitus: systematic review and meta-analysis *Molecules* **27** 5232

[60] Sharma S, Nair N, Majeed J, Patel B, Mandal V and Dhobi M 2023 Critically analyzing the resilience of alternative and complementary medicines as possible COVID-19 intervention: a cross-sectional study based on CTRI database *J. Herb. Med.* **41** 100730

[61] Rangnekar H, Patankar S, Suryawanshi K and Soni P 2020 Safety and efficacy of herbal extracts to restore respiratory health and improve innate immunity in COVID-19 positive patients with mild to moderate severity: a structured summary of a study protocol for a randomised controlled trial *Trials* **21** 943

Chapter 11

Plasma therapy

Pralhad Wangikar, M V S Sandhya, Pratyusha Janaswamy and Aditi Wangikar

Serotherapy or plasma therapy involves the transfer of sera/plasma containing the neutralizing antibody (Ig) obtained from an immunized individual recovered from an infection to an actively infected patient. The use of blood components, especially plasma, has been used in the treatment of not only viral and bacterial infection but also rare genetic conditions involving the loss of certain plasma proteins treating life-threatening conditions. Human convalescent plasma (CP) as a source of antiviral neutralizing antibodies was revolutionized as a clinical strategy for treatment since the H1N1 Spanish flu outbreak. Since then, CP has been an efficient immunization strategy against pandemic influenza and other viral diseases. In 2019, when COVID-19 emerged as a pandemic, the potential of plasma therapy became a beacon of hope in the face of initial uncertainties in vaccine development and a lack of therapeutic modalities. The antiviral Ig, along with anti-inflammatory cytokines and immunomodulatory plasma proteins from the COVID-19 survivors, proved to alleviate the cytokine storm efficiently and reduce the mortality in critically ill patients. This chapter focuses on the role of blood plasma as an immunization strategy for viral diseases, especially for novel coronavirus disease 2019 (COVID-19), summarizing the clinical data on the immunological response of patients to plasma therapy, and understanding the knowledge gaps in its clinical application, which may improve future research.

11.1 Introduction

11.1.1 Efficacy of plasma therapy in diseases

In 1880, the principle of serotherapy was established. Immunity against Diphtheria was shown, and then tetanus toxins primarily relied on antibodies in the blood of animals intentionally immunized with non-lethal doses of toxins, which could be transferred to naïve animals experiencing active infection. This was applied successfully to humans suffering from Diphtheria. Sera from diverse species (horses, sheep, goats) were subjected to a flourishing pharma industry between 1920 and 1940. Despite the occasional side effects due to treatment defined as 'serum sickness,'

doi:10.1088/978-0-7503-4987-1ch11

this saved numerous lives against the deadly effects of bacterial toxins. CP, a passive immunization strategy, has been used to treat and prevent epidemic infections for over 100 years. In 1916, it was tried as a treatment for acute paralysis in the New York outbreak of poliomyelitis. The same year, it was also applied to contain a small measles epidemic in Tunis. In 1907, in an Italian journal, Francesco Cenci was finally credited as the first to use serum as a therapeutic tool to protect children exposed to measles.

Around 1950, plasma fractionation into plasma-derived therapeutic factors was made available. Immunoglobulins (Igs) were purified and concentrated from highly immunized donors who have fully recovered from past clinical infection, constituting the hyperimmune immunoglobulin fractions. This human immunoglobulin, and some specific Igs, progressively replaced animal sera and are still in use, notably for neutralizing the HBV, rubella, rabies, pertussis, and tetanus toxin. The polyclonal Igs from plasma offered by blood donors under the form of intravenous Igs (IVIGs) conferred some degree of protection to eliminate or reduce infected patients with bacterial sepsis and has been proposed to help patients and children who have not yet developed infection, such as with human immunodeficiency virus type 1 (Lee *et al* 2021, Cohen 2023).

In 2002–03, during the SARS-CoV outbreak, there were rapid produced convalescent therapy initiatives and reports were made available. All recent publications claimed that this therapy was followed by a drop in viral load and improved patient symptoms (Franchini 2021). The study reports and meta-analyses or look-back studies show a specific efficacy when applied early (before five days after exposure) during the H1N12009p flu infection. Experimental studies done with material collected during the outbreak also conclude that this procedure promises to reduce the viral burden and morbidity/mortality (Axfors *et al* 2021).

CP is efficient in Ebolavirus (EBV) disease and was brought in an experimental model. The intensity of the 2013–15 outbreak in West-Central Africa has encouraged diverse consortia in the US and Europe to set up protocols for collecting plasma from convalescent individuals on the existence and sustainability of protective neutralizing antibodies (Abs). A study conducted on 84 patients from Guinea receiving CP confirmed the safety of the blood component but failed to demonstrate a survival benefit in the CP treatment arm. Another study conducted in Sierra Leone evaluated CP for Ebola treatment in 44 subjects versus 25 non-treated patients. It showed an improvement in death rate in patients receiving CP compared to the control group (27.9% versus 44%) with a 2.3 odds ratio (OR) for survival in CP-treated arm (Peng *et al* 2020; Johns Hopkins Bloomberg School of Public Health 2022).

A study has also reported using CP in addition to an antiviral drug in two patients; both recovered without noticeable sequelae. The authors concluded that the role of CP versus other support care is challenging to delineate.

11.1.2 Procedure

Plasma is the liquid component of blood, and CP refers to plasma collected from individuals who have recovered from infections such as COVID-19. This plasma may contain antibodies and proteins the immune system produces that help neutralize or eliminate viruses. In the case of COVID-19, CP therapy has been explored as a potential treatment, utilizing plasma from recovered patients to support the recovery of others.

Plasmapheresis is a standard technique for separating and collecting plasma from whole blood. During this process, blood is drawn from a vein and passed through a machine where plasma is isolated, and the remaining blood components are returned to the body. This procedure takes around 40 min and is widely used to treat various blood disorders, neurological disorders, and blood cancers and in organ transplant recovery (Senefeld *et al* 2023).

Plasma therapy has also been applied to neurological conditions such as multiple sclerosis, myasthenia gravis, and Guillain–Barré syndrome, as well as certain blood disorders like cryoglobulinemia and thrombotic thrombocytopenic purpura. CP comprises numerous essential elements, including immunoglobulins, albumin, and cytokines. The neutralizing antibodies (NAbs) found in CP can block interactions between pathogens and host cells, such as how SARS-CoV-2 binds to human ACE2 receptors via the spike protein's receptor-binding domain (RBD) (Everts *et al* 2020).

These NAbs can prevent viral entry into cells by targeting and binding to critical parts of the virus, reducing its ability to infect new cells. Moreover, natural IgM and high-affinity IgG antibodies in plasma provide additional defense by binding to various antigens or clumping viral particles together, such as seen with the poliovirus.

While CP therapy holds promise, it has not yet consistently proven effective as a treatment for COVID-19. Early studies have shown that some patients improved with this therapy, and large blood centers in the U.S. have begun collecting plasma to help in the COVID-19 pandemic response. The U.S. FDA granted emergency use authorization for CP with high antibody levels to treat COVID-19 in hospitalized patients, particularly those early in their illness or with compromised immune systems (U.S. Food and Drug Administration 2023). However, more research is needed to determine its efficacy fully.

Neutralizing antibodies are critical for eliminating viral infections and key to preventing viral diseases. In CP therapy, these antibodies are transferred from recovered individuals to boost the immune response in patients with active infections. The effectiveness of CP therapy largely depends on the concentration of neutralizing antibodies in the donor's plasma. In viruses like MERS and SARS-CoV, neutralizing antibodies bind to specific domains on the spike protein, inhibiting viral replication and helping control the infection. Studies have shown that IgG antibodies, which develop in response to the virus, can persist for years, and other antibodies, such as IgM and non-neutralizing antibodies, may aid recovery without directly interfering with viral replication. CP therapy also enhances processes like antibody-dependent cellular cytotoxicity, offering a multifaceted approach to supporting recovery and potentially preventing further infection (figure 11.1) (Piyush *et al* 2020).

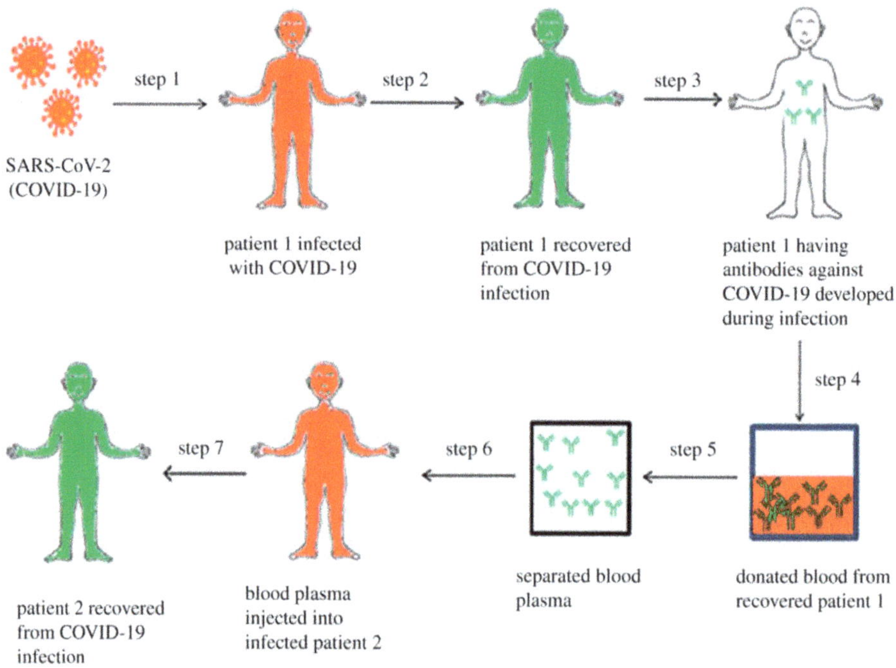

Figure 11.1. Schematic of plasma therapy. When the COVID-19-infected individuals recover, their blood plasma contains antibodies against the COVID-19-causing SARS-CoV-2 virus. The recovered individuals donate their blood, from which the plasma containing the required antibodies is extracted. This plasma is then administered to the infected individual(s) via transfusion. Adapted from Piyush *et al* (2020) CC BY 4.0.

11.1.3 Strategy for COVID-19

Blood donated by individuals who have recovered from COVID-19 contains antibodies that help fight the virus. After donation, the blood is processed to remove cells, leaving behind plasma and antibodies. This plasma can be transfused to people with COVID-19 to strengthen their immune response against the virus. Hyperimmune IgG antibodies, collected from individuals who have recovered from the virus, are preferred because they tend to have a higher concentration of antibodies, making them more effective at neutralizing the virus.

Since the virus has multiple strains that vary across regions, it is recommended that donors and recipients be from the same geographical area. This helps ensure the antibodies target the specific strain prevalent in the region. In combination with antiviral treatments, antibody therapy can modulate immune responses, such as cytotoxicity and phagocytosis, to help neutralize the virus. The duration of treatment and the concentration of antibodies required often depend on the illness's severity and the patient's viral load.

Before donation, potential plasma donors undergo a standard assessment to ensure safety and compliance with donation regulations. Eligible donors are typically between 18 and 65 years old, must test negative for COVID-19 at least 14 days post-recovery, and should be symptom-free. Follow-up tests are conducted

48 h later and again at the time of donation (U.S. Food and Drug Administration 2023).

Plasma is typically collected through apheresis, which continuously separates plasma from whole blood using a centrifuge. This method allows for collecting 400–800 ml of plasma per donation. The plasma is then stored in 200 or 250 ml units and frozen within 24 h to preserve its potency. Procedures like pathogen neutralization using UV light or riboflavin safeguard the plasma before further transfusion.

11.1.4 Mechanism of convalescent plasma therapy against SARS-COV-2

The neutralizing antibody of MERS and SARS-CoV was observed to inhibit the viral amplification after binding the spike protein S1-N-terminal domain (S1-NTD), which helped control the infection. Further, the CP administration enhances antibody-dependent cytotoxicity. After infection with SARS-CoV, in response to the nucleoprotein of the virus, the IgG antibodies are produced, mainly detected on the 14th day or the 4th day after the beginning of the disease. Around 89% of the patients displayed neutralizing and IgG-specific antibodies, even after two years of the infection, of the convalesced. Some non-neutralizing antibodies were observed to have interacted with the virus by binding to it, contributing to an enhanced recovery rate or promoting prophylaxis. At the same time, it did not intervene in the viral replication (Weiqian *et al* 2020; Piyush *et al* 2020).

11.1.5 Accomplishments using therapy

Without a definitive treatment for COVID-19, researchers continue to explore potential therapies and strategies to combat the disease. One option that has shown promise is CP therapy, a technique that has been used successfully in previous viral epidemics. The rationale behind using CP against COVID-19 is based on past experiences and early studies that indicate its potential effectiveness.

In one study involving ten critically ill patients who had tested positive for COVID-19, each received a 200 ml dose of CP from individuals who had recently recovered from the virus. The plasma had high virus-neutralizing antibody titers (above 1:640) and was given with other antiviral treatments. After three days, patients showed noticeable improvements: oxygen saturation increased, clinical symptoms diminished, and the lymphocyte count rose from 0.65×10^9 per liter to 0.76×10^9 per liter. Additionally, levels of C-reactive protein, a marker of inflammation, dropped significantly from 55.98 to 18.3 mg l^{-1}. Imaging via chest CT scans also revealed a reduction in lung lesions. Notably, no severe side effects were reported, leading researchers to suggest that CP therapy could help neutralize the virus in severely ill patients, potentially improving outcomes in critical COVID-19 cases (Lindemann *et al* 2021).

This research points to CP as a potential therapeutic option for those battling severe forms of COVID-19, offering hope in the fight against the pandemic.

11.1.6 Ongoing clinical trials

After the outbreak of COVID-19 as a global pandemic, scientists worldwide began searching for effective treatments and preventive measures. Among these efforts, CP therapy emerged as a potential option, with approximately 69 studies registered on http://clinicaltrials.gov/ focusing on its use against COVID-19.

One such study, titled 'Convalescent Plasma as Therapy for COVID-19 Severe SARS-CoV-2 Disease (CONCOVID Study)' (clinical trial no. NCT04342182), is a randomized trial aimed at evaluating the safety and efficacy of plasma from recovered COVID-19 patients as a treatment for hospitalized individuals with COVID-19. Another study, 'Early Transfusion of Convalescent Plasma in Elderly COVID-19 Patients to Prevent Disease Progression' (clinical trial no. NCT04374526), hypothesizes that administering CP early in infection can help prevent the inflammatory response triggered by SARS-CoV-2, to halt pneumonia progression, boosting antibody levels, and lower viral loads in elderly patients (Davenport *et al* 2015; Rajendran *et al* 2020; Estcourt and Callum 2022).

Further, the study 'Convalescent Plasma Trial in COVID-19 Patients' (clinical trial no. NCT04356534) focuses on comparing CP therapy with SARS-CoV-2-specific antibodies in patients with pneumonia and hypoxia to evaluate improvements in their clinical outcomes. Similarly, 'Efficacy of Convalescent Plasma Therapy in Severely Sick COVID-19 Patients' (clinical trial no. NCT04346446) is another randomized trial investigating the effectiveness of CP in severely ill COVID-19 patients. This study involves collecting 500 ml of CP from recovered patients after confirmed recovery and analyzing the plasma for COVID-19-specific antibodies (Duan *et al* 2020; Herrera 2020).

Additionally, the study 'Convalescent Plasma for Treatment of COVID-19: An Exploratory Dose Identifying Study' (clinical trial no. NCT04384497) focuses on treating high-risk individuals with detectable viral loads before they develop severe pulmonary infections, aiming to prevent reliance on supplemental oxygen therapy.

These ongoing studies provide valuable insights into how CP therapy may help combat COVID-19, though more research is needed to confirm its overall efficacy (Humphrey 2022; Facher 2020).

11.1.7 Concluding remarks: old or new therapies?

Plasma therapy has long been a debated intervention, particularly for severely ill patients. While it has been considered a last-resort, compassionate treatment for critical cases like organ failure or severe bleeding, many experts agree that it works best when administered early, before the disease progresses too far.

Researchers emphasize different aspects of plasma therapy's efficacy. For example, technologists focus on the specific Igs extracted from plasma, which are thought to be the primary mode of action. Meanwhile, physiologists acknowledge additional factors, such as healing agents that prevent excess vascular leakage and regulate coagulation, which may play a crucial role in treatment outcomes. For diseases without hemorrhagic features, such as COVID-19, purifying antibodies and even developing monoclonal antibodies is highly desirable—as seen in other viral infections like HIV, where many attempts at antibody-based therapies have been pursued (Piyush *et al* 2020, Garraud *et al* 2016).

In the case of SARS-CoV-2, its high transmission rate demands an immediate therapeutic approach. CP therapy has emerged as a promising option. It has been used successfully in past viral epidemics and has been considered by the World Health Organization (WHO) as part of its COVID-19 control strategy. Despite its potential, CP therapy requires further investigation and optimization to ensure its efficacy in COVID-19 cases (Piyush *et al* 2020).

Significantly, CP therapy relies on the generosity of individuals who have recovered from COVID-19 or have been exposed to the virus without developing symptoms. These donors are essential to the process, and their contributions highlight the generous nature of plasma donation, which must remain free from commercial interests. Ensuring the safety of the donated plasma is crucial, typically done through pathogen reduction technologies—standard practice in economically developed nations. However, it is critical to make these technologies accessible to developing countries, as shown during the Ebola crisis (Piyush *et al* 2020).

In conclusion, CP therapy represents a significant therapeutic approach for combating viral infections, including COVID-19. By directly targeting the SARS-CoV-2 virus, it has demonstrated the potential to save lives and reduce the impact of the global pandemic (Piyush *et al* 2020).

Abbreviations

Abs	Antibodies
CT	Computerized tomography
CP	Convalescent plasma
COVID-19	Coronavirus-19
EBV	Ebolavirus
FDA	Food and Drug Administration
HFs	Hemorrhagic Fevers
hACE2	Human ACE2
Igs	Immunoglobulins
IVIGs	Intravenous Igs
MERS	Middle Eastern Respiratory Syndrome
OR	Odds ration
RBD	Receptor-binding domain
S1-NTD	S1-N-terminal domain

References

Axfors C *et al* 2021 Association between convalescent plasma treatment and mortality in COVID-19: a collaborative systematic review and meta-analysis of randomized clinical trials *BMC Infect. Dis.* **21** 1170

Cohen E 2023 Study shows convalescent plasma works for immune-compromised COVID-19 patients, but it can be hard to find *CNN Health* https://edition.cnn.com/2023/01/12/health/convalescent-plasma-immune-compromised-covid/index.html

Davenport K L, Campos J S, Nguyen J, Saboeiro G, Adler R S and Moley P J 2015 Ultrasound-guided intratendinous injections with platelet-rich plasma or autologous whole blood for treatment of proximal hamstring tendinopathy: a double-blind randomized controlled trial *J. Ultrasound in Med.* **34** 1455–63

Duan K *et al* 2020 Effectiveness of convalescent plasma therapy in severe COVID-19 patients *Proc. Natl Acad. Sci.* **117** 9490–6

Estcourt L and Callum J 2022 Convalescent plasma for COVID-19—making sense of the inconsistencies *New Engl. J. Med.* **386** 1753–4

Everts P, Onishi K, Jayaram P, Lana J F and Mautner K 2020 Platelet-rich plasma: new performance understandings and therapeutic considerations in 2020 *Int. J. Mol. Sci.* **21** 7794

Facher L 2020 Is convalescent plasma safe and effective? We answer the major questions about the COVID-19 treatment *Statnews* https://statnews.com/2020/08/23/is-convalescent-plasma-safe-and-effective

Franchini M 2021 Convalescent plasma therapy for managing infectious diseases: a narrative review *Ann Blood* **6** 17

Garraud O, Heshmati F, Pozzetto B, Lefrere F, Girot R, Saillol A and Laperche S 2016 Plasma therapy against infectious pathogens, as of yesterday, today and tomorrow *Transfus. Clin. Biol.* **23** 39–44

Herrera T 2020 What is convalescent blood plasma, and why do we care about it? *The New York Times* https://nytimes.com/2020/04/24/smarter-living/coronavirus-convalescent-plasma-antibodies.html

Humphrey N 2022 Convalescent plasma doesn't help severely ill COVID patients: study https://news.vumc.org/2022/07/07/convalescent-plasma-doesnt-help-severely-ill-covid-patients-study/

Johns Hopkins Bloomberg School of Public Health 2022 An update on convalescent plasma for COVID-19. https://jhsph.edu/news/stories/2022/an-update-on-convalescent-plasma-for-covid-19.html

Lee W T *et al* 2021 Neutralizing antibody responses in COVID-19 convalescent sera *J. Infect. Dis.* **223** 47–55

Lindemann M *et al* 2021 Convalescent plasma treatment of critically ill intensive care COVID-19 patients *Transfusion* **61** 1394–403

Peng H *et al* 2020 A synergistic role of convalescent plasma and mesenchymal stem cells in the treatment of severely ill COVID-19 patients: a clinical case report *Stem Cell Res. Ther.* **11** 291

Piyush R, Rajarshi K, Khan R and Ray S 2020 Convalescent plasma therapy: a promising coronavirus disease 2019 treatment strategy *Open Biol.* **10** 200174

Rajendran K *et al* 2020 Convalescent plasma transfusion for the treatment of COVID-19: a systematic review *J. Med. Virol.* **92** 1475–83

Senefeld J W *et al* 2023 COVID-19 convalescent plasma for the treatment of immunocompromised patients: a systematic review and meta-analysis *JAMA Netw. Open* **6** e2250647

U.S. Food and Drug Administration 2023 Donate COVID-19 plasma https://fda.gov/emergency-preparedness-and-response/coronavirus-disease-2019-covid-19/donate-covid-19-plasma

U.S. Food and Drug Administration 2023 Investigational COVID-19 convalescent plasma https://fda.gov/regulatory-information/search-fda-guidance-documents/investigational-covid-19-convalescent-plasma (accessed 2 May 2023)

Weiqian D, Haihui G and Sha H 2020 Potential benefits, mechanisms, and uncertainties of convalescent plasma therapy for COVID-19 *Blood Sci.* **2** 71–5

Chapter 12

RNAi in viral control and diagnostics

Arvind K Singh Chandel, Bhakti Tanna, Amisha Parmar, Gopal Patel and Neeraj S Thakur

This chapter explores the potential of RNA interference (RNAi) in the treatment and diagnosis of viral diseases. It discusses the mechanisms of RNAi, including siRNA and miRNA, and their applications in inhibiting viral replication and disrupting essential viral proteins. The chapter highlights successful case studies and clinical trials of RNAi-based therapies against various viruses, including respiratory syncytial virus (RSV), influenza, and Hepatitis B virus (HBV). It also examines the advantages of RNAi in diagnostic approaches, comparing it with traditional methods and addressing the challenges posed by rapidly evolving viruses. The chapter further delves into the challenges and limitations of RNAi therapeutics, such as off-target effects and delivery issues, while also discussing future prospects and potential breakthroughs in the field. Finally, it provides an overview of the evolving landscape of viral disease treatment and diagnostics, emphasizing the integration of RNAi with other advanced technologies like next-generation sequencing (NGS) and digital polymerase chain reaction (PCR). Overall, the chapter presents RNAi as a promising frontier in virology, with significant potential to revolutionize both treatment and diagnostic strategies for viral infections.

12.1 Introduction

The fight to develop novel treatments is never-ending in the hopes of conducting safe, effective clinical trials that preserve therapeutic efficacy [1]. Traditionally, most medications are tiny compounds with protein-binding capabilities that frequently have harmful side effects. On the other hand, RNA treatments hold the potential to specifically target the individual nucleic acids implicated in a given disease, exhibiting enhanced potency, reduced toxicity, and increased specificity. With hereditary illnesses, when targeting the RNA rather than the protein is more favorable, this could be very effective [2]. Up until the advent of monoclonal antibody therapy, small-molecule medications were thought to be the panacea for all

doi:10.1088/978-0-7503-4987-1ch12

illnesses. Although monoclonal antibody therapy has shown promise in treating a wide range of illnesses, tissue penetration, production, and purification issues persist. In cases where existing medication technology is ineffective, RNAi treatments offer an alternate course of treatment. Furthermore, because of mutational escape, viral disease treatments are soon outdated. Since RNAi techniques are being developed to meet both demands, they could be the next big thing to change the pharmaceutical industry [1].

Cells employ RNAi, a naturally occurring mechanism, to control gene expression and stop genes from being translated into proteins. Furthermore, as a defense mechanism against invading nucleic acids from bacteria and viruses, RNAi is employed in cells' innate immunological response [2]. The process of silencing genes at the mRNA level under the guidance of tiny complementary non-coding RNA species is known as RNAi [3].

Three important factors to examine are delivery, efficacy, and toxicity. In addition to any harmful effects brought on by the delivery technique, RNAi therapeutic toxicity can also result from incorrect target recognition or immunogenic effects from exogenously delivered RNA. Poor annealing of the guide strand to the target mRNA or the choice of the passenger strand by RNA-induced silencing complex (RISC) instead of the guide strand causes improper target identification. Asymmetrical siRNAs can be used to bias the selection of the guide strand, as can chemically modifying the ends of the molecule to reduce thermodynamic stability at the guide strand's 5′end. This boosts efficacy and decreases toxicity from off-target effects. Chemical alterations limit the activation of the immune system by activating Toll-like receptors, such as those made possible by substituting 2-O-methyl pyrimidines for pyrimidines. Many delivery mechanisms, such as liposomes, expose RNA to Toll-like receptors, RIG-I, PKR, and other inflammatory pathways that activate innate immunity, frequently resulting in delivery-induced toxicity. This problem is resolved by either utilizing different delivery techniques or chemically altering the RNA [1].

The clinical trials for RNAi are going well. RNAi therapies are expected to receive FDA approval in the coming years, with multiple trials currently in Phase III research. Furthermore, new RNAi targets can be created and authorized more quickly using the authorized delivery technology. The potential for RNAi treatments is vast, with a wide range of illness targets, including cancer, viral diseases, cardiometabolic diseases, and orphan diseases. However, present delivery technology is limiting this promise. Future treatment approaches will face difficulties in delivering treatments to harder-to-reach locations and controlling the side effects of non-cell-type-specific therapies. Thus far, RNAi therapies appear to have a bright future ahead of them [1].

12.2 Mechanism of RNAi

12.2.1 Overview of the RNAi pathway

Small RNA duplexes, such as miRNA mimics, siRNAs, shRNAs, and dsiRNAs, are delivered using RNAi to provide therapeutic effects. The most upstream method, shRNA, needs to be processed nuclearly. The dsiRNA, on the other hand, needs to be processed by a dicer. The most direct routes, from delivery to RISC loading, are those taken by siRNA and miRNA mimics. The distinction is that siRNAs are 100% complementary to the target sequences, while miRNAs are not. This distinction influences the silencing process: siRNAs cause Argonaute 2-mediated degradation, while miRNAs cause translational repression (figure 12.1) [1].

siRNAs are one of the several kinds of RNAi mediators that help plants, fungi, and invertebrates develop antiviral immunity and are produced from the viral genome or its replicative intermediates [3]. Following more than ten years of clinical research, RNAi therapy is starting to fulfill its potential in several disease areas, such as cancer, viral infections, genetic abnormalities, and many more. By 1995, the first animal RNAi event was documented in *Caenorhabditis elegans*. They can also be

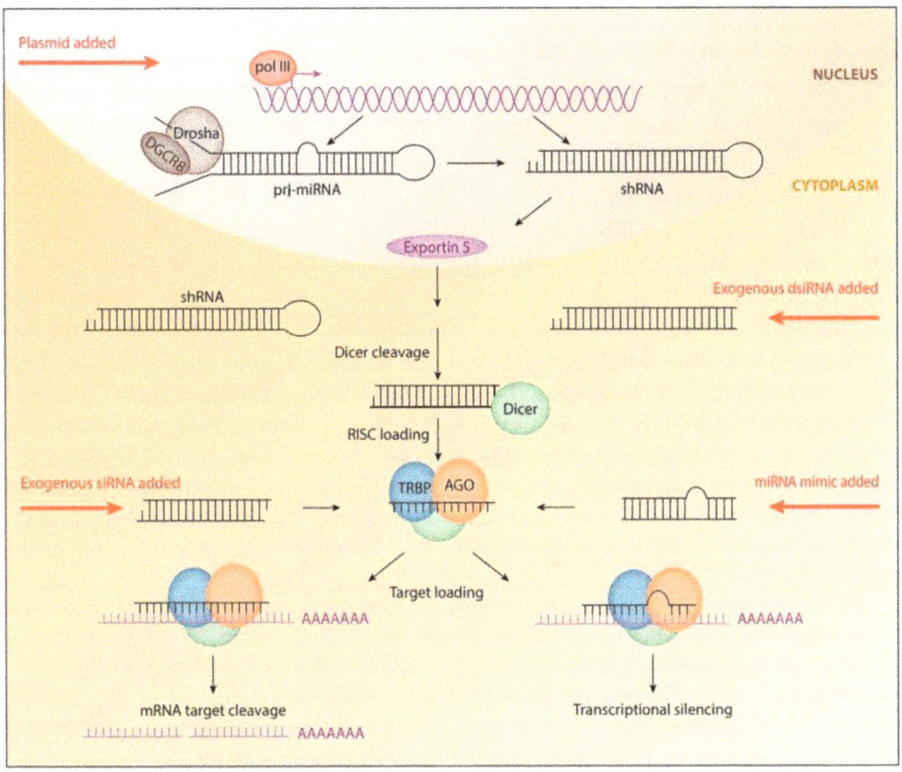

Figure 12.1. RNA interference (RNAi) pathway. One of four sites on the RNAi pathway is where RNAi medicines enter. The insertion of primary microRNA (pri-miRNA) or short hairpin RNA (shRNA) via plasmid is the most advanced of these processes. This needs to be processed nuclearly and then exported into the cytoplasm. Canonical short interfering RNA (siRNA) or microRNA (miRNA) are produced there via the processing of shRNA and Dicer substrate RNA (dsiRNA). The messenger RNA (mRNA) target is cleaved and degraded due to the shRNAs' binding to target regions through the RNA-induced silencing complex (RISC). If miRNA is supplied, RISC binds to the target sequence, causing translational repression and subsequent segregation into p-bodies for destruction. Here polymerase III (pol III). Adapted from reference [1].

employed therapeutically to knock down genes linked to disease. The majority of synthetic siRNAs have been made chemically up to this point [4].

The siRNAs are derived from viral double-stranded RNA (dsRNA), which is broken down into 19–27 base pair (bp) long molecules with a precisely complementary middle region and 2-nt overhangs on both 3′ end by the cytoplasmic RNAse III family enzyme Dicer during infection. A multiprotein RISC is formed by incorporating these siRNAs. After the separation of strands, the antisense strand directs the RISC to identify and cleave target RNA transcripts [3]. Researchers discovered that RISC, which is made up of Ago2, Dicer, and TRBP (the HIV-1 TAR RNA-binding protein), is necessary for RNAi events. Ago2 and the Dicer complex are recruited by TRBP, forming a ternary complex that triggers RNAi activities. siRNAs made synthetically are an essential tool for studying the function of genes in eukaryotic cells [4, 5].

12.2.2 Key molecules involved: siRNA and miRNA

I. siRNA: Dicer transforms dsRNA—transcribed or intentionally introduced into siRNA, which is then fed into the RISC. The RISC component AGO2 cleaves the siRNA's passenger strand. The active RISC is subsequently directed to the target mRNA by the guide strand. The cleavage of mRNA occurs when the guide strand of siRNA fully complements the target mRNA.

II. miRNA: RNA polymerase II in the nucleus carries out the transcription of the miRNA gene to produce pr-miRNA, which Drosha cleaves to produce pre-miRNA. Exportin 5 carries the pre-miRNA to the cytoplasm, where Dicer converts it into miRNA. The miRNA is inserted into the RISC, where the passenger strand is eliminated. Then, by partially complementary binding, the miRISC is directed to the target mRNA by the remaining guide strand. By means of translational repression, degradation, or cleavage, the target mRNA is inhibited. The difference between siRNA and miRNA listed in table 12.1.

Table 12.1. Difference between siRNA and miRNA.

	SiRNA	miRNA
Before Dicer processing	RNA that is double-stranded and has between 30 and more nucleotides	Precursor miRNA, also known as pre-miRNA, is a chain of 70–100 nucleotides with a hairpin structure with mismatches strewn throughout.
Complementary	Perfectly matched to mRNA	Partially complementary to mRNA, usually focusing on the mRNA's 3′ untranslated region
Structure	RNA duplex of 21–23 nucleotides with a 3′ overhang of two nucleotides	RNA duplex of 19–25 nucleotides with a 3′ overhang of two nucleotides
mRNA target	One	Multiple

12.3 RNAi applications in viral disease

12.3.1 Inhibition of viral replication

12.3.1.1 Targeting viral RNA

By targeting and degrading viral RNA molecules or inhibiting their translation, RNAi can effectively suppress virus replication within the host cell. This mechanism is particularly effective against RNA viruses, as their genomes and replication intermediates are composed of RNA molecules that can be targeted by the RNAi machinery [3, 6].

RNAi is a natural cellular mechanism that can inhibit virus replication by targeting and degrading viral RNA molecules. Mechanistically, viruses, during their replication cycle, produce dsRNA molecules or dsRNA intermediates. These dsRNA molecules are recognized as foreign by the host cell's RNAi machinery. The dsRNA molecules are cleaved by an enzyme called Dicer into small fragments called siRNAs, typically 20–25 nucleotides long. Further, the siRNAs are incorporated into a multiprotein complex called RISC. One strand of the siRNA called the guide strand, remains associated with the RISC, while the other strand, called the passenger strand, is degraded. Then the RISC, guided by the siRNA sequence, recognizes and binds to complementary viral RNA sequences present in the cell. Finally, the RISC can either cleave and degrade the target viral RNA molecules or prevent their translation into proteins, effectively silencing the expression of viral genes.

12.3.1.2 Disruption of essential viral proteins

The ability of RNAi to specifically target and disrupt the expression of essential viral proteins make it a powerful tool for antiviral research and potential therapeutic applications. By selectively silencing critical viral proteins, RNAi can impair virus replication and potentially mitigate viral infections or diseases [3, 6].

RNAi can be involved in the disruption of essential viral proteins through the targeted degradation or translational repression of viral mRNA transcripts encoding these proteins. The identification of essential proteins for virus virus's replication cycle or pathogenesis is a critical step. These proteins can be involved in various processes, such as viral entry, genome replication, protein synthesis, assembly, or release of new viral particles. After, identifying the specific viral protein, small siRNAs or shRNAs that are complementary to the mRNA sequences encoding these proteins are designed. The designed siRNAs or shRNAs are then introduced into the host cells using various delivery methods, such as transfection, viral vectors, or nanoparticle-based delivery systems. Within the host cells, the siRNAs or shRNAs are recognized by the RNAi machinery and incorporated into the RISC. The RISC, guided by the siRNA or shRNA sequence, binds to the complementary viral mRNA transcripts encoding the essential proteins. This binding leads to either the cleavage and degradation of the viral mRNA or the inhibition of its translation into protein. By degrading or preventing the translation of viral mRNA transcripts, RNAi effectively reduces or eliminates the expression of essential viral proteins. This disruption can interfere with various stages of the viral replication cycle, ultimately inhibiting virus propagation within the host cells.

12.3.2 Specific examples of successful RNAi applications against viral diseases

12.3.2.1 Case studies and clinical trials

RNAi has been explored as a potential therapeutic approach to prevent viral infections, and several case studies have been conducted to evaluate its efficacy. Here are some notable case studies on the use of RNAi to prevent viral infections:

Respiratory syncytial virus (RSV): A clinical trial evaluated the safety and efficacy of ALN-RSV01, an RNAi-based therapeutic targeting the RSV nucleocapsid gene [7]. The study involved healthy adults challenged with RSV and demonstrated that ALN-RSV01 significantly reduced viral load and symptom severity compared to placebo when administered prophylactically. The study provided evidence that RNAi-based therapies can prevent RSV infection in humans. Further, ALN-RSV01 was also found safe in lung transplant (LTX) recipients infected with RSV [8].]

Influenza virus: A preclinical study in mice evaluated the prophylactic and therapeutic efficacy of siRNAs targeting the influenza virus nucleoprotein (NP) gene [9]. Intranasal administration of NP-specific siRNAs before or after the influenza virus challenge significantly reduced viral titers in the lungs and protected mice from lethal infection. The study suggested that RNAi-based therapies could be effective in preventing or treating influenza virus infections.

Hepatitis B virus (HBV): The clinical trials evaluated the safety and efficacy of VIR-2218, an RNAi-based therapy targeting the HBV X protein. The studies involved patients with chronic HBV infection and demonstrated that VIR-2218 led to significant reductions in HBV surface antigen levels, suggesting its potential to prevent HBV replication and spread [10]. It also showed favorable pharmacokinetics in healthy volunteers supportive of subcutaneous dosing and continued development in patients with chronic HBV infection [11].

Coronaviruses (CoVs): SARS-CoV and SARS-CoV-2 are severe respiratory viruses that can cause life-threatening complications like viral pneumonia and acute respiratory distress syndrome (ARDS). The current SARS-CoV-2 pandemic has renewed interest in developing RNAi therapeutics for coronavirus treatment. One such RNAi therapeutic, using combined siRNAs (siSC2 and siSC5) targeting the Spike protein and ORF1b (NSP12) regions of SARS-CoV, progressed to *in vivo* macaque studies and demonstrated significant virus suppression [12].

Ebola virus: A preclinical study in non-human primates evaluated the efficacy of siRNAs targeting the Ebola virus L polymerase gene [13]. Prophylactic treatment with siRNAs prior to Ebola virus challenge provided complete protection against lethal infection in the study animals. The study highlighted the potential of RNAi-based therapies for preventing Ebola virus infections.

Human immunodeficiency virus (HIV): A preclinical study in humanized mice evaluated the efficacy of a combinatorial RNAi approach targeting multiple HIV genes [14, 15]. Prophylactic treatment with the combined siRNAs prior to HIV challenge significantly reduced viral load and protect mice from infection. The study suggested that RNAi-based therapies could be effective in preventing HIV infection.

These case studies demonstrate the potential of RNAi-based therapeutics in preventing viral infections by targeting specific viral genes and inhibiting viral replication. While further research and clinical trials are necessary, these studies provide promising evidence for the potential of RNAi as a preventive strategy against various viral diseases.

12.3.2.2 Challenges and advancements

The development of RNAi-based antiviral therapeutics has shown promising potential, but there are several challenges that need to be addressed for their successful clinical application. Overcoming these challenges will require advancements in various aspects of RNAi technology and delivery strategies. Here are some key challenges and advancements required [16–19]:

Delivery and cellular uptake: Efficient delivery of siRNAs or shRNAs to the target cells and tissues is a major hurdle, as these molecules are prone to degradation and poor cellular uptake. Development of effective delivery systems, such as nanoparticles, lipid-based carriers, or viral vectors, that can protect the RNAi molecules, facilitate cellular uptake and target specific cell types or tissues.

Off-target effects and specificity: RNAi molecules can potentially interact with and silence unintended targets, leading to off-target effects and potential toxicity. Improved design algorithms and screening methods to ensure high specificity and minimization of off-target effects, as well as chemical modifications to enhance stability and reduce immune stimulation.

Viral resistance and escape mechanisms: Viruses can evolve mechanisms to counteract or escape RNAi-based therapies, such as mutating the target sequences or expressing viral suppressors of RNAi. Development of strategies to target multiple viral genes simultaneously, use of pooled or combinatorial RNAi molecules, and identification of highly conserved viral targets less prone to mutations.

Effective dosing and duration of action: Determining the optimal dosing regimen and achieving sustained therapeutic levels of RNAi molecules in target tissues can be challenging due to their relatively short half-life and potential for saturation of the RNAi machinery. Development of formulations or delivery systems that can provide controlled and sustained release of RNAi molecules, as well as exploration of strategies to enhance the stability and persistence of RNAi molecules *in vivo*.

Preclinical and clinical development: Translating promising preclinical results into successful clinical trials and obtaining regulatory approval for RNAi-based antiviral therapeutics can be complex and challenging. Comprehensive preclinical studies to assess safety, efficacy, and pharmacokinetics, as well as well-designed clinical trials to evaluate the therapeutic potential, dosing, and potential side effects in various patient populations.

Manufacturing and scalability: Large-scale production of RNAi molecules with consistent quality and purity can be challenging and costly. Optimization of manufacturing processes, development of cost-effective and scalable production methods, and establishment of quality control and regulatory standards for RNAi-based therapeutics.

12.4 RNAi in diagnostics

12.4.1 Detection of viral RNA using RNAi-based assays

In virology research and diagnostics, the detection of viral RNA using RNA interference (RNAi)-based assays could be an effective technique. RNAi is a natural practice in which small RNA molecules reduce gene expression or translation, efficiently silencing specific genes [16]. Here's an overview of how RNAi can be utilized for viral RNA detection:

12.4.1.1 Principle and designing of RNAi

RNA interference involves the use of siRNAs (small interfering RNAs) or miRNAs (microRNAs) that bind to complementary RNA sequences, causing it to degrade or inhibit translation. This mechanism can be used to target viral RNA for detection and quantification as follows [17].

siRNA design and vector construction: Specific siRNAs are designed to target sequences in viral RNA. SiRNAs should be carefully selected to ensure that they complement the viral genome and have minimal off-target effects. siRNAs can be cloned into plasmid vectors that express short hairy membrane RNA (SiRNA) to receptor cells, resulting in siRNA production in transcription.

Transfection and stabilization: First host cells (e.g., HEK293, HeLa) could be transfected with the synthetic siRNAs or constructed plasmids. Then stable cell lines can be developed to express the RNAi constructs, providing a consistent platform for viral RNA detection.

12.4.1.2 Assays

RT-qPCR: RT-qPCR (reverse transcription quantitative PCR) can be used to determine the levels of viral RNA. A decrease in viral RNA levels with RNAi shows successful silencing. **Northern blotting:** This technique can be used to imagine the viral RNA directly. The intensity of viral RNA can be measured comparative to a control to assess the efficiency of RNAi. This can be done by measuring the fold change in viral RNA levels. These results could be confirmed using some other techniques, like assessing viral replication or quantifying viral protein levels. In virology research and clinical diagnostics RNAi-based assays for detecting viral RNA recommend a potent tool. Researchers can precisely measure viral infections and investigate therapeutic avenues though designing specific siRNAs and utilizing susceptible detection methods [18].

12.4.2 Advantages of RNAi in diagnostic approaches

In diagnostic approaches for viral infections and other diseases RNA interference (RNAi) provide numerous advantages. Some key benefits are mentioned here [19].

12.4.2.1 High specificity and sensitivity
RNAi could be designed to particular target and humiliate viral RNA sequences, reducing off-target effects and increased the specificity of the assay. This elevated specificity helps decrease false positives and negatives, leading to further trustworthy diagnostic results. **Amplification of signal** RNAi methods can magnify the silencing effect, allowing for the exposure of low levels of viral RNA that can be missed by conventional techniques. Higher sensitivity makes RNAi predominantly valuable for detecting infections in their initial stages.

12.4.2.2 Rapid and cost-effective detection
RNAi-based diagnostics can give rapid results, which is significant for timely diagnosis and treatment decisions, particularly in acute viral infections. **Adaptability:** RNAi can be incorporated into a variety of investigative platforms, such as microarrays, RT-qPCR, or even point-of-care tests, increasing its utility across different settings. **Multiplexing potential:** RNAi assays can be designed to concurrently goal different pathogens or multiple viral strains, allowing for widespread diagnostics. **Low input needs:** RNAi-based assays often work with tiny amounts of biological samples, making them suitable for those samples that are difficult to obtain or inadequate.

RNAi-based diagnostic approaches influence the sensitivity and specificity of RNA interference to advancement in the detection of viral RNA and additional nucleic acids. These advantages could lead to rapid, more precise diagnostics, eventually enhancing patient outcomes and contributing to better public health responses to viral outbreaks.

12.4.3 Comparison with traditional diagnostic methods

Numerous differences and advantages come out, when comparing RNA interference (RNAi) in diagnostics with traditional diagnostic methods [18].

12.4.3.1 Specificity and sensitivity
RNAi is highly specific; it can be designed to target unique viral or pathogen sequences, reducing cross-reactivity with non-target organisms or host RNA. While traditional methods like antigen assays or PCR may have less specificity, particularly if antibodies or primers are not completely matched to the target, leading to potential false positives. RNAi improved sensitivity due to the capability to sense and degrade even less amount of viral RNA, making it appropriate for before time detection of infections. Whereas traditional methods like RT-PCR are sensitive, they may not sense extremely low viral loads as effectively, mainly if the virus RNA is degraded or fragmented [18].

12.4.3.2 Quantitative capability and speed of results

RNAi allows for precise quantification of viral RNA levels, offering insights into infection severity and progression. In traditional methods quantitative PCR methods can also measure viral loads but may lack the granularity that RNAi approaches can provide, particularly if looking for dynamic changes in RNA levels. RNAi can provide rapid results, particularly with optimized assays or point-of-care applications, enabling timely clinical decisions. However, in traditional techniques like culture-based methods can take long time (days to weeks) although PCR-based techniques usually give results within hours, but may not be identical with the speed of well-optimized RNAi assays [18].

12.4.3.3 Complexity and cost-effectiveness

RNAi may require more difficult design and confirmation of siRNAs, along with dedicated knowledge for implementation, even though this is becoming more comprehensible with advancements. While techniques like PCR or ELISA (enzyme-linked immunosorbent assays) or are normally well-established, with widespread protocols and kits available, making them easier for regular use. The initial arrangement (designing, validating siRNAs, and developing the assay) can be expensive, but the potential for before time detection and modified treatment may lead to overall savings in RNAi. While tradition methods are frequently extra cost-effective in terms of availability of reagent and well-known workflows, particularly for broadly used tests like rapid antigen tests or PCR [18].

12.4.3.4 Adaptability to emerging pathogens

RNAi can be speedily adapted to target strains by designing highly specific siRNAs, providing a flexible response to emerging infectious diseases. Nevertheless, traditional techniques often require the development of new primers or antibodies for different strains which can be a time-taking process. RNAi-based treatment and diagnosis may provide numerous advantages over traditional processes, mainly in terms of sensitivity, adaptability and specificity to new pathogens. However, traditional methods remain precious due to their widespread availability and established protocols. The selection between traditional techniques and RNAi will depend on the specific circumstance, including available resources, the type of infection, and time required for turnaround. As RNAi technologies continue to progress, their incorporation into regular diagnostics could improve the correctness and rapidity of viral recognition appreciably [18].

12.4.4 Addressing challenges of rapidly evolving viruses

Due to the interconnected nature of the world, the threat of rapidly evolving viruses is unavoidable. The emerging and re-emerging viruses are introduced to naïve people via vectors, such as mosquitoes, or due to spillovers from animals to humans. Several factors contribute to the emergence of new viruses, such as changes in land use, urbanization, and ecological disruption—which in turn disrupts delicate balance between humans and wildlife. For instance, repeated emergence of novel

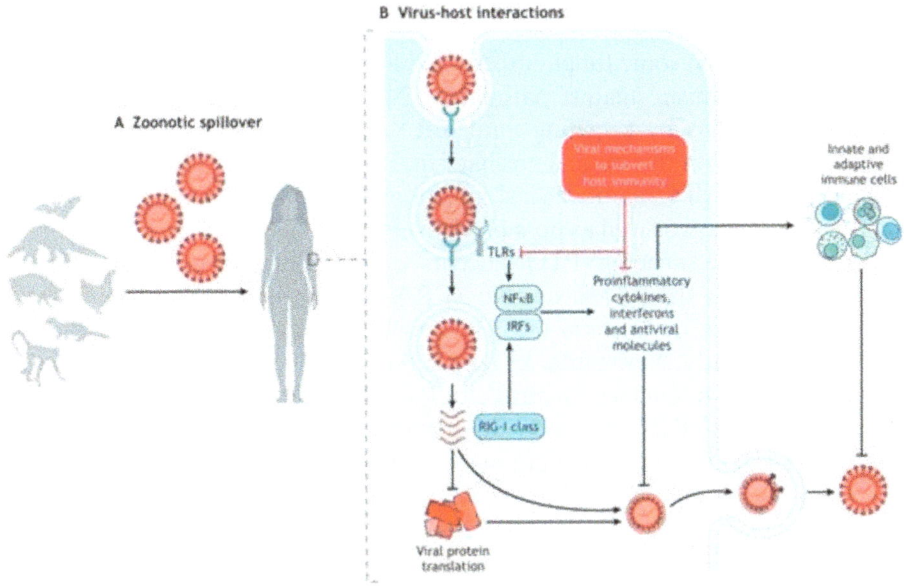

Figure 12.2. Emerging and re-emerging viruses: a challenge on global health. In combating the threat of emerging and re-emerging viruses, in part (A) zoonotic spillovers from animals to humans and (B) virus–host interactions are factors to be considered. (The intracellular replication of an RNA virus is shown here in red. Host TLRs and RIG-I class receptors detect the intracellular virus and activate transcription factors NFκB and IRFs, which initiate the production of proinflammatory cytokines, interferons and antiviral molecules. This directly inhibits viral replication and recruits innate and adaptive immune cells to help clear the viral infection. Consequently, viruses have developed mechanisms to subvert these host immune responses. IRF, interferon response factor; NFκB, nuclear factor-κB; RIG-I, retinoic acid-inducible gene I; TLR, Toll-like receptor.). Adapted from reference [21]. Copyright (2023) Published by The Company of Biologists Ltd. CC BY 4.0.

coronaviruses in the past two decades resulting in widespread outbreaks in human populations has been linked to spillovers from bats to humans via intermediary animals [20]. Another reason could be climate change which alters the geographic locality of virus-carrying vectors leading to the emergence of viruses in new regions (figure 12.2) [21].

Our limited knowledge and unpredictability of viral attacks are key challenges associated with emerging and re-emerging viruses. In this situation, a constant surveillance of human and animal populations, research and development and a robust global public health infrastructure are critical. In-depth knowledge of viral genomics, evolution, ecology and host interactions of these viruses will help understand virus origins, potential transmission dynamics, and treatment strategies [21]. Vaccines are still widely accepted approach in combating viral infections, but there are some limitations associated with them, too. For instance, influenza virus (highly evolving), which necessitates annual vaccine updates. In other cases, such as dengue, developing an effective vaccine has proved challenging on account of the complex interactions of the pathogen with the immune system [22]. Moreover, antiviral therapeutics has shown potential in combating many deadly virus infections [23].

12.4.5 Customization of RNAi for novel viral strains

In plants as well as in some fungi, insects, and lower eukaryotes, RNAi is a primary self defence mechanism against pathogens [24]. RNAi inhibits the expression of crucial viral proteins by targeting viral mRNA for degradation through cellular enzymes [6]. Based on this critical mechanism, RNAi is now considered a promising therapeutic approach to combat viral infections in humans. Figure 12.1 represents basic RNAi pathways as well as possible delivery approaches. Classic RNAi or post-transcriptional gene silencing (PTGS) occurs via RISC machinery initiating specific mRNA cleavage in the cytoplasm. Novel RNAi or transcriptional gene silencing (TGS) occurs in the nucleus via the RITS complex initiating repressive epigenetic modifications. Ago1, Argonaute 1; Ago2, Argonaute 2; shRNA, short hairpin RNA; RISC, RNA-induced silencing complex; RITS, RNA-induced transcriptional silencing complex; TRBP, transactivating response (TAR) RNA-binding protein; TNRC6, trinucleotide repeat containing 6 protein (figure 12.3) [25].

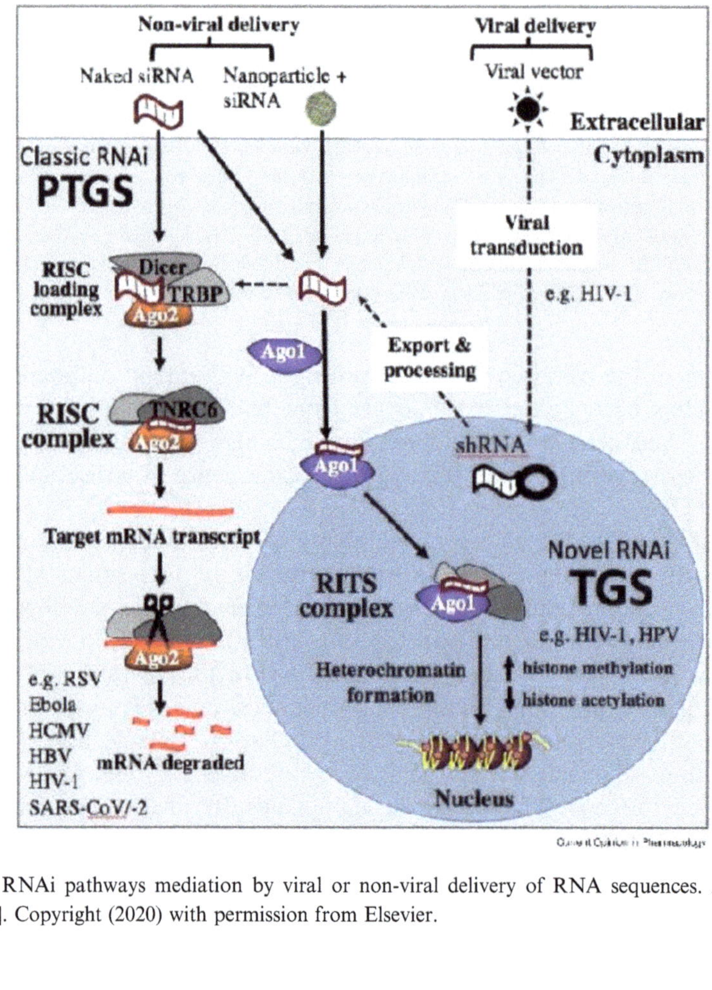

Figure 12.3. RNAi pathways mediation by viral or non-viral delivery of RNA sequences. Adapted from reference [25]. Copyright (2020) with permission from Elsevier.

12.4.6 Prospects and potential breakthroughs

Although there are currently no approved RNAi-based antiviral therapeutics, ever since the discovery of the potentially natural defense mechanisms of RNAi, there has been progressive advancement. The journey of RNAi therapeutic began with the approval of the first RNAi therapeutic, patisiran (Onpattro, Alnylam Pharmaceuticals), a liver-targeting siRNA. Patisiran was approved by the US Food and Drug Administration (FDA) in August 2018 for the treatment of hereditary transthyretin amyloidosis (hATTR) [26]. Later in November 2019, a second RNAi therapeutic-givosiran (Givlaari, Alnylam) was approved to treat a rare genetic condition called acute hepatic porphyria [27]. Further, RNAi-based therapeutic list expanded by the approval of lumasiran (Oxlumo, 2020) [28], and inclisiran (Leqvio, 2021) [29]. Aside from this, many other RNAi therapeutic candidates are currently in clinical trials. Altogether, the ongoing success of approved RNAi therapeutics in recent years exhibits the enormous potential for its therapeutic use in all human diseases, including present and emerging virus infections.

Moreover, there is always a challenge for RNA viruses since they frequently mutate their genomic sequence to evade host immune responses. For example, human immunodeficiency virus type 1 (HIV-1) and hepatitis C virus (HCV) have high mutation rates. Early RNAi therapeutics relied on a single siRNA sequence to induce effective gene silencing. Still, more recent RNAi therapies overcome this problem by using multiple siRNA sequences in a process called multiplexing [25]. Another approach is the use of novel RNAi that acts via the nuclear, transcriptional gene silencing pathway to target the virus promoter, which, in theory, has less opportunity for effective mutations to arise, as the driver of gene expression is silenced upstream of the error-prone transcription process [30].

12.5 Challenges and limitations

Despite RNAi being a promising therapeutic in theory for many diseases, some noteworthy limitations need to be overcome for translational efforts, which include the following.

12.5.1 Off-target effects and unintended consequences

Poor construction of siRNAs can alter the expression profiles of several non-targets, therefore, unanticipated phenotypes, and complicate the interpretation of the therapeutic benefits of siRNAs. The off-target effects associated with siRNA delivery fall into three broad categories: siRNA-induced sequence-dependent regulation of unintended transcripts through partial sequence complementarity to their 3′ UTRs (microRNA-like off-target effects); an inflammatory response through activation of Toll-like receptors triggered by siRNAs and their delivery vehicles (such as cationic lipids); and widespread impact on microRNA processing and function through saturation of the endogenous RNAi machinery by exogenous siRNAs [31].

Jackson *et al* emphasized that using siRNA sequences that partially match other transcripts can unintentionally silence those transcripts in addition to the targeted gene, leading to ambiguous results and potential harm [32]. Off-target effects of siRNA can be avoided by performing homology and specificity analyses [33]. In addition, Elmén *et al* demonstrated that a locked nucleic acid, a synthetic high-affinity RNA-like analog, was compatible with the intracellular siRNA machinery and mitigated undesired, sequence-related off-target effects [34]. Moreover, this group demonstrated that locked nucleic acid-modified siRNAs targeting the SARS-CoV-1 genome exhibited higher efficiency than unmodified siRNAs. Because the antisense strand in siRNA guides the RISC, precise sequence complementarity of this strand is pivotal for on-target RNAi and minimized off-target effects [35]. Employing cutting-edge technological tools has significantly increased siRNA recognition by the RISC and reduced off-target effects. Any clear matches between target and whole-genome sequences in the host cell should be carefully analyzed to rule out the possibility of off-target silencing [36].

12.5.2 Delivery challenges for RNAi-based therapeutics

Delivery of naked RNAi therapeutic is prone to enzymatic cleavage and rapid clearance through liver accumulation and renal filtration in the system [37]. Therefore, safe delivery is crucial to attain the maximum therapeutic benefit of RNAi. Viral vector-based delivery approaches are common for RNAi delivery but lack efficiency. For example, lentivirus vector-based formulations have reduced safety profiles and achieved modest outcomes *in vivo* [25]. Therefore, multiple ways are considered to improve siRNA delivery outcomes, including avoiding target effects and enhancing efficacy: (a) siRNA can be chemically modified, conjugated to a macromolecule, or formulated within a nanoparticle. These non-viral vector-based formulations encapsulate, complex, or conjugate with siRNA to improve their biodistribution and facilitate cell entry and endosomal escape, leading to enhanced gene silencing. (b) Administration routes for the delivery of nanoparticle formulation with RNAi cargo (figure 12.4).

Chemical-based modified formulations have indeed improved the delivery of RNAi, but superior delivery and highly efficient cell transfection through viral vectors are attractive for RNAi therapy. Therefore, further investigations in this direction are ongoing. Interestingly, viral vectors manufacture the drug in the host target cell while keeping delivery aside. Moreover, self-replicating RNA viruses directly amplify RNA in the cytoplasm, generating enhanced gene silencing efficacy [38]. Self-replicating RNA virus vectors can be delivered as naked or encapsulated RNA and DNA plasmids due to their RNA amplification at significantly lower concentrations than synthetic mRNAs or conventional DNA plasmids. Along with all these advantages, ensuring safety related to viral vector-based formulations is essential. Today, several studies have confirmed the feasibility of RNAi-based gene silencing and inhibition of replication of pathogenic viruses by viral vectors in various animal models [39]. To obtain the maximum efficacy and safety of RNAi therapeutics, studies are carried out

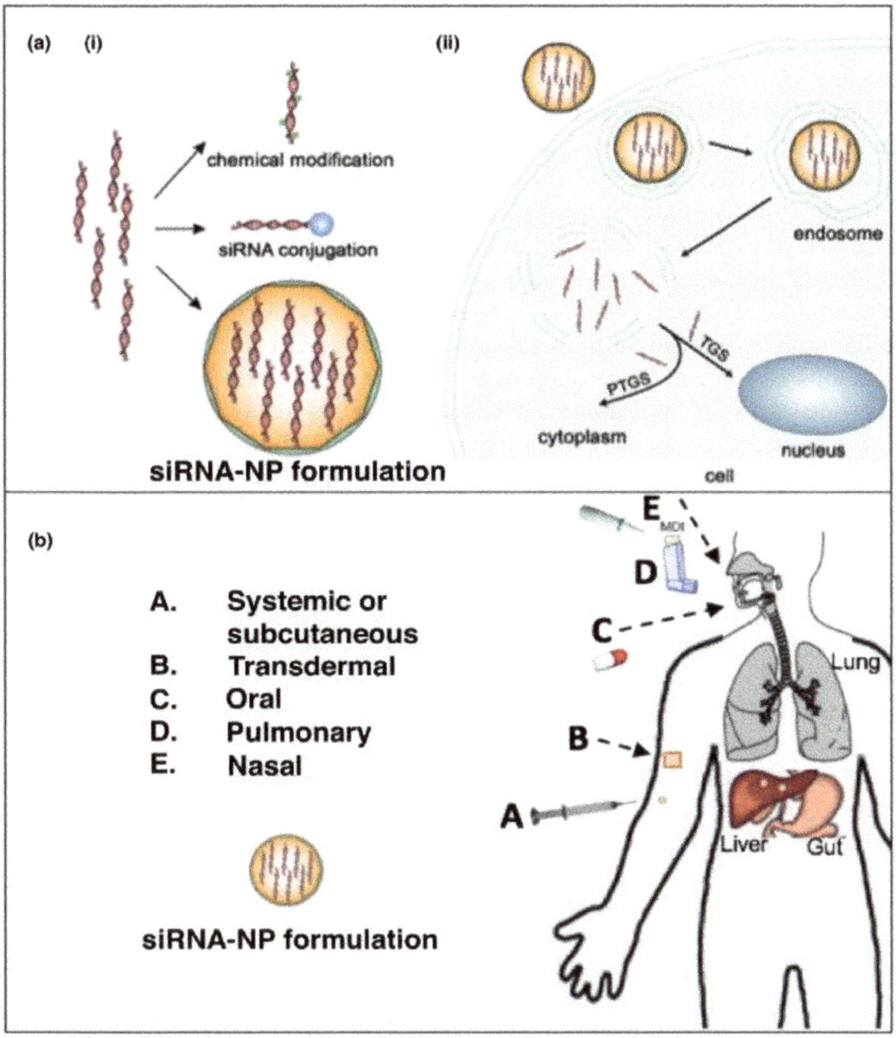

Figure 12.4. RNA therapeutics and administration routes for nanoparticle delivery of RNAi cargo. Adapted from reference [25]. Copyright (2020) with permission from Elsevier.

with viral vector delivery and far more studies with naked RNAi molecules, DNA-based vectors or liposome/polymer-based nanoparticles [39].

12.6 Future prospective of viral disease treatment and cure

In recent years, technological advancements have revolutionized how we detect and count virus genomes in clinical samples. This has not only helped identify susceptibility to certain antiviral medications but has also allowed us to pinpoint specific molecular sequences linked to the severity of infections. Moreover, these technologies help identify viral and host-related factors that influence whether infections are resolved or become chronic. Consequently, diagnostic virology laboratories have become indispensable for patient care, playing a vital role in managing various illnesses. This shift in approach has rendered some traditional infectious disease diagnostic methods obsolete, as they were primarily focused on detecting entire viruses or specific viral components in specimens [40].

Over the past 30 years, the clinical virology laboratory has undergone significant transformations, especially in directly diagnosing viral infections. Previously, the primary method for direct diagnosis involved detecting virus particles or their components (such as viral antigens or nucleic acids) in clinical specimens [41]. This was typically done retrospectively by isolating viral pathogens in cell culture, which could take days or weeks to yield results. However, with the continuous advancements in diagnostic assays, virus culture has taken a backseat to a wide array of molecular techniques designed to swiftly detect the virus genome, measure its quantity, identify its genotype, and identify specific molecular patterns within the genome. Consequently, the importance of diagnostic virology has surged, leading to changes in laboratory operations, including shifts and operating hours, as well as a shift in clinical decision-making, which is now heavily reliant on laboratory findings. The expedited and accurate diagnosis facilitated by these methods has resulted in improved patient management, personalized antiviral therapies, and cost savings due to reduced unnecessary drug use, quicker recovery, and shorter hospital stays. It's important to note that no single diagnostic approach, whether molecular detection, antigen identification, or virus isolation, can meet all the needs of virology laboratories, as each method has its limitations and applicability depending on the clinical scenario and virus type. Virologists are mindful of these constraints and choose the method that best suits the specific clinical situation, yielding the most valuable results. This shift has led to a change in the concept of the reference standard, which is now seen as an overarching approach encompassing a variety of tests tailored to the specific diagnostic context [42–44].

Novel and repurposed technologies are crucial in enhancing the detection, quantification, and sequencing of virus genomes in clinical specimens. Since viruses exist in minuscule quantities within clinical samples, and their nucleic acids constitute only a tiny fraction of the total nucleic acids present, enrichment of virus genome molecules is necessary. Traditionally, this enrichment has been achieved through target-specific amplification utilizing PCR. For RNA viruses, this process is preceded by reverse transcription. Subsequently, DNA sequencing has been conducted using Sanger-based technology [45, 46].

Since its inception in 1987, PCR has become an indispensable tool for detecting virus genomes, provided their nucleotide sequences are known. Initially, PCR assays were primarily utilized to identify single virus species or closely related groups, offering diagnostic opportunities for viruses that exhibited antigenic diversity or could not grow in cell cultures, impeding traditional *in vitro* diagnostics. Despite its potential, PCR faced several limitations that hindered its integration into routine processes for many years [47–49].

The breakthrough came with the development of real-time quantitative PCR (qPCR), which revolutionized virus diagnosis by accurately quantifying the number of virus genome molecules, known as 'virus load,' in clinical specimens. qPCR swiftly emerged as the gold standard method for analyzing infection progression, disease evolution, and response to therapy across various viral infections. Recent advancements, including full automation, high-throughput analysis, shortened reaction times, reduced hands-on labor, standardization, and real-time monitoring for clinically significant viruses like HIV, hepatitis C (HCV), and hepatitis B (HBV), have overcome remaining barriers. Consequently, qPCR has firmly established itself as the primary technique in virus diagnosis.

During the early stages of PCR's development, numerous alternative methods emerged, some initially showed promise but eventually faded due to technical challenges, limited versatility, or inadequate company support. However, certain old technologies have resurfaced and found renewed relevance, exceptionally when outperforming qPCR. Transcription-mediated amplification, loop-mediated isothermal amplification, ligase chain reaction, rolling circle amplification, and others have carved out their niche or have become the foundation for various companies' product portfolios [50, 51].

The demand for technical enhancements has not only revitalized old methods but has also spurred the invention and repurposing of molecular technologies. A notable example of novel technology is digital PCR (dPCR). In droplet dPCR, the reaction occurs within water–oil emulsion droplets, enabling absolute quantification of the target template. Unlike qPCR, dPCR does not rely on an external curve for template quantification, unaffected by linearity range limitations. Additionally, dPCR offers precise quantitation even at meager template copy numbers and for virus variants with high sequence diversity. This capability is particularly significant for detecting drug-resistant variants, as dPCR can identify rare variants amidst numerous irrelevant ones. The ability to detect minute amounts of template enhances the prevention of drug-resistant variant emergence, allows for precise timing in therapy adjustments, facilitates accurate measurement of residual viremia in HIV patients, and overall improves patient management.

Among the new technologies vying for a place in the *in vitro* diagnostic market, NGS and microbial clustered regularly interspaced short palindromic repeats (CRISPR) are rapidly gaining traction. NGS enables the parallel sequencing of millions of DNA templates in a single reaction, offering the capability to sequence the entire genomes of hundreds of microbial samples rapidly and cost-effectively. In virology, NGS is pivotal in managing viral infections, identifying infection sources, analyzing host immune responses, and devising treatment strategies. NGS offers three main approaches for sequencing viral genetic material: amplification and sequencing of a specific target, metagenomic sequencing of all genetic material within a sample, and enrichment of virus genetic material followed by sequencing. Depending on the approach, NGS can be used for automated high-throughput workflows to identify drug-resistance mutations, target multiple viruses, or detect known and novel microbes [52–54].

Currently, the detection and characterization of low-abundance drug-resistance variants in HIV and HBV infections are among the most critical applications of NGS in clinical virology. While the clinical significance of detecting these previously undetectable variants remains uncertain, experience with resistance testing suggests a growing impact on routine clinical practice, particularly for patients with low virus levels and rare mutations.

Moreover, the widespread use of NGS across various biological samples has led to the discovery of numerous novel virus types and expanded the tropism of known viruses. NGS has challenged conventional beliefs by revealing higher variability in genetically stable viruses, demonstrating that many body sites previously thought to be sterile harbor their flora, and uncovering many virus elements in biological samples unrelated to disease and often outnumber pathogenic viruses. This realization has introduced the concept, initially met with skepticism or reluctance, that some viruses are commensal and not necessarily harmful, ultimately leading to the development of the virome concept—the viral component of the human microbiome, defined as the community of microorganisms inhabiting the human body.

The demand for molecular diagnostic tests is being driven by improvements in speed and accuracy, even in the face of declining disease prevalence. Specifically, the market for molecular diagnostics in infectious diseases has experienced rapid growth in recent years, outpacing the overall diagnostic market by 60%.

These tests comprise over 25% of the diagnostic market share worldwide. In the laboratory market, about one-third of total profits come from tests detecting infectious agents, focusing on influenza, papillomaviruses, and emerging viruses.

The growth in demand for molecular diagnostics is primarily fueled by emerging economies, which require affordable and straightforward assays due to changing demographics, global prosperity, advances in genetic pathogen evolution knowledge, personalized medicine, climate change, globalization, and travel. These factors have reshaped the geographic distribution of infectious diseases and therapies, resulting in two significant markets.

Firstly, wealthy countries demand cutting-edge assays to identify virus genetic traits associated with virulence and drug responsiveness and to identify host genes linked to resistance and resilience against pathogens, facilitating personalized medicine. Secondly, developing countries require simple, low-cost, and rapid assays. Although the profit margin in these regions may be low, the vast geographical area and potential market, along with the benefits for wealthy countries in controlling epidemics and rapidly spreading infections, are prompting many companies to focus their efforts on low-income countries.

Overall, the dynamic growth and evolving world market suggest that molecular diagnostics may lead to future eradication of infectious diseases. Understanding microbial interactions, particularly viruses, has evolved significantly in recent years. It's now recognized that viruses coexist with other microbes in the host and directly and indirectly interact with them, influencing each other's presence. For example, intestinal bacteria have been shown to promote the replication and transmission of enteric viruses, impacting specific aspects of host immunity. This phenomenon, known as transkingdom interaction, affects explicitly the host's response to viral infection and may explain variations in virus-associated pathogenesis between individuals.

Several key points should be considered regarding these interactions:

- Viruses present in human samples are not always associated with disease. Many viruses, collectively known as the virome, inhabit various human body regions without causing illness.
- Non-pathogenic viruses can lead to severe illness in healthy individuals under certain circumstances, such as transient immunosuppression, medical interventions, or the emergence of virus variants. The natural course of viral infections and associated diagnostic methods may vary depending on the host, virus, and other factors.
- Viruses interact functionally and genetically with the host and the microbiome. They can be regulated by different microorganisms and their products, establishing transkingdom communication.

While we are still in the early stages of understanding these microbial relationships, these findings represent a significant breakthrough in understanding the pathogenesis, immunity, and diagnosis of viral infections. For instance, torquetenovirus, a component of the human virome, is emerging as a valuable parameter for monitoring immune system efficiency in transplant recipients.

It's crucial to remember these considerations when using susceptible methods to detect minute amounts of viruses and when employing multiplex assays that may detect bystander microorganisms unrelated to the disease process. Careful interpretation of results is essential to avoid misinterpretation and ensure accurate diagnosis and treatment decisions [53, 54].

12.7 Conclusion

RNA interference (RNAi) has emerged as a promising frontier in treating and diagnosing viral diseases. As our understanding of RNAi mechanisms deepens, its potential applications expand, offering new avenues for combating established and emerging viral threats. RNAi-based approaches' high specificity and sensitivity present significant advantages over traditional methods, particularly in rapidly evolving viral landscapes. However, the path to widespread clinical application is not without challenges. Issues such as off-target effects, delivery obstacles, and the complexity of viral–host interactions remain active research and development areas. Despite these hurdles, the progress made in RNAi therapeutics, exemplified by recent FDA approvals in other disease areas, suggests a bright future for antiviral applications.

Parallel advancements in diagnostic technologies, including NGS and dPCR, are revolutionizing our ability to detect, quantify, and characterize viral infections with unprecedented precision. Combined with RNAi-based approaches, these tools reshape our understanding of the human virome and the complex interactions between viruses, hosts, and other microorganisms. As we move forward, integrating RNAi technologies with other cutting-edge approaches in virology promises to yield more effective, personalized strategies for managing viral infections. The ongoing research in this field not only advances our scientific knowledge but also holds the potential to significantly impact public health, particularly in the face of future pandemics and emerging viral threats.

Abbreviations

Ago1	Argonaute 1
Ago2	Argonaute 2
ARDS	Acute respiratory distress syndrome
bp	Base pair
CoVs	Coronaviruses
CRISPR	Clustered regularly interspaced short palindromic repeats
dPCR	Digital PCR
dsRNA	Double-stranded RNA
dsiRNA	Dicer substrate RNA
hATTR	Hereditary transthyretin amyloidosis
HBV	Hepatitis B virus
HCV	Hepatitis C virus
HIV	Human immunodeficiency virus
HIV-1	Human immunodeficiency virus type 1 IRF interferon response factor
LTX	Lung transplant
mRNA	Messenger RNA
miRNA	microRNA
NGS	Next-generation sequencing
NFκB	Nuclear factor-kappa B
NP	Nucleoprotein
Pri-miRNA	Primary microRNA
PTGS	Post-transcriptional gene silencing
qPCR	Quantitative PCR
RIG-I	Retinoic acid-inducible gene I
RISC	RNA-induced silencing complex
RITS	RNA-induced transcriptional silencing complex
RNAi	RNA interference
siRNA	Interfering RNA
shRNA	Short hairpin RNA
TAR	Transactivating response
TGS	Transcriptional gene silencing
TLR	Toll-like receptor
TNRC6	Trinucleotide repeat containing 6 protein
TRBP	Transactivating response RNA-binding protein

References

[1] Bobbin M L and Rossi J J 2016 RNA interference (RNAi)-based therapeutics: delivering on the promise? *Annu. Rev. Pharmacol. Toxicol.* **56** 103–22

[2] Chery J 2016 RNA therapeutics: RNAi and antisense mechanisms and clinical applications *Postdoc J.* **4** 2151

[3] Levanova A and Poranen M M 2018 RNA interference as a prospective tool for controlling human viral infections *Front. Microbiol.* **9** 409222

[4] Aneja K K, Dixit N and Kumar A 2020 Can RNAi be used as a weapon against COVID-19/SARSCoV-2? *Microbiol. Discov.* **8** 1

[5] Lam J K W, Chow M Y T, Zhang Y and Leung S W S 2015 siRNA versus miRNA as therapeutics for gene silencing *Mol. Ther. Nucleic Acids* **4** e252

[6] Tan F L and Yin J Q 2004 RNAi, a new therapeutic strategy against viral infection *Cell Res* **14** 460

[7] DeVincenzo J, Lambkin-Williams R, Wilkinson T, Cehelsky J, Nochur S, Walsh E, Meyers R, Gollob J and Vaishnaw A 2010 A randomized, double-blind, placebo-controlled study of an RNAi-based therapy directed against respiratory syncytial virus *Proc. Natl. Acad. Sci. USA* **107** 8800–5

[8] Zamora M R *et al* 2011 RNA interference therapy in lung transplant patients infected with respiratory syncytial virus *Am. J. Respir. Crit. Care Med.* **183** 531–8

[9] Tompkins S M, Lo C Y, Tumpey T M and Epstein S L 2004 Protection against lethal influenza virus challenge by RNA interference *in vivo Proc. Natl Acad. Sci. USA* **101** 8682–6

[10] Gane E *et al* 2023 Evaluation of RNAi therapeutics VIR-2218 and ALN-HBV for chronic hepatitis B: results from randomized clinical trials *J. Hepatol.* **79** 924–32

[11] Gupta S V, Fanget M C, MacLauchlin C, Clausen V A, Li J, Cloutier D, Shen L, Robbie G J and Mogalian E 2021 Clinical and preclinical single-dose pharmacokinetics of VIR-2218: an RNAi therapeutic targeting HBV infection *Drugs RD* **21** 455–65

[12] Donia A and Bokhari H 2021 RNA interference as a promising treatment against SARS-CoV-2 *Int. Microbiol.* **24** 123–4

[13] Geisbert T W *et al* 2010 Postexposure protection of non-human primates against a lethal Ebola virus challenge with RNA interference: a proof-of-concept study *Lancet* **375** 1896–905

[14] Spanevello F, Calistri A, Del Vecchio C, Mantelli B, Frasson C, Basso G, Palù G, Cavazzana M and Parolin C 2016 Development of lentiviral vectors simultaneously expressing multiple siRNAs against CCR5, VIF and TAT/REV Genes for an HIV-1 gene therapy approach *Mol. Ther. Nucleic Acids* **5** e312

[15] Bennett M S and Akkina R 2013 Gene therapy strategies for HIV/AIDS: preclinical modeling in humanized mice *Viruses* **5** 3119–41

[16] Traber G M and Yu A M 2023 Special section on non-coding RNAs in clinical practice: from biomarkers to therapeutic tools-minireview RNAi-based therapeutics and novel RNA bioengineering technologies *J. Pharmacol. Exp. Ther.* **384** 133–54

[17] Chinnappan M *et al* 2014 Key elements of the RNAi pathway are regulated by hepatitis B virus replication and HBx acts as a viral suppressor of RNA silencing *Biochem. J.* **462** 347–58

[18] Myhrvold C *et al* 2018 Field-deployable viral diagnostics using CRISPR-Cas13 *Science (80)* **360** 444–8

[19] Aagaard L and Rossi J J 2007 RNAi therapeutics: principles, prospects and challenges *Adv. Drug Deliv. Rev.* **59** 75–86

[20] Ruiz-Aravena M *et al* 2022 Ecology, evolution and spillover of coronaviruses from bats *Nat. Rev. Microbiol.* **20** 299–314

[21] Sanyal S 2023 Crossroads in virology: current challenges and future perspectives in the age of emerging viruses *Dis. Model. Mech.* **16** dmm050476

[22] van Leur S W, Heunis T, Munnur D and Sanyal S 2021 Pathogenesis and virulence of flavivirus infections *Virulence* **12** 2814–38

[23] Meganck R M and Baric R S 2021 Developing therapeutic approaches for twenty-first-century emerging infectious viral diseases *Nat. Med.* **27** 401–10
[24] Rosa C, Kuo Y W, Wuriyanghan H and Falk B W 2018 RNA interference mechanisms and applications in plant pathology *Annu. Rev. Phytopathol.* **56** 581–610
[25] Kelleher A D, Cortez-Jugo C, Cavalieri F, Qu Y, Glanville A R, Caruso F, Symonds G and Ahlenstiel C L 2020 RNAi therapeutics: an antiviral strategy for human infections *Curr. Opin. Pharmacol.* **54** 121–9
[26] Hoy S M 2018 Patisiran: first global approval *Drugs* **78** 1625–31
[27] Scott L J 2020 Givosiran: first approval *Drugs* **80** 335–9
[28] Scott L J and Keam S J 2021 Lumasiran: first approval *Drugs* **81** 277–82
[29] Lamb Y N 2021 Inclisiran: first approval *Drugs* **81** 389–95
[30] Suzuki K, Ahlenstiel C, Marks K and Kelleher A D 2015 Promoter targeting RNAs: unexpected contributors to the control of HIV-1 transcription *Mol. Ther. Nucleic Acids* **4** e222
[31] Jackson A L and Linsley P S 2010 Recognizing and avoiding siRNA off-target effects for target identification and therapeutic application *Nat. Rev. Drug Discov.* **9** 57–67
[32] Jackson A L *et al* 2006 Position-specific chemical modification of siRNAs reduces 'off-target' transcript silencing *RNA* **12** 1197–205
[33] Zhang Y, Almazi J G, Ong H X, Johansen M D, Ledger S, Traini D, Hansbro P M, Kelleher A D and Ahlenstiel C L 2022 Nanoparticle delivery platforms for RNAi therapeutics targeting COVID-19 disease in the respiratory tract *Int. J. Mol. Sci.* **23** 2408
[34] Elmén J *et al* 2005 Locked nucleic acid (LNA) mediated improvements in siRNA stability and functionality *Nucleic Acids Res.* **33** 439–47
[35] Reynolds A, Leake D, Boese Q, Scaringe S, Marshall W S and Khvorova A 2004 Rational siRNA design for RNA interference *Nat. Biotechnol.* **22** 326–30
[36] Shawan M M A K *et al* 2021 Designing an effective therapeutic siRNA to silence RdRp gene of SARS-CoV-2 *Infect. Genet. Evol.* **93** 104951
[37] Huang Y, Hong J, Zheng S, Ding Y, Guo S, Zhang H, Zhang X, Du Q and Liang Z 2011 Elimination pathways of systemically delivered siRNA *Mol. Ther.* **19** 381–5
[38] Lundstrom K 2020 Self-amplifying RNA viruses as RNA vaccines *Int. J. Mol. Sci.* **21** 5130
[39] Lundstrom K 2020 Viral vectors applied for RNAi-based antiviral therapy *Viruses* **12**
[40] Maggi F, Pistello M and Antonelli G 2019 Future management of viral diseases: role of new technologies and new approaches in microbial interactions *Clin. Microbiol. Infect.* **25** 136–41
[41] Souf S 2016 Recent advances in diagnostic testing for viral infections *Biosci. Horizons Int. J. Student Res.* **9** hzw010
[42] Boonham N, Kreuze J, Winter S, van der Vlugt R, Bergervoet J, Tomlinson J and Mumford R 2014 Methods in virus diagnostics: from ELISA to next generation sequencing *Virus Res* **186** 20–31
[43] Hodinka R L and Kaiser L 2013 Is the era of viral culture over in the clinical microbiology laboratory? *J. Clin. Microbiol.* **51** 2
[44] Leland D S and Ginocchio c c 2007 Role of cell culture for virus detection in the age of technology *Clin. Microbiol. Rev.* **20** 49
[45] Vemula S V, Zhao J, Liu J, Xue X W, Biswas S and Hewlett I 2016 Current approaches for diagnosis of influenza virus infections in humans *Viruses* **8** 96
[46] Poljak M, Kocjan B J, Oštrbenk A and Seme K 2016 Commercially available molecular tests for human papillomaviruses (HPV): 2015 update *J. Clin. Virol.* **76** S3–13

[47] Andrews D, Chetty Y, Cooper B S, Virk M, Glass S K, Letters A, Kelly P A, Sudhanva M and Jeyaratnam D 2017 Multiplex PCR point of care testing versus routine, laboratory-based testing in the treatment of adults with respiratory tract infections: a quasi-randomised study assessing impact on length of stay and antimicrobial use *BMC Infect. Dis.* **17** 671

[48] Gubbins P O, Klepser M E, Adams A J, Jacobs D M, Percival K M and Tallman G B 2017 Potential for pharmacy-public health collaborations using pharmacy-based point-of-care testing services for infectious diseases *J. Public Health Manag. Pract.* **23** 593–600

[49] Sasaki T *et al* 2012 Reliability of a newly-developed immunochromatography diagnostic kit for pandemic influenza A/H1N1pdm virus: implications for drug administration *PLoS One* **7** e50670

[50] Josko D 2010 Molecular virology in the clinical laboratory *Clin. Lab. Sci.* **23** 231–6

[51] Yee C, Suarthana E, Dendukuri N, Nicolau I, Semret M and Frenette C 2016 Evaluating the impact of the multiplex respiratory virus panel polymerase chain reaction test on the clinical management of suspected respiratory viral infections in adult patients in a hospital setting *Am. J. Infect. Control* **44** 1396–8

[52] Lowe C F, Merrick L, Harrigan P R, Mazzulli T, Sherlock C H and Ritchie G 2016 Implementation of next-generation sequencing for hepatitis B virus resistance testing and genotyping in a clinical microbiology laboratory *J. Clin. Microbiol.* **54** 127–33

[53] Moscona R, Ram D, Wax M, Bucris E, Levy I, Mendelson E and Mor O 2017 Comparison between next-generation and Sanger-based sequencing for the detection of transmitted drug-resistance mutations among recently infected HIV-1 patients in Israel, 2000–2014 *J. Int. AIDS Soc.* **20** 21846

[54] Quiñones-Mateu M E, Avila S, Reyes-Teran G and Martinez M A 2014 Deep sequencing: becoming a critical tool in clinical virology *J. Clin. Virol.* **61** 9

Chapter 13

MicroRNA (miRNA) therapeutic modalities

Amisha Parmar and Luca Ghigliotti

The discovery of potential regulatory functions of microRNAs (miRNAs) in health and diseases has attracted growing attention in biomedical research. After the discovery of the critical role of miRNAs in cancer in 2002, extensive data has been published focusing on their physiological role, dysregulation in various diseases, and potential in diagnostics and therapeutics. Emerging evidence points to the immense potential of miRNAs present in the host in responding to infections. As a result, presently miRNAs are being explored for their clinical applications as biomarkers [1] and therapeutics [2] in infectious diseases. The role played by miRNAs in the ongoing battle between host and viruses has been extensively studied in the last decade. This chapter summarizes the promising role of miRNAs in response to viruses in host—preventing, diagnosing, and treating viral infections.

13.1 miRNA biology

It all started in 1993 when Lee *et al* made a surprise discovery of these short RNA sequences regulating gene expression in the nematode. They discovered a 22 nucleotide RNA sequence that controlled the expression of a protein-encoding gene [3]. Following that, hundreds of 20–24 nucleotide RNA molecules were discovered in viruses, plants, animals, and humans. Moreover, the exclusive function of these small RNA molecules was identified: their ability to regulate the expression of genes [4]. miRNAs fine-tune protein production after a gene has been transcribed [2]. miRNA biogenesis and mechanism of action is shown in figure 13.1. miRNAs are endogenous, small, 18–25 nucleotides long single-stranded RNAs that derive from the non-coding region of DNA. These small RNAs are derived from longer primary transcripts that fold back on themselves to produce stem-loop structures. These are recognized and processed by Drosha and co-factors in the nucleus followed by Dicer and co-factors in the cytoplasm, resulting in a ~22 nucleotide duplex RNA [5]. One strand of the duplex is preferentially incorporated into the RNA-induced silencing complex (RISC), which then mediates binding to target

doi:10.1088/978-0-7503-4987-1ch13

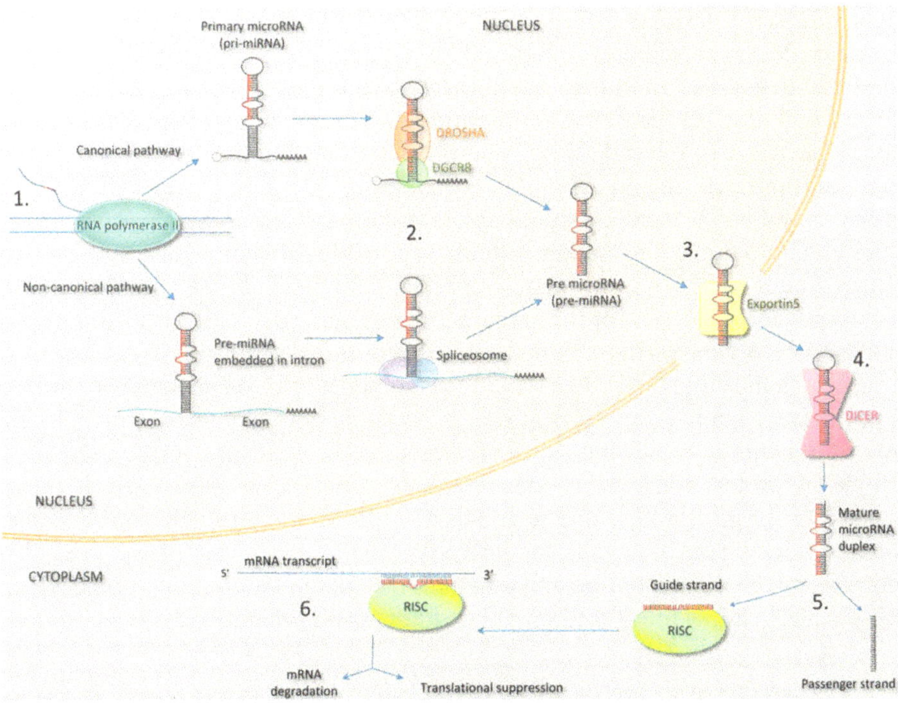

Figure 13.1. miRNA biogenesis and mechanism of action. Original taken from [2] Copyright (2017) CC BY 4.0.

messenger RNAs (mRNAs). miRNAs act by binding to the complementary 3′-untranslated regions (3′UTR) of specific mRNAs, to prevent translation, either through mRNA degradation or translational repression [5]. The miRNA registry, miRbase, lists 2558 human miRNAs at present [6]. In total, >45 000 miRNA target sites within human 3′UTRs are conserved above background levels, and >60% of human protein-coding genes have been under selective pressure to maintain pairing to miRNAs [7].

miRNA genes are either localized within introns, and sometimes exons of other genes or as an independent transcriptional unit. In the canonical pathway, RNA polymerase II (and occasionally RNA polymerase III) plays a role in miRNAs transcription, primarily as long primary miRNA transcripts (pri-miRNAs). Pri-miRNAs can be several kilobases long and can contain the stem-loops of several mature miRNAs. In the non-canonical pathway, miRNA precursors lie in mRNA introns (‘miRtrons’), are transcribed by RNA Polymerase II into a primary precursor, called pri-miRNA. Pri-miRNAs are processed by the nuclear protein DGCR8 (DiGeorge syndrome critical 8 region) and the enzyme DROSHA into hairpin-shaped structures called pre-miRNA transcripts. In the non-canonical pathway, miRNA precursors in mRNA introns are spliced out and bypass DGCR8/DROSHA. Pre-miRNAs are exported to the cytoplasm by exportin-5. The enzyme DICER cleaves the pre-miRNA hairpin loop to produce a mature miRNA duplex. One strand of the miRNA duplex (the guide strand) associates with Argonaut (AGO) protein in the RISC. The remaining strand (termed the passenger strand) is degraded. In most cases, there is a preference for which strand is incorporated due to factors like thermodynamic stability. The mature single-stranded miRNA in the miR-RISC complex binds to complementary sequences in the 3′ untranslated region of mRNA molecule, preventing translation. Bound mRNA may be degraded or stored for translation later. Bound mRNA may be sequestered into processing bodies (p-bodies) possibly for later release figure 13.1 [2].

Interestingly, miRNAs only require perfect complementarity with only the first 2–7 nucleotides on mRNA for the binding to occur, termed as 'seed' site [8]. Therefore, a single miRNA can bind to hundreds of different mRNAs [9]. miRNA binding sites are present in most human protein-coding genes under selective pressure [7]. miRNAs are post-transcriptional repressors of gene expression, but functionally miRNA can be involved in pathway repression or enhancement by the direct and indirect effects. For example, if protein's repressors are targets of miRNA, in that case, there is an upregulation of that protein due to miRNAs [10]. Multiple proteins in the same or related pathways can be targets for miRNAs [10, 11]. miRNAs play a critical role in controlling cell differentiation and functions including various cellular processes (for instance, mechanisms integral to innate and adaptive immunity) [2].

13.2 Host miRNA–virus interactions

Viruses are obligate intracellular parasites, intimately interconnected with their host cells. By virus–host cell interactions, viruses exclusively rely on host cellular machinery for their replication and infectivity. But, in the same process, they also provide an advantage of combating viral infection to the host cell [12]. The invading viruses constantly develop defence mechanisms to avoid detection and clearance by the host immune response. In mammals, innate immunity is a primary defence system, which is initiated by the recognition of foreign material detected in the presence of invading viruses. In vertebrates, when cells sense a specific pathogen-associated molecular pattern, such as double-stranded (ds) RNA or the presence of a 5′ triphosphate group, a cascade of a signaling pathway is activated resulting in the initiation of expression of type I interferon (IFN). This leads to the transcription of hundreds of interferon-stimulated genes (ISGs), known as pro-inflammatory cytokines [13]. In this manner, the host defence inhibits viral replication and protein synthesis, induces cellular RNA degradation, and eventually leads to apoptosis of the infected cell [14].

In plants, arthropods, and nematodes, RNA interference (RNAi) represents their major antiviral defence system in the presence of exogenous long ds RNA [15]. In vertebrates, the machinery which is involved in the biogenesis of miRNAs has the previously known role of clearing unwanted nucleic acids in cells [16]. miRNAs interfere in viral attachment to viral multiplication to eventually disease progression in the event of a viral infection [17]. miRNAs directly target viral genes or indirectly regulate host genes which are involved in causing infection [16]. The microRNA Response Elements (MRE) are generally located in the 5′UTR and 3′UTR of the viral genome, which corroborates the antiviral roles of miRNA [18, 19]. miRNAs exhibit multiple mechanisms in combating viral infections. *In vitro* studies show that host miRNAs inhibit viral replication of influenza; vesicular stomatitis virus; human papillomavirus; human T-cell leukemia virus 1; and enterovirus [2]. By directly targeting viral transcripts, miRNAs may be act as direct contributors of innate immunity [2].

Contrary to this, some studies show enhanced viral genome stability and translation upon direct binding of miRNA to the viral genome. For instance, Jopling *et al* demonstrated that miR-122, a liver-specific miRNA contributes to Hepatitis C virus (HCV) liver tropism [18]. miR-122 forms an oligomeric complex which stabilizes the HCV genome. Here, miR-122 binds to two closely target sites (S1 and S2) in the 5′ UTR of the HCV genome, and thus protects the HCV genome from degradation [20, 21]. Interestingly, when miR-122 inhibitor, miravirsen was administered to chimpanzees chronically infected with HCV9, it successfully reduced viremia *in vivo* [22], and currently, in clinical trials for the treatment of HCV infection. Interestingly, miRNAs are also expressed by some viruses, which may contribute repressing host-cell mRNAs which have a role in diminishing viral infection [23].

13.2.1 Cellular miRNAs directly regulate viral genes

miRNAs directly target viral RNAs at 3′UTR, 5′UTR, or coding sequences. Interaction of miRNAs with viral RNAs results in impaired viral genome replication, RNA stabilization, and enhanced translation (figure 13.2) [15]. Studies have shown miRNA–virus interaction in a human retrovirus: Human Immunodeficiency Virus 1 (HIV-1) production is suppressed by five miRNAs in CD4+ T cells [24]. miR-29a is involved in suppression of viral replication by interfering with the HIV-1 3′UTR [25, 26]. Moreover, miRNA–virus interactions have been witnessed in human viruses belonging to Orthomyxoviridae, Flaviviridae, Hepadnaviridae, and Rhabdoviridae families. Excepting miR-122-HCV interaction, the rest of the viral–miRNA interactions reduce viral replication by suppressing the expression of viral gene. Up- and down-regulation of antiviral miRNAs are observed during the infection: for example, IFNβ induces miRNA which is responsible for the suppression of HCV replication [27].

13.2.2 Indirect effects of cellular miRNAs on viruses

Even though it has been an incredible advancement in this field, to date, there is scarce knowledge on exactly how miRNAs exert their antiviral properties. At the same time, hundreds of proteins can be regulated by miRNAs [28, 29] and rather than regulating individual genes, miRNAs can play a role by targeting host networks rather than individual genes [30, 31]. Reports suggest that the expression of host protein-encoding transcripts required for the viral cycle for one or multiple steps can be modulated by mRNAs indirectly. Moreover, mRNAs can inhibit viral tropism by regulating the expression of the receptor that controls entry of the virus (figure 13.2) [15]. To identify whether miRNAs target viral genomes or host gene networks, Santhakumar *et al* explored the direction of identifying cellular miRNAs

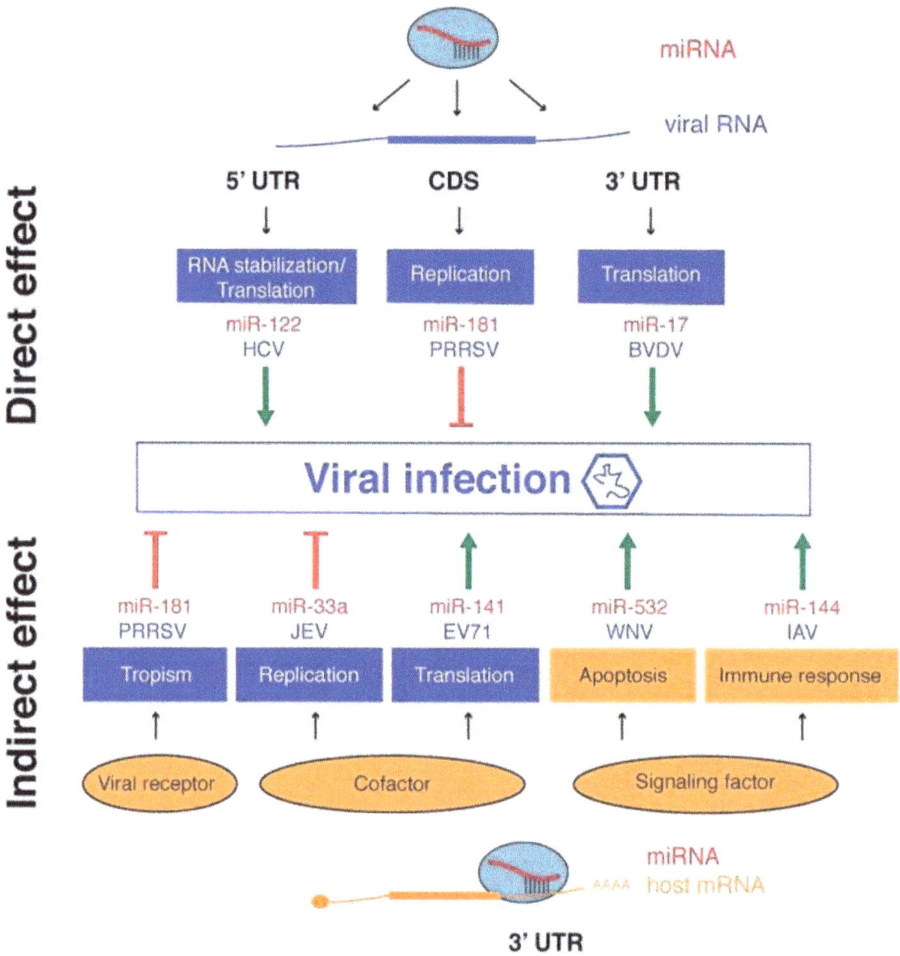

Figure 13.2. Mechanism by which miRNA regulates viral infection. Blue represents steps of viral cycle which orange represents host factors and pathways associated. Original illustration taken from [15]. Copyright (2018) CC BY 4.0.

with broad-spectrum viral inhibitory activities and developed a global functional screening method [32]. Their exploration revealed the role of miR-199a-3p as a broad-spectrum inhibitor of viral load, observed in CMV (both murine and human), herpes simplex virus-1, and mouse gamma herpesvirus [32]. In this case, miR- 199a-3p is likely to be targeting host factors rather than interactions with viral genes or pathways [16]. Moreover, when global mRNA analysis was applied to cells treated with miR-199a-3p mimics versus inhibitors, the method identified numerous miR-199a-3p-regulated genes, therefore the enrichment of a couple of pathways commonly activated by many viruses. The pathways include ERK/MAPK signalling, PI3K/AKT signalling, prostaglandin synthesis, oxidative stress signalling and viral entry [32].

13.2.3 miRNAs and viral genome: potential interactions

As shown in figure 13.3, the viral genome is sequestered by host miRNAs to stabilize it by interfering with miRNA targets present in the cell, which in turn results in the modulation of viral infection associated cellular pathways. On the other hand, the virus can also alter the transcriptome and modulate miRNA expression by interacting directly with the host genes in order to exert pro- or antiviral activities. This is apparent from the observations that some viruses are capable of encoding viral miRNAs targeting host and viral RNA [33].

13.2.4 Influence of viral miRNAs

To date, at least 66 distinct miRNAs are identified which are produced by mammalian viruses [34]. Amongst those are dsDNA viruses belonging to the herpesvirus family. When this possibility was explored in RNA viruses (retroviruses or flaviviruses), or the papillomavirus which is a dsDNA virus, there was no detection of miRNAs [35, 36]. Evidence suggests that these viral-encoded miRNAs may be involved in virus pathogenesis in terms of promoting replication, and latency control [2]. Interestingly, it is discovered that HIV, Ebola, Adenoviridae, Herpesviridae, and the BK polyomavirus born miRNA need host-cell machinery to exert functional effects [2]. Since, these miRNAs do not have an orthologue in the human genome they can be utilized as potential therapeutic targets [37]. The pro-viral mechanism adopted by viral miRNAs against the immune response during infection is the regulation of the major histocompatibility complex class I chain-related molecule B (MICB) expression, a natural killer cell ligand [38]. Epstein–Barr virus (EBV), Kaposi's sarcoma-associated herpesvirus (KSHV) and human

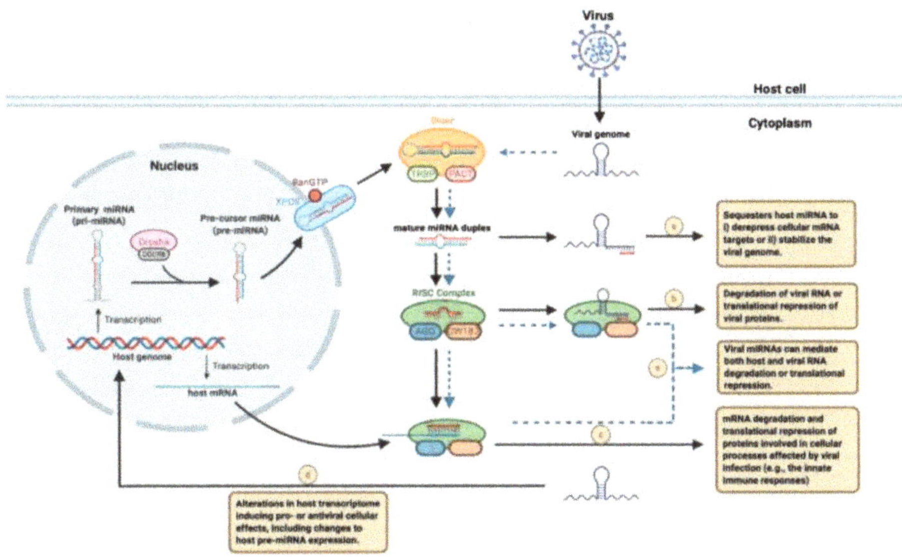

Figure 13.3. miRNAs and viral infection: potential interactions. Original taken from [33]. Copyright (2021) with permission from Springer Nature.

cytomegalovirus (HCMV) express miRNAs which inhibit MICB expression by targeting two different sites on MICB mRNA [15]. Furthermore, in the case of KSHV miR-9, Bellare *et al* revealed that miR-9 targets the protein that controls viral reactivation from latency by binding to 32 UTR of the major lytic-switch mRNA [39].

13.3 Identification of host miRNAs in the regulation of viral infection and their targets

To determine diagnostic markers and potential therapeutic targets, the identification of miRNAs involved in viral pathogenesis or inhibition of viral infection is prerequisite. The role of miRNAs in health and disease is studied by increasing and decreasing miRNA function or abundance. This is possible through transfection or viral transduction of mature miRNA or miRNA duplex (figure 13.4(A)); small interfering RNA duplex (figure 13.4(B)); short hairpin RNA (figure 13.4(C)); pre-miRNA (figure 13.4(D)); pri-miRNA (figure 13.4(E)); modified single-stranded RNA (figure 13.4(F)) [34].

Antisense oligonucleotides (ASOs) are single-stranded RNA or DNA molecules, short in length, binding other nucleic acids by Watson–Crick base pairing. Traditional ASOs target a specific mRNA either by blocking its protein translation or demolishing it by recruiting RNase H which is responsible for the hydrolysis of the RNA strand of an RNA:DNA duplex. ASOs are widely used to discover gene function *in vitro* and *in vivo*. ASOs were identified to inhibit specific miRNAs in cultured cells and invertebrates back in 2004. Presently, modified ASOs are utilized to study the molecular function of an individual miRNA, which is discovered by inhibiting individual miRNA-specific ASO and evaluating the resulting changes mRNA or protein expression levels in the cell, other functional changes, such as developmental defects, physiology of organs, cell proliferation and differentiation, lipid metabolism, or behaviour [34]. ASOs are designed in a way that they remain intact from the degradation by extra- and intracellular nucleases to effectively inhibit miRNAs in the whole animal [40, 41]. The first anti-miRNA ASOs were composed of 22-O-methyl ribose-modified RNA. Such 2′-O-methyl oligonucleotides are introduced

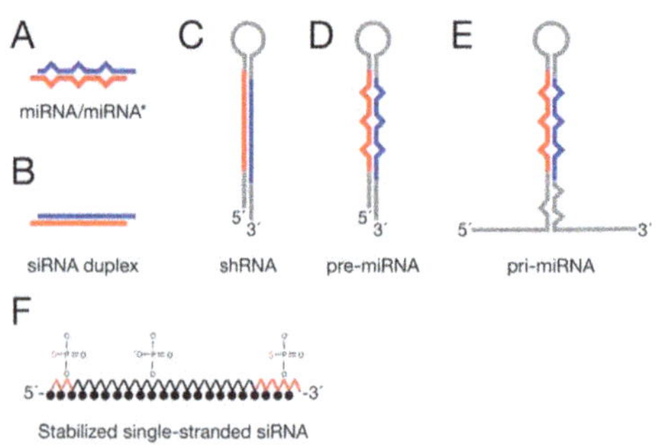

Figure 13.4. miRNA replacement strategies. Reproduced from [34] with permission from Springer Nature.

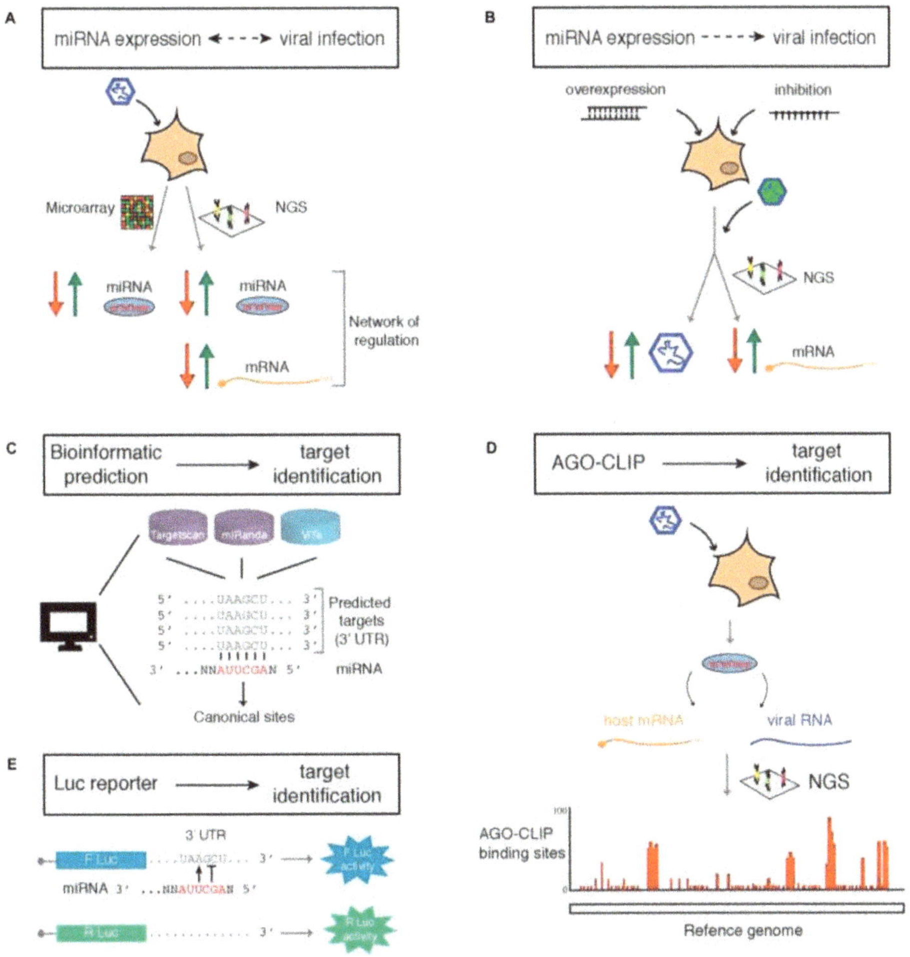

Figure 13.5. Current approaches available for the identification of miRNAs involved in the regulation of viral infection (A, B) and their targets (C–E). Adapted from [15] CC BY 4.0.

by lipid-mediated transfection into cultured human cells or by injection in *Caenorhabditis elegans*, this approach made them effective miRNA inhibitors [34].

As shown in figures 13.5(A) and (B), there are diverse experimental approaches utilized to study viral infection and its impact on miRNA expression. To obtain the complete profile of miRNA expression in a cell at a given time and condition, techniques such as multiplexed RT-qPCR, microarray, or next-generation sequencing (NGS)-based genome-wide approaches are used. Viral infection-impacted regulation of miRNA allows the identification of upregulated (green arrow) or downregulated (red arrow) candidate miRNAs by miRNA profiling through microarray [15]. The regulated targets and resulting networks of gene regulation are deciphered by NGS (figure 13.5(A)). Moreover, a reporter virus (green colour) is used for the screenings of candidate miRNA in the context of viral infection based on miRNA overexpression or inhibition approach. The usage of the reporter virus gives visuals of increase or decrease of virus load. If this method is coupled with transcriptome profiling, it makes possible identifying the target genes of candidate miRNA (figure 13.5(B)) [15].

In computational analysis for target identification of a specific miRNA, the seed matches in the 3′ UTRs of cellular mRNAs are identified. Specific target prediction tools such as Targetscan or miRanda for cellular targets or ViTa for viral genomes and transcripts are utilized (figure 13.5(C)). Moreover, AGO crosslinked to the miRNA and bound target are isolated using biochemical methods and deep sequencing (AGO-CLIP) is applied followed by that. AGO-CLIP allows the identification of miRNA-specific targets in the whole genome and reveals the precise binding sites on the target (figure 13.5(D)). The functional validation of an miRNA binding site is detected by Luciferase (Luc) reporter assays. As an end point, luciferase enzymatic activity is measured when a potential binding site is present on the 3′UTR. Variants of luciferase (F, firefly; or R, Renilla) with or without the binding site are used to estimate differential regulation (figure 13.5(E)) [15].

13.4 miRNA therapeutics: development and challenges

Deregulation of miRNAs in various viral diseases has indeed made miRNAs a potential therapeutic in the context of viral infection. miRNAs show low immunogenicity and an advantage of cross-species conservation, which makes them widely accepted in *in vivo* preclinical research [15]. There are two novel approaches to target miRNAs, inhibition of overexpressed miRNAs or replacement of miRNAs that are downregulated to treat clinical conditions driven by miRNA dysregulation. miRNA-based antiviral therapy includes miRNA mimics (as therapeutics) or anti-miRs (as targets of therapeutics) [42]. Anti-miRs are formulated by the chemical modification of a single-stranded oligonucleotide or chemical modification of a ds nucleic acid molecule when its miRNA mimics [43].

In the development of miRNA-based therapeutics, as a first step, patient samples are analysed and miRNA candidates are systemically selected. Then the relevance of these candidate miRNAs to a specific disease and its biology is elucidated by *in vivo*, *ex vivo* and *in vitro* approaches [44]. Even though it is straight forward to inhibit [45] or overexpress a given miRNA [46], ribonucleotide-based therapeutics comes with a challenge for *in vivo* applications due to their degradation by nucleases and endosomal escape [44]. For *in vivo* use, limited efficacy is obtained for miRNA-based therapies due to difficulty in delivery system [44]. In initial efforts to develop miRNA-based formulations, miRNA mimics in naked or viral vectors-encoded forms were injected at target tissue sites (local or systemic delivery). For miRNA therapeutics, pharmacological difficulties related to poor bioavailability caused by systemic delivery and degradation and the local delivery associated failures in clinical setting were faced. Despite these hurdles, miRNA therapeutics is now in clinics due to advanced knowledge in RNA chemistry and delivery technologies! The chemical modification approaches such as the addition of a 2′-*O*-methyl group or locked nucleic acids (LNAs) are proven to be a useful approach to increase stability.

Moreover, several encapsulation methods have shown improved delivery to the target sites. Lipid nanoparticles such as neutral lipid emulsions (NLEs) or dendrimer complexes with a targeting moiety attached are commonly used delivery systems [44]. However, immunogenicity and lack of accuracy for target hitting, the translation of these delivery systems into the clinic are far-fetched [44]. Finally, in this process, successful miRNA therapeutic candidates are tested in disease-specific *in vivo* rodent or non-human primate models manner (figure 13.6) [44].

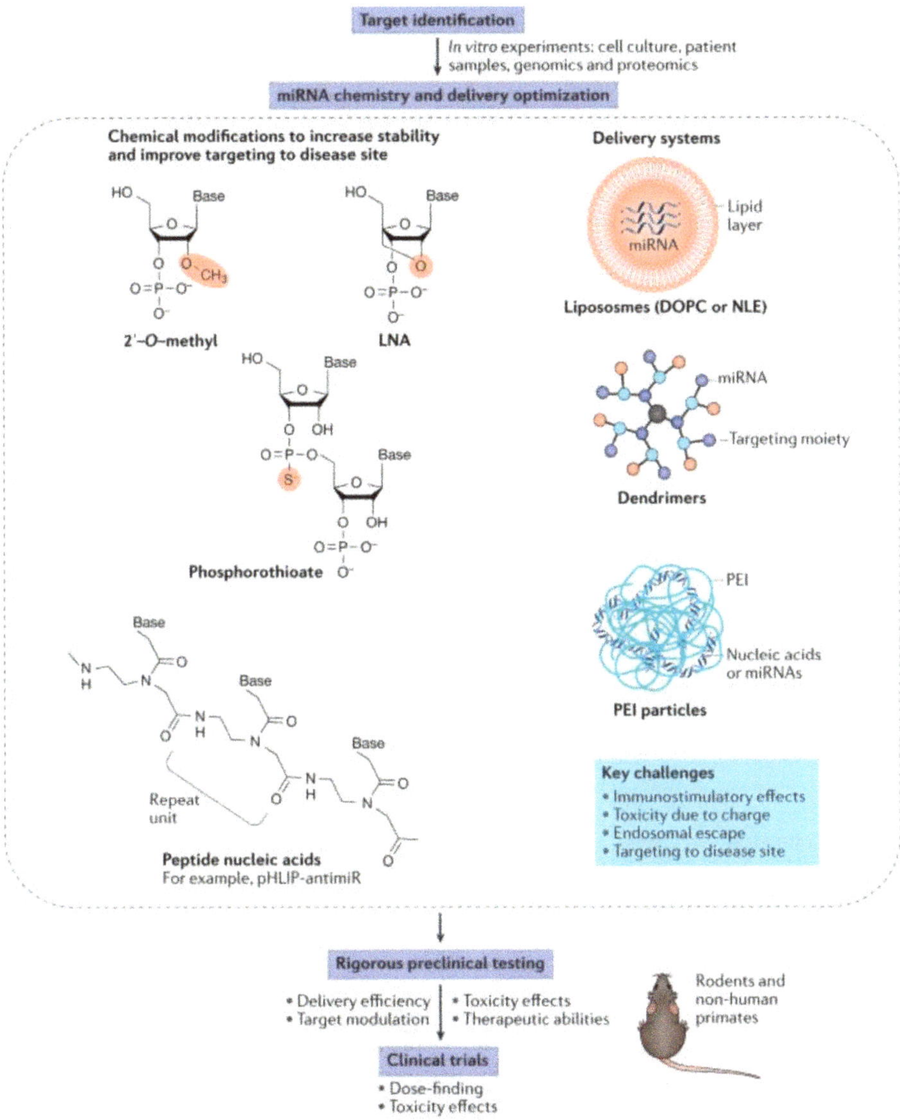

Figure 13.6. Summary of miRNA-based therapeutics development strategies. Reproduced from [44] with permission from Springer Nature.

13.5 miRNA targets and therapeutic exploration in various viral infections

The most interesting example of an miRNA agent is Miravirsen (an ASO), miR-122 inhibitor in the infection of HCV which is currently being explored in the clinic. A previous study showed Miravirsen-based miR-122 silencing in HCV-infected chimpanzees, along with long-lasting suppression of viral load [22]. Later, patients with chronic HCV infection treated with Miravirsen injections (5-weekly) in a phase 2a study [47] exhibited a prolonged and dose-dependent reduction in HCV RNA levels [47, 48]. RG-101 (*N*-acetylgalactosamine conjugated ASO)-based miR-122 inhibition led to a notable viral suppression in all treated patients within 4 weeks in a phase 1b trial [49].

Aside from that, in various recent studies, miRNA therapeutics have shown significant potential in *in vivo* studies. In a recent study, mice with H1N1 infection were treated with a combination of five chemically-modified miRNA mimics, which showed synergistic suppression of replication of H1N1 and protection from viral infection [50]. In another study, the inhibitor of miR-301, modified miR-301a morpholino was administered by intracranial injection in mice with neurotropic virus Japanese encephalitis virus (JEV) infection. The study discovered induction in miR-301 expression in infected neuronal cells associated with impaired antiviral host response in JEV infection. *In vivo* inhibition of miR-301 restored the interferon (IFN) response, thus improving the survival of mice with JEV infection by the production of IFNβ, thereby restricting viral spread [51]. Moreover, miRNAs are also found to affect dengue virus (DENV) pathogenesis. miRNAs currently identified for DENV mostly supress replication, either via modulation of host mediators which are required for the multiplication of DENV or directly attacking the viral genome [17].

Interestingly, in SARS-CoV-2, SARS-CoV, and MERS-CoV genomes, several miRNA binding sites are located. Among them, promisingly SARS-CoV-2 infection is shown to be modulated by miR-24, miR-200, and miR-16 [33]. In severe COVID-19 patients, miRNAs are found to downregulate viral replication, modulate viral infectious progress, and enhance survival rates [52].

13.5.1 Attenuated vaccines

The advantage of the natural capacity of cellular miRNAs to stop viral infection by targeting viral RNAs can be taken to generate live attenuated vaccines [53]. The new attenuated vaccines can be created by incorporating cell-specific miRNA target sequences into respective viral genomes making them tissue-specific. This is the most exciting invention in the current era to fight against viruses. Based on this, the proof of principle was established a few years ago. The complementary sequences for miR-124 (neuronal specific) were inserted into the genome of poliovirus, limited its tissue-based tropism in mice and prevented the attenuated viral strain pathogenicity [54]. After this, another approach was tried, in which attenuation was performed using miRNA-based silencing of responsible gene/s and improvement of safety for influenza A virus vaccine [55]. Recent advances in vaccine research have demonstrated the potential of miR-21 knockout cells as a platform for vaccine to engineer and grow miR-21 targeted viruses and replace the usual egg-based vaccine production approaches [56].

13.6 Conclusion

The continued efforts of the research groups seeking therapies against deadly viral attacks are praiseworthy, however, currently, very limited effective antiviral options are available in the market. The unravelling of the intrinsic regulatory role of miRNAs in viral infections has opened vistas into various diagnostic therapeutic strategies. In multiple viral infections, cellular miRNAs are identified and shown to interact with the viral genome, directly and/or indirectly. To date, the knowledge is limited in this direction and warrants further investigation of molecular interactions between host and viral genome. The knowledge of viral infection pathogenesis and elucidation of the fundamental role of miRNAs is crucial for the development efficient antiviral therapies.

Moreover, as discussed earlier, even though many miRNA targets are discovered in various viral infections, the effective delivery of miRNA-based formulations to a target site is still a huge challenge. Future research should focus on seeking better delivery systems that help improve efficacy and reduce unwanted side effects.

Abbreviations

ASOs	Antisense oligonucleotides
DENV	Dengue virus
DGCR8	DiGeorge syndrome critical 8 region
ds	Double-stranded
EBV	Epstein–Barr virus
HCMV	Human cytomegalovirus
HCV	Hepatitis C virus
HIV-1	Human immunodeficiency virus 1
IFN	Interferon
ISGs	Interferon-stimulated genes
JEV	Japanese encephalitis
KSHV	Kaposi's sarcoma-associated herpesvirus
LNAs	Locked nucleic acids
MICB	Major histocompatibility complex class I chain-related molecule B
miRNAs	microRNAs
MREs	microRNA response elements
mRNAs	messenger RNAs
NLEs	Neutral lipid emulsions
NGS	Next generation sequencing
p-bodies	Processing bodies
pri-miRNA	Primary miRNA
RISC	RNA-induced silencing complex
RNAi	RNA interference
3'UTR	3′-untranslated regions

References

[1] Reid G, Kirschner M B and van Zandwijk N 2011 Circulating microRNAs: association with disease and potential use as biomarkers *Crit. Rev. Oncol./Hematol.* **80** 193–208
[2] Drury R E, O'Connor D and Pollard A J 2017 The clinical application of MicroRNAs in infectious disease *Front. Immunol.* **8** 1182
[3] Lee R C, Feinbaum R L and Ambros V 1993 The *C. elegans* heterochronic gene lin-4 encodes small RNAs with antisense complementarity to lin-14 *Cell* **75** 843–54
[4] He L and Hannon G J 2004 MicroRNAs: small RNAs with a big role in gene regulation *Nat. Rev. Genet.* **5** 522–31
[5] Bartel D P 2004 MicroRNAs: genomics, biogenesis, mechanism, and function *Cell* **116** 281–97
[6] Kozomara A, Birgaoanu M and Griffiths-Jones S 2019 miRBase: from microRNA sequences to function *Nucleic Acids Res.* **47** D155–62
[7] Friedman R C, Farh K K H, Burge C B and Bartel D P 2009 Most mammalian mRNAs are conserved targets of microRNAs *Genome Res* **19** 92–105
[8] Bartel D P 2009 MicroRNAs: target recognition and regulatory functions *Cell* **136** 215–33
[9] Lewis B P, Burge C B and Bartel D P 2005 Conserved seed pairing, often flanked by adenosines, indicates that thousands of human genes are microRNA targets *Cell* **120** 15–20
[10] Ebert M S and Sharp P A 2012 Roles for microRNAs in conferring robustness to biological processes *Cell* **149** 515–24
[11] Mehta A and Baltimore D 2016 MicroRNAs as regulatory elements in immune system logic *Nat. Rev. Immunol.* **16** 279–94
[12] Hoenen T and Groseth A 2022 Virus–host cell interactions *Cells* **11** 804
[13] Nakhaei P, Genin P, Civas A and Hiscott J 2009 RIG-I-like receptors: sensing and responding to RNA virus infection *Semin. Immunol.* **21** 215–22
[14] Barber G N 2001 Host defense, viruses and apoptosis *Cell Death Differ.* **8** 113–26
[15] Girardi E, López P and Pfeffer S 2018 On the importance of host microRNAs during viral infection *Front. Genet.* **9** 439
[16] Laqtom N N 2014 microRNA manipulation as a host-targeted antiviral therapeutic strategy *Eur. Pharmaceut. Rev.* **16** 52–5
[17] Wong R R, Abd-Aziz N, Affendi S and Poh C L 2020 Role of microRNAs in antiviral responses to dengue infection *J. Biomed. Sci.* **27** 4
[18] Jopling C L, Yi M, Lancaster A M, Lemon S M and Sarnow P 2005 Modulation of hepatitis C virus RNA abundance by a liver-specific microRNA *Science* **309** 1577–81
[19] Trobaugh D W, Gardner C L, Sun C, Haddow A D, Wang E, Chapnik E *et al* 2014 RNA viruses can hijack vertebrate microRNAs to suppress innate immunity *Nature* **506** 245–8
[20] Henke J I, Goergen D, Zheng J, Song Y, Schüttler C G, Fehr C *et al* 2008 microRNA-122 stimulates translation of hepatitis C virus RNA *EMBO J.* **27** 3300–10
[21] Shimakami T, Yamane D, Jangra R K, Kempf B J, Spaniel C, Barton D J *et al* 2012 Stabilization of hepatitis C virus RNA by an Ago2-miR-122 complex *Proc. Natl Acad. Sci. USA* **109** 941–6
[22] Lanford R E, Hildebrandt-Eriksen E S, Petri A, Persson R, Lindow M, Munk M E *et al* 2010 Therapeutic silencing of microRNA-122 in primates with chronic hepatitis C virus infection *Science* **327** 198–201
[23] Umbach J L and Cullen B R 2009 The role of RNAi and microRNAs in animal virus replication and antiviral immunity *Genes Dev* **23** 1151–64

[24] Huang J, Wang F, Argyris E, Chen K, Liang Z, Tian H *et al* 2007 Cellular microRNAs contribute to HIV-1 latency in resting primary CD4+ T lymphocytes *Nat. Med.* **13** 1241–7
[25] Ahluwalia J K, Khan S Z, Soni K, Rawat P, Gupta A, Hariharan M *et al* 2008 Human cellular microRNA hsa-miR-29a interferes with viral nef protein expression and HIV-1 replication *Retrovirology* **5** 117
[26] Nathans R, Chu C Y, Serquina A K, Lu C C, Cao H and Rana T M 2009 Cellular microRNA and P bodies modulate host-HIV-1 interactions *Mol Cell* **34** 696–709
[27] Pedersen I M, Cheng G, Wieland S, Volinia S, Croce C M, Chisari F V *et al* 2007 Interferon modulation of cellular microRNAs as an antiviral mechanism *Nature* **449** 919–22
[28] Baek D, Villén J, Shin C, Camargo F D, Gygi S P and Bartel D P 2008 The impact of microRNAs on protein output *Nature* **455** 64–71
[29] Selbach M, Schwanhäusser B, Thierfelder N, Fang Z, Khanin R and Rajewsky N 2008 Widespread changes in protein synthesis induced by microRNAs *Nature* **455** 58–63
[30] Giraldez A J, Mishima Y, Rihel J, Grocock R J, Van Dongen S, Inoue K *et al* 2006 Zebrafish MiR-430 promotes deadenylation and clearance of maternal mRNAs *Science* **312** 75–9
[31] Cancer Genome Atlas Research Network 2017 Comprehensive and integrative genomic characterization of hepatocellular carcinoma *Cell.* **169** 1327–41
[32] Santhakumar D, Forster T, Laqtom N N, Fragkoudis R, Dickinson P, Abreu-Goodger C *et al* 2010 Combined agonist-antagonist genome-wide functional screening identifies broadly active antiviral microRNAs *Proc. Natl Acad. Sci. USA* **107** 13830–5
[33] Hum C, Loiselle J, Ahmed N, Shaw T A, Toudic C and Pezacki J P 2021 MicroRNA mimics or inhibitors as antiviral therapeutic approaches against COVID-19 *Drugs* **81** 517–31
[34] Broderick J A and Zamore P D 2011 MicroRNA therapeutics *Gene Ther.* **18** 1104–10
[35] Cullen B R 2009 Viral and cellular messenger RNA targets of viral microRNAs *Nature* **457** 421–5
[36] Cullen B R 2010 Five questions about viruses and microRNAs *PLoS Pathog.* **6** e1000787
[37] Hammond S M 2015 An overview of microRNAs *Adv. Drug Deliv. Rev.* **87** 3–14
[38] Stern-Ginossar N, Elefant N, Zimmermann A, Wolf D G, Saleh N, Biton M *et al* 2007 Host immune system gene targeting by a viral miRNA *Science* **317** 376–81
[39] Bellare P and Ganem D 2009 Regulation of KSHV lytic switch protein expression by a virus-encoded microRNA: an evolutionary adaptation that fine-tunes lytic reactivation *Cell Host Microbe.* **6** 570–5
[40] Davis M E, Zuckerman J E, Choi C H J, Seligson D, Tolcher A, Alabi C A *et al* 2010 Evidence of RNAi in humans from systemically administered siRNA via targeted nano-particles *Nature* **464** 1067–70
[41] Lennox K A and Behlke M A 2010 A direct comparison of anti-microRNA oligonucleotide potency *Pharm. Res.* **27** 1788–99
[42] Saliminejad K, Khorram Khorshid H R, Soleymani Fard S and Ghaffari S H 2019 An overview of microRNAs: biology, functions, therapeutics, and analysis methods *J. Cell. Physiol.* **234** 5451–65
[43] Gibson N W 2014 Engineered microRNA therapeutics *J. R. Coll. Phys. Edinb.* **44** 196–200
[44] Rupaimoole R and Slack F J 2017 MicroRNA therapeutics: towards a new era for the management of cancer and other diseases *Nat. Rev. Drug Discov.* **16** 203–22
[45] Li Z and Rana T M 2014 Therapeutic targeting of microRNAs: current status and future challenges *Nat. Rev. Drug Discov.* **13** 622–38

[46] Yang N 2015 An overview of viral and nonviral delivery systems for microRNA *Int. J. Pharm. Investig.* **5** 179–81

[47] Janssen H L A, Reesink H W, Lawitz E J, Zeuzem S, Rodriguez-Torres M, Patel K *et al* 2013 Treatment of HCV infection by targeting microRNA *N. Engl. J. Med.* **368** 1685–94

[48] van der Ree M H, van der Meer A J, de Bruijne J, Maan R, van Vliet A, Welzel T M *et al* 2014 Long-term safety and efficacy of microRNA-targeted therapy in chronic hepatitis C patients *Antiviral Res.* **111** 53–9

[49] van der Ree M H, de Vree J M, Stelma F, Willemse S, van der Valk M, Rietdijk S *et al* 2017 Safety, tolerability, and antiviral effect of RG-101 in patients with chronic hepatitis C: a phase 1B, double-blind, randomised controlled trial *Lancet* **389** 709–17

[50] Peng S, Wang J, Wei S, Li C, Zhou K, Hu J *et al* 2018 Endogenous cellular microRNAs mediate antiviral defense against influenza A virus *Mol. Ther. Nucleic Acids* **10** 361–75

[51] Hazra B, Kumawat K L and Basu A 2017 The host microRNA miR-301a blocks the IRF1-mediated neuronal innate immune response to Japanese encephalitis virus infection *Sci. Signal* **10** eaaf5185

[52] Schultz I C, Bertoni A P S and Wink M 2021 Mesenchymal stem cell-derived extracellular vesicles carrying miRNA as a potential multi target therapy to COVID-19: an in silico analysis *Stem Cell Rev. Rep.* **17** 341–56

[53] Minor P D 2015 Live attenuated vaccines: historical successes and current challenges *Virology* **479–80** 379–92

[54] Barnes D, Kunitomi M, Vignuzzi M, Saksela K and Andino R 2008 Harnessing endogenous miRNAs to control virus tissue tropism as a strategy for developing attenuated virus vaccines *Cell Host Microbe* **4** 239–48

[55] Perez J T, Pham A M, Lorini M H, Chua M A, Steel J and tenOever B R 2009 MicroRNA-mediated species-specific attenuation of influenza A virus *Nat. Biotechnol.* **27** 572–6

[56] Waring B M, Sjaastad L E, Fiege J K, Fay E J, Reyes I, Moriarity B *et al* 2018 MicroRNA-based attenuation of influenza virus across susceptible hosts *J Virol* **92** 1128

IOP Publishing

Viral Diseases
History and new developments in diagnostics and therapeutics
Arvind K Singh Chandel, Bhakti Tanna, Amisha Parmar, Gopal Patel and Neeraj S Thakur

Chapter 14

Novel targets: host proteins, nucleic acid, and antibodies

Amisha Parmar and Bhakti Tanna

The development of specific antiviral drugs has become a huge challenge due to the constant threat of viral infections to all living organisms and the rapid evolution of viral genes. Antiviral agents are discovered based on two approaches: (i) drugs targeting viral proteins that play a key role in the viral life cycle; and (ii) drugs targeting indispensable host factors, thereby indirectly inhibiting viral infections [1]. Based on these approaches, in recent years, myriad viral and host targets have been exploited to discover antiviral agents; along with this significant progress, it remains an unsolved puzzle regarding the complete elimination of infection! This chapter aims to briefly explain novel antiviral targets such as host proteins, viral nucleic acids, and antibodies.

14.1 Host proteins

So far, more than 80 antiviral agents targeting viral proteins have been approved, but most inhibitors are prone to drug resistance. Therefore, targeting the host factor/s approach has become an interest of research with the possibility of discovering broad-spectrum inhibitors, that is, by targeting host proteins, interfering with cellular functions required by multiple viruses and reducing the risk of drug resistance. This is based on the principle that viruses require host factors to translate their transcripts; targeting the host factor/s offers a unique opportunity to develop novel antiviral drugs. Classical antiviral agents combat viral infections by inhibiting the biological activities of viral structural proteins [2] such as capsid, nucleocapsid, envelope, etc, and replication enzymes such as RNA methyltransferase, capping enzyme [3], protease [4], RNA-dependent RNA polymerase (RdRp), helicase [5] etc. With the disadvantage of drug resistance due to the continuous evolution of viruses, it is now considered to design molecules targeting the host pathways hijacked by viruses for pathogenesis and immune evasion inside the host. This includes the host

doi:10.1088/978-0-7503-4987-1ch14

metabolic pathways (lipid [6], glucose [7], and polyamine [8]), ubiquitin-proteasome system [9], glycosylations [10], inflammatory cascades [11], programmed ribosomal frameshifting (PRF), etc [12, 13].

The survival of the virus in the host cells depends upon the host factors that render the infected cell amenable to viral genome replication. Therefore, identifying these host–viral interactions is fundamental for developing host-targeted antiviral drugs.

14.1.1 Advantages and disadvantages

This approach comes with the major advantage of the broad-spectrum inhibitory activity of antivirals against multiple viruses and an increased threshold for the emergence of drug resistance. This is because of the relatively low genetic variability and mutation rate of humans when compared to viruses. Therefore, the probability of host-directed antiviral agents losing their efficiency against rapidly evolving and mutating viruses is also quite low. However, host-targeted antivirals are associated with the disadvantage of being more prone to have side effects compared with viral-targeted antivirals [1, 13].

14.1.2 Host targets for antiviral therapy

Some of the key approaches used for identifying host–viral interactions are RNA interference-based methods [14, 15], a drug combination approach [16], transcriptome and proteomic analysis of virus-infected cells [17], and CRISPR/Cas9 screens [14, 18]. Small interfering RNA screens are used for high-throughput screening of host factors required for replication and pathogenesis of viruses [19, 20]. The drug combination approach uses a suitable combination of drugs to target multiple host proteins and signaling enzymes that aid in viral pathogenesis [16]. CRISPR/Cas9 is an improved approach to identify exploitable host factors for the development of antivirals [21].

So far, many host targets have been discovered and FDA-approved for different viral infections, which are arbitrarily mainly categorized into four groups: (i) host chemokine receptors, (ii) host glycoproteins, (iii) host kinases, and (iv) other host proteins [1]. Hepatitis C virus (HCV) depends on the vesicle-associated membrane protein-associated protein, 33-kDa human homolog (hVAP-33), and HIV exploits C-C chemokine receptor type 5 (CCR5) to facilitate its successful infection [22, 23]. Similarly, the influenza virus also exploits host proteases and other important nuclear components to evade host antiviral responses and to establish its infection successfully [24–27].

14.1.2.1 Host chemokine receptors

CCR5 from the beta chemokine receptor family is expressed as an integral membrane protein on the surface of various immune cells such as CD4+ T cells, dendritic cells, macrophages, monocytes, and microglia [28]. HIV gp120 on the viral surface binds to the chemokine receptor CCR5 or CXCR4, thereby triggering viral entry. The first CCR5 antagonist, maraviroc, was approved by the FDA in August 2007, and later, a few other CCR5 inhibitors (e.g., leronlimab, GRL-117C) [29]. But they only prevent the CCR5-mediated entry; HIV can develop resistance by switching viral tropism from CCR5 (R5-tropism) to CXCR4 (X4-tropism) [1]. For this reason, dual antagonists that inhibit both CCR5 and CXCR4 are currently under development (e.g. GUT-70, NF297, diterpene derivatives) [30].

14.1.2.2 Host glycoproteins

CD4

Cluster of differentiation 4 (CD4), a membrane glycoprotein highly expressed on the surface of immune cells such as T-helper cells, dendritic cells, and macrophages. HIV viral entry is initiated by the gp120–CD4 interactions that make CD4 host-directed drug targets when developing HIV entry inhibitors [1]. The first CD4 inhibitor approved by the FDA, ibalizumab, shows broad-spectrum activity against HIV-1 resistant strains. Moreover, ibalizumab is a nonimmunosuppressive, humanized monoclonal antibody that binds to CD4, thereby competing with HIV-1 gp120 to block viral entry [31]. Fostemsavir in a phase 3 trial (NCT02362503) is a novel inhibitor that targets HIV-1 gp120 and blocks the gp120–CD4 interaction [32].

NTCP

Sodium taurocholate co-transporting polypeptide (NTCP) is a transmembrane glycoprotein that mediates the transport of liver-specific bile acids [33]. NTCP is highly expressed in human hepatocytes and interacts with the preS1 protein of HBV and HDV for viral entry [34]. Therefore, NTCP as host factor novel compounds (e.g. myrcludex B) have been developed to inhibit HBV or HDV infections [33].

LAMP1

Lysosomal-associated membrane protein 1: LAMP1 and LAMP2 proteins are widely distributed mammalian proteins that line the lysosome limiting membrane and protect it from lysosomal hydrolase action [35]. Lysosomal membrane glycoprotein, which is crucial for autophagy, cholesterol homeostasis, lysosomal pH regulation, and lysosome biogenesis, plays a crucial role in controlling the pH of the lysosomal lumen by directly inhibiting the proton channel Transmembrane protein 175 (TMEM175) and promoting lysosomal acidification for maximum hydrolase activity [36] promotes the virus's fusion with the host membrane in endosomes that are less acidic [37].

14.1.2.3 Host kinases

The control of virus entry into cells has been linked to several host kinases [38]. A thorough understanding of this interaction between the host kinase and the influenza virus is needed to map out all aspects of influenza virus replication inside the host cellular milieu. It could additionally clear the way for the development of kinase inhibitors as innovative anti-influenza medications in the future [39]. Many host kinases play different roles in viral infections. As an example: (1) Protein kinase R (PKR) detects double-stranded RNA (dsRNA) during viral infection; (2) during endoplasmic reticulum stress, PERK is activated, initiating the unfolded protein response (UPR); (3) heme-regulated eIF2α kinase (HRI) measures changes in hemoglobin levels; (4) general control nonderepressible 2 kinase (GCN2) detects amino acid deficiency, ultraviolet damage, and viral infection. During the viral infection process, several eIF2α kinases are activated by dsRNA or viral proteins produced by viral growth. This leads to eIF2α phosphorylation, which prevents the formation of ternary tRNA Met-GTP-eIF2 complexes and limits the synthesis of host or viral proteins. Nonetheless, a lot of viruses have developed a matching escape [40].

Other host proteins

Viral helicases: Helicases are motor proteins that catalyze the unwinding of duplex nucleic acids by utilizing the free energy of NTP hydrolysis. Helicases are involved in nearly every nucleic acid-related process. Based on the substrates they require, helicases can be roughly categorized into two groups: RNA helicases and DNA helicases. Among the most well-researched and structurally well-characterized helicases are Superfamily 1, 2 (SF1 and SF2) helicases. The first crucial step in unwinding the duplex substrate is the helicase's binding to the nucleic acid. Because of the helicase's directed translocation on its nucleic-acid substrate, the nucleic acid binding site must likewise be polarized with respect to the sugar-phosphate backbone [41].

Viral polymerases: Viral polymerases are essential for the transcription and replication of viral genomes. RNA-dependent RNA polymerase, RNA-dependent DNA polymerase, DNA-dependent RNA polymerase, and DNA-dependent RNA polymerases are found in different viruses, depending on the genome type and the special requirements of that virus. In most cases, viral polymerases function as a single, active protein that can perform a variety of tasks associated with the synthesis of the viral genome. The primary job of polymerase is to replicate a parent nucleic acid strand to create a daughter strand [42].

14.1.3 Host-directed therapeutic monoclonal antibodies

It has been widely known that monoclonal antibodies (mAbs) are directed against viral proteins; recently, mAbs have been designed to direct against host factors to treat viral infections [65]. Antiviral mAbs are immunoglobulins that have defined specificity and, with the help of antigen-binding fragments (Fab), exhibit therapeutic effects [43]. Antiviral mAbs, similar to passive immunotherapy, directly target viral agents. Further explorations revealed that antiviral mAbs can interact with different constituents of the immune system, both directly and indirectly [44]. Direct interaction includes antibody-dependent, cell-mediated virus inhibition (ADCVI), while the involvement of the immune response of the host, etc are the indirect mechanisms (table 14.1) [13].

14.2 Nucleic acids

CRISPR/Cas (Clustered Regularly Interspaced Short Palindromic Repeats–CRISPR-associated protein) and RNA interference (RNAi) are two well-established nucleic acid(NA)-based antiviral mechanisms. These therapies leverage synthetic nucleic acid molecules to recognize and modulate specific target gene sequences, ultimately helping to combat diseases. In bacteria and archaea, the CRISPR/Cas system works by capturing DNA fragments from invading bacteriophages and

Table 14.1. Antiviral mAbs acting against host factors in various viral infections. Reprinted from [13], copyright (2021) with permission from Elsevier.

Monoclonal antibodies	Host target	Viral infection
Anti-occludin, anti-claudin1 (CLDN1)	Entry receptors- claudin and occludin	HCV infection [45, 46]
Tocilizumab, sarilumab, siltuximab, sirukumab, clanakinumab, olokizumab, and levilimab	IL-6	SARS-CoV-2 [47]
Ly-CoV1404	Angiotensin-converting enzyme (ACE2) receptor of host cell	SARS-CoV-2 [48]
Oral anti-CD3 antibody	CD3 T-cell receptor	HCV infection [49]
Anti-SR-BI mAb	Human scavenger receptor class B, type I (SR-BI)	HCV infection [50]

incorporating them into the host genome, forming what is known as clustered, regularly interspaced short palindromic repeats (CRISPR) [51]. These viral DNA fragments are then transcribed into CRISPR RNAs (tracrRNAs), which help Cas proteins identify and destroy similar viral DNA during future infections. In plants and insects, RNAi mechanisms utilize double-stranded RNA produced during viral replication, which is then processed into short interfering RNAs (siRNAs) by the Dicer enzyme. These siRNAs guide the RNA-induced silencing complex (RISC) to direct the Argonaute protein (Ago2) to break down viral RNA [52, 53].

Therapeutic nucleic acids (TNAs) are emerging as a significant platform for drug discovery alongside small molecules and antibody-based therapies. They are highly specific, easy to design, and often require less development time than conventional therapies [54]. Because TNAs can target conserved viral sequences, they have the potential to combat multiple viral strains and reduce the risk of drug resistance. Current TNA approaches include antisense oligonucleotides (ASOs), CRISPR-Cas, and other gene-editing and regulatory tools like siRNAs, mRNAs, ribozymes, and aptamers [8]. These molecules work differently—some modulate gene expression via RNAi, others catalytically degrade target RNA, while others disrupt protein interactions by binding specific peptide regions [55]. Additionally, NA-based technology is used in vaccine development, where viral proteins encoded in TNAs serve as antigens to stimulate immune responses.

TNA therapies are being explored for various applications, including treating cancers, central nervous system disorders, and viral infections. Given the promise of NA-based therapies, there are many ongoing clinical trials, and as of now, ten NA-based drugs have received FDA approval [8, 56].

An ideal therapeutic approach might combine multiple NA-based drugs in a 'cocktail' to target one or several viral sequences, potentially enhancing their antiviral effectiveness [57]. Recently, targeting multiple sequences from swine enteric CoVs (SECoVs) and multiple virus types has shown promising results [58]. Such cocktails can also be designed to target both viral and host factors and used alongside other antiviral drugs, like nucleoside analogs (e.g., remdesivir, EIDD-2801), protease inhibitors (e.g., ritonavir/lopinavir), and cysteine protease inhibitors (e.g., MDL-28170, ONO 5334) [54]. This combined approach can improve therapeutic efficacy at lower doses, reducing side effects and lowering the risk of drug resistance through synergistic effects [54].

14.2.1 Nucleic acid-based vaccines

Nucleic acid (NA) vaccines are based on either DNA or RNA that encodes antigenic proteins from a specific pathogen. These vaccines use the host's own cellular machinery to produce disease-specific antigens, which then stimulate an immune response [59]. For DNA vaccines, the plasmids carrying the antigen-encoding genes are delivered into host cells, where they are transcribed in the nucleus under the guidance of eukaryotic promoters and translated into proteins in the cytoplasm [60]. On the other hand, mRNA vaccines are created by *in vitro* transcription from DNA templates encoding the antigen. Once these mRNAs are delivered into cells, they are directly translated into proteins in the cytoplasm to produce the target antigens [60]. In both cases, the proteins generated are processed and presented to the immune system, initiating a strong antibody (humoral) and T-cell response [61].

To improve the delivery and stability of mRNAs, they are typically encapsulated in carriers like lipid nanoparticles (LNPs) and administered via intramuscular injection. When these LNP-encased mRNAs enter host cells, the mRNAs are released and translated using the cell's protein synthesis machinery. Proteins produced from these mRNAs are then broken down into peptides, which associate with MHC class I molecules and are displayed on the surface of antigen-presenting cells. These peptide-MHC I complexes are recognized by CD8+ T cells, activating cellular immune responses (figure 14.1, [54]).

Extensive studies have shown that NA vaccines offer greater safety, tolerance, and potency than traditional vaccines. They can deliver multiple antigens in a single immunization and effectively trigger antibody and cellular immune responses [60, 62, 63]. Among NA vaccines, mRNA vaccines present several advantages over DNA vaccines, making them a more promising alternative [60]. Self-amplifying RNA (saRNA) vaccines, for instance, encode both the antigen and additional proteins, allowing for strong immune responses with much lower mRNA quantities [63].

Recently, a nucleoside-modified mRNA vaccine targeting multiple conserved influenza virus antigens was developed as a potential universal flu vaccine. In animal models, this multi-targeting mRNA vaccine triggered robust immune responses, protecting mice from a range of group 1 influenza A viruses [64].

For COVID-19, FDA-approved mRNA vaccines include Comirnaty (Pfizer-BioNTech COVID-19 Vaccine, mRNA, BioNTech Manufacturing GmbH), Pfizer-BioNTech COVID-19 Vaccine (Pfizer Inc.), Spikevax (Moderna COVID-19 Vaccine, mRNA, ModernaTX Inc.), and Moderna COVID-19 Vaccine (ModernaTX Inc.) (FDA).

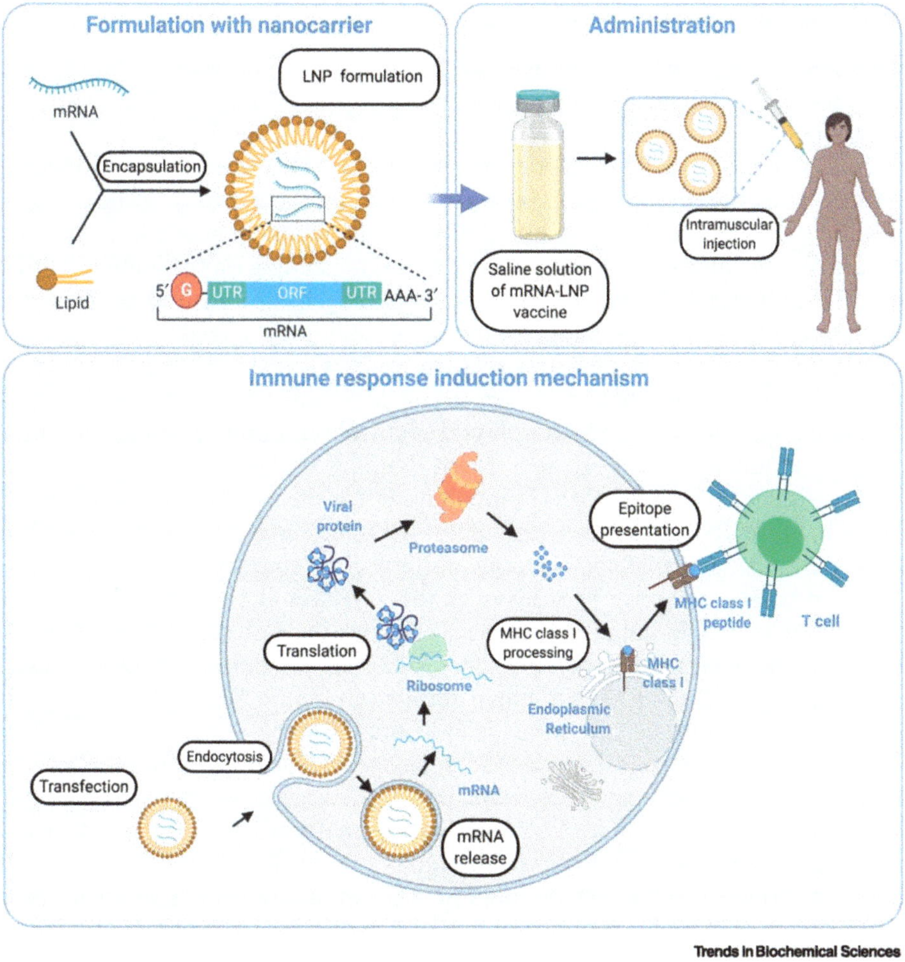

Figure 14.1. Basic mechanism of action of mRNA vaccines. Adapted from [54]. Copyright (2020) with permission from Elsevier.

14.3 Antibodies

14.3.1 Introduction

The deadly COVID-19 pandemic led to intense efforts to develop neutralizing mAbs that target severe acute respiratory syndrome coronavirus 2 (SARS-CoV-2) to treat and prevent COVID-19. As a result, more than 20 mAbs entered clinical development. So far, several of these mAbs have received emergency use authorization (EUA) from the FDA and other regulatory agencies worldwide [65]. The neutralizing activity of mAbs against coronaviruses in the development stage shows promise. As of now, in 2022, advances in vaccine research are booming, and vaccines can be used to develop mAbs against other viral infections.

14.3.2 Antibody structure and function

Antibodies (Abs), known as immunoglobulins, are natural proteins circulating in the blood and lymph. They are produced by plasma cells or memory B cells activated through infection or vaccination. Structurally, immunoglobulins are *Y*-shaped molecules made of two light chains, each about 25 kDa, and two heavy chains of at least 50 kDa, depending on the antibody's isotype. These chains are held together by multiple disulfide bridges and non-covalent interactions (figure 14.2), with slight variations in the number and type of connections depending on the immunoglobulin class. The Fab regions of antibodies bind to pathogens and neutralize them. Fabs are connected to the Fc (crystallizable fragment) region by a flexible hinge, allowing the Fabs to adopt various positions relative to the Fc and efficiently interact with antigens from any angle [65].

The glycosylated Fc region also plays a vital role in immune defense by linking pathogens to immune cells. It does so by binding to Fcγ receptors (FcγRs) on effector cells, which helps alert the immune system to the presence of pathogens. The expression of FcγRs varies across different types of immune cells, with each cell type and activation state displaying a unique pattern of receptors [65, 66].

IgG antibodies comprise two heavy chains (HCs) and two light chains (LCs), connected at a flexible hinge region that separates the Fab and Fc domains. The heavy chain is a larger polypeptide with four immunoglobulin domains: two in the Fab region (VH and CH1), a hinge, and two in the Fc region (CH2 and CH3). The light chain comprises two domains (VL and CL) [66].

Each antibody isotype is determined by the specific recombination of alpha, mu, gamma, epsilon, or delta gene segments, with the variable region playing a unique role in the immune response. The IgG isotype, particularly IgG1, is extensively studied because of its crucial role in immunity, especially in immunotherapeutics and viral defense [65]. IgG1 is the predominant antibody in human serum and is primarily responsible for protection against infections [65]. Most therapeutic

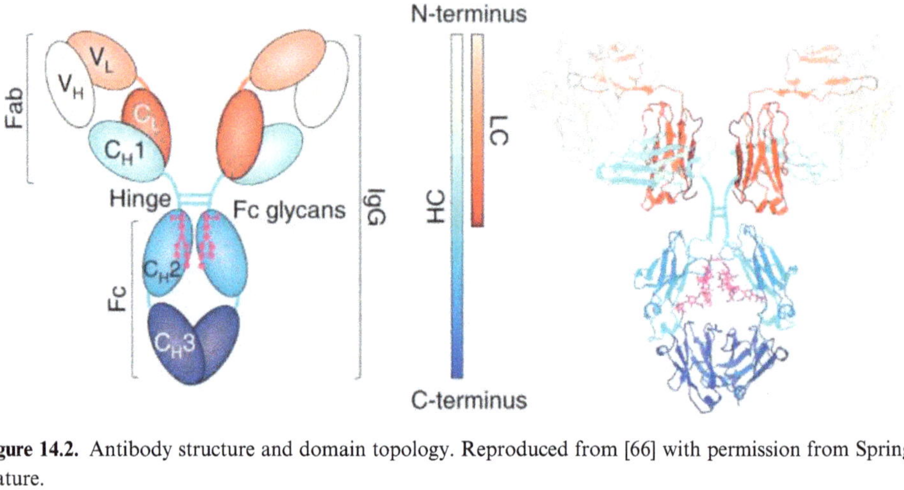

Figure 14.2. Antibody structure and domain topology. Reproduced from [66] with permission from Springer Nature.

monoclonal antibodies (mAbs) currently used or under development to treat infectious diseases are of the human IgG1 type, known for their ability to activate FcγRs and aid in infection control [65, 67].

14.3.3 Mechanisms by which antibodies combat various viral infections

Passive immunization with monoclonal or polyclonal antibodies has been essential in treating and preventing infectious diseases for decades. Antibodies can help by blocking viral glycoproteins in enveloped viruses or the protein shells in non-enveloped viruses from attaching to host cells [68, 69]. These viral proteins are essential for a virus's life cycle, either by binding to cellular receptors to enable fusion with cell membranes (in enveloped viruses) or by penetrating the cytosol (in non-enveloped viruses) [68, 69]. A good example is SARS-CoV-2, which enters host cells by interacting with its spike (S) glycoprotein and the ACE2 receptor on host cells [65].

Antibodies can also aid in fighting infections by engaging complement protein C1q or Fcγ receptors on immune cells [65]. This can activate the complement system, leading to the destruction of the virus or infected host cells. Additionally, antibodies can stimulate the release of cytokines and reactive oxygen species or enhance phagocytosis [65, 70].

Recently, there's been a growing focus on neutralizing monoclonal antibodies (mAbs) for passive immunization against infectious diseases. These mAbs are designed to be highly specific and effective, eliminating the risk of blood-borne infections. Thanks to established manufacturing processes, large-scale production of neutralizing mAbs is feasible within a reasonable timeframe [65].

14.4 Conclusion

By combining various treatments, researchers can create effective techniques to treat viral infections with lower side effects, more resilience against viral resistance, and higher efficacy. Understanding host proteins is crucial for viral entry or replication and can impact vaccine development. Vaccines can be designed to induce immune responses against these host proteins, preventing viral attachment or replication. Additionally, targeting host proteins alongside vaccination may enhance vaccine efficacy by modulating host responses to improve vaccine-induced immunity. Nucleic acid-based vaccines utilize genetic material to encode antigens from the target pathogen, typically a virus. These vaccines work by introducing the genetic material into the body, where cells then produce the antigen, stimulating an immune response. This approach offers advantages such as rapid development and potential scalability compared to traditional vaccine methods. In the context of viral infections, researchers may develop antibodies either as therapeutic agents or for use in diagnostic tests. Therapeutic antibodies can neutralize viruses by binding to specific viral proteins, preventing them from infecting cells or marking them for destruction by other immune cells. Each of these targets presents unique opportunities for developing interventions to combat viral infections, and often researchers explore combinations of these approaches to enhance effectiveness. In some cases, researchers may explore triple combination therapies involving host protein targeting, nucleic acid vaccines, and antibodies. This comprehensive approach aims to disrupt viral infection at multiple levels, including host–virus interactions, viral replication, and immune response modulation. Such therapies have the potential to achieve higher efficacy and reduce the likelihood of viral escape mutants. By integrating multiple approaches, researchers can develop robust strategies to combat viral infections with improved efficacy, reduced side effects, and enhanced resilience against viral resistance.

Abbreviations

Abs	Antibodies
ACE2	Angiotensin-converting enzyme
ADCVI	Antibody dependent, cell-mediated virus inhibition
Ago2	Argonaute protein 2
ASOs	Antisense oligonucleotides
CCR5	C-C chemokine receptor type 5
CD4	Cluster of differentiation 4
CLDN1	Anti-claudin1
CRISPR/Cas	Clustered regularly interspaced short palindromic repeats–CRISPR-associated protein
dsRNA	double-stranded RNA
EUA	Emergency use authorization
Fab	Antigen-binding fragment
Fc	Crystallizable fragment (Fc)
FcγRs	Fcy receptors
GCN2	General control nonderepressible 2 kinase
HC	Heavy chains
HCV	Hepatitis C virus
HRI	Heme-regulated eIF2α kinase
hVAP-33	Vesicle-associated membrane protein associated protein, 33-kDa human homologue
IgG	Ig gamma
LAMP1	Lysosomal-associated membrane protein 1
LNP	Lipid nanoparticle
mAbs	Monoclonal antibodies
MHC	Major histocompatibility complex
NTCP	Sodium taurocholate co-transporting polypeptide
NA	Nucleic acid
ORF	Open reading frame
PKR	Protein kinase R
PRF	Programmed ribosomal frameshifting
RdRp	RNA dependent RNA polymerase
RISC	RNA-induced silencing complex
RNAi	RNA interference
saRNA	Self-amplifying RNA
SARS-CoV-2	Severe acute respiratory syndrome coronavirus 2
SECoVs	Swine enteric CoVs

siRNAs	Short interfering RNAs
SR-BI	Human scavenger receptor class B, type I
TMEM175	Transmembrane protein 175
TNAs	Therapeutic nucleic acids
TracrRNAs	Trans-activating CRISPR RNAs
UPR	Unfolded protein response
UTR	Untranslated region

References

[1] Li G and De Clercq E 2021 Overview of antiviral drug discovery and development: viral versus host targets *Antiviral Discovery for Highly Pathogenic Emerging Viruses* ed C Muñoz-Fontela and R Delgado (London: The Royal Society of Chemistry) pp 1–27

[2] Fatma B, Kumar R, Singh V A, Nehul S, Sharma R, Kesari P *et al* 2020 Alphavirus capsid protease inhibitors as potential antiviral agents for Chikungunya infection *Antiviral Res* **179** 104808

[3] Mudgal R, Mahajan S and Tomar S 2020 Inhibition of Chikungunya virus by an adenosine analog targeting the SAM-dependent nsP1 methyltransferase *FEBS Lett.* **594** 678–94

[4] Dhindwal S, Kesari P, Singh H, Kumar P and Tomar S 2017 Conformer and pharmacophore based identification of peptidomimetic inhibitors of chikungunya virus nsP2 protease *J. Biomol. Struct. Dyn.* **35** 3522–39

[5] Tomar S and Aggarwal M 2017 Chapter 5—Structure and function of alphavirus proteases *Viral Proteases and their Inhibitors* ed S P Gupta (New York: Academic) pp 105–35 https://sciencedirect.com/science/article/pii/B9780128097120000058

[6] Kielian M, Chatterjee P K, Gibbons D L and Lu Y E 2000 Specific roles for lipids in virus fusion and exit. Examples from the alphaviruses *Subcell Biochem* **34** 409–55

[7] Su C, Hou Z, Zhang C, Tian Z and Zhang J 2011 Ectopic expression of microRNA-155 enhances innate antiviral immunity against HBV infection in human hepatoma cells *Virol J.* **8** 354

[8] Weng Y, Huang Q, Li C, Yang Y, Wang X, Yu J *et al* 2020 Improved nucleic acid therapy with advanced nanoscale biotechnology *Mol. Ther. Nucleic Acids* **19** 581–601

[9] Amaya M, Keck F, Lindquist M, Voss K, Scavone L, Kehn-Hall K *et al* 2015 The ubiquitin proteasome system plays a role in venezuelan equine encephalitis virus infection *PLoS One* **10** e0124792

[10] Yang N 2015 An overview of viral and nonviral delivery systems for microRNA *Int. J. Pharm. Investig.* **5** 179–81

[11] Sun X, Wang T, Cai D, Hu Z, Chen J, Liao H *et al* 2020 Cytokine storm intervention in the early stages of COVID-19 pneumonia *Cytokine Growth Factor Rev.* **53** 38–42

[12] Chang K C and Wen J D 2021 Programmed-1 ribosomal frameshifting from the perspective of the conformational dynamics of mRNA and ribosomes *Comput. Struct. Biotechnol. J.* **19** 3580–8

[13] Mahajan S, Choudhary S, Kumar P and Tomar S 2021 Antiviral strategies targeting host factors and mechanisms obliging +ssRNA viral pathogens *Bioorg. Med. Chem.* **46** 116356

[14] Kumar N, Sharma S, Kumar R, Tripathi B N, Barua S, Ly H *et al* 2020 Host-directed antiviral therapy *Clin. Microbiol. Rev.* **33** 00168-19

[15] Ketzinel-Gilad M, Shaul Y and Galun E 2006 RNA interference for antiviral therapy *J. Gene Med.* **8** 933–50

[16] Bean B 1992 Antiviral therapy: current concepts and practices *Clin. Microbiol. Rev.* **5** 146–82

[17] Woodhouse S D, Narayan R, Latham S, Lee S, Antrobus R, Gangadharan B *et al* 2010 Transcriptome sequencing, microarray, and proteomic analyses reveal cellular and metabolic impact of hepatitis C virus infection *in vitro Hepatology* **52** 443–53

[18] Deans R M, Morgens D W, Ökesli A, Pillay S, Horlbeck M A, Kampmann M *et al* 2016 Parallel shRNA and CRISPR-Cas9 screens enable antiviral drug target identification *Nat. Chem. Biol.* **12** 361–6

[19] Zhou R and Rana T M 2013 RNA-based mechanisms regulating host-virus interactions *Immunol. Rev.* **253** 97–111

[20] Perwitasari O, Bakre A, Tompkins S M and Tripp R A 2013 siRNA genome screening approaches to therapeutic drug repositioning *Pharmaceuticals (Basel)* **6** 124–60

[21] Perreira J M, Meraner P and Brass A L 2016 Functional genomic strategies for elucidating human-virus interactions: will CRISPR knockout RNAi and haploid cells? *Adv. Virus Res.* **94** 1–51

[22] Gao L, Aizaki H, He J W and Lai M M C 2004 Interactions between viral nonstructural proteins and host protein hVAP-33 mediate the formation of hepatitis C virus RNA replication complex on lipid raft *J. Virol.* **78** 3480–8

[23] Rottman J B, Ganley K P, Williams K, Wu L, Mackay C R and Ringler D J 1997 Cellular localization of the chemokine receptor CCR5. Correlation to cellular targets of HIV-1 infection *Am. J. Pathol.* **151** 1341–51

[24] Rajendran M, Krammer F and McMahon M 2021 The human antibody response to the influenza virus neuraminidase following infection or vaccination *Vaccines (Basel)* **9** 846

[25] Martín-Vicente M, González-Riaño C, Barbas C, Jiménez-Sousa M Á, Brochado-Kith O, Resino S *et al* 2020 Metabolic changes during respiratory syncytial virus infection of epithelial cells *PLoS One* **15** e0230844

[26] Keshavarz M, Solaymani-Mohammadi F, Namdari H, Arjeini Y, Mousavi M J and Rezaei F 2020 Metabolic host response and therapeutic approaches to influenza infection *Cell. Mol. Biol. Lett.* **25** 15

[27] Zhou Y, Pu J and Wu Y 2021 The role of lipid metabolism in influenza A virus infection *Pathogens* **10** 303

[28] Xu G G, Guo J and Wu Y 2014 Chemokine receptor CCR5 antagonist maraviroc: medicinal chemistry and clinical applications *Curr. Top. Med. Chem.* **14** 1504–14

[29] Nakata H, Maeda K, Das D, Chang S B, Matsuda K, Rao K V *et al* 2019 Activity and structural analysis of GRL-117C: a novel small molecule CCR5 inhibitor active against R5-tropic HIV-1s *Sci. Rep.* **9** 4828

[30] Grande F, Occhiuzzi M A, Rizzuti B, Ioele G, De Luca M, Tucci P *et al* 2019 CCR5/CXCR4 dual antagonism for the improvement of HIV infection therapy *Molecules* **24** 550

[31] Bettiker R L, Koren D E and Jacobson J M 2018 Ibalizumab *Curr. Opin. HIV AIDS* **13** 354–8

[32] Meanwell N A, Krystal M R, Nowicka-Sans B, Langley D R, Conlon D A, Eastgate M D *et al* 2018 Inhibitors of HIV-1 attachment: the discovery and development of Temsavir and its prodrug Fostemsavir *J. Med. Chem.* **61** 62–80

[33] Yu Y, Li S and Liang W 2018 Bona fide receptor for hepatitis B and D viral infections: Mechanism, research models and molecular drug targets *Emerg. Microbes Infect.* **7** 134

[34] Fukano K, Tsukuda S, Watashi K and Wakita T 2019 Concept of viral inhibitors via NTCP *Semin. Liver Dis.* **39** 78–85

[35] Li J and Pfeffer S R 2016 Lysosomal membrane glycoproteins bind cholesterol and contribute to lysosomal cholesterol export *eLife* **5** e21635

[36] Zhang J, Zeng W, Han Y, Lee W R, Liou J and Jiang Y 2023 Lysosomal LAMP proteins regulate lysosomal pH by direct inhibition of the TMEM175 channel *Mol. Cell.* **83** 2524–39.e7

[37] Hulseberg C E, Fénéant L, Szymańska K M and White J M 2018 Lamp1 increases the efficiency of lassa virus infection by promoting fusion in less acidic endosomal compartments *mBio* **9** e01818-17

[38] Yang X, Dickmander R J, Bayati A, Taft-Benz S A, Smith J L, Wells C I *et al* 2022 Host kinase CSNK2 is a target for inhibition of pathogenic SARS-like β-coronaviruses *ACS Chem. Biol.* **17** 1937–50

[39] Dey S and Mondal A 2024 Unveiling the role of host kinases at different steps of influenza A virus life cycle *J. Virol.* **98** e01192-23

[40] Liu Y, Wang M, Cheng A, Yang Q, Wu Y, Jia R *et al* 2020 The role of host eIF2α in viral infection *Virol. J.* **17** 112

[41] Cameron C E, Raney K D and Götte M 2009 *Viral Genome Replication* (New York: Springer) pp 1–636

[42] Choi K H 2012 Viral polymerases *Adv. Exp. Med. Biol.* **726** 267–304

[43] Vlahava V M, Murrell I, Zhuang L, Aicheler R J, Lim E, Miners K L *et al* 2021 Monoclonal antibodies targeting nonstructural viral antigens can activate ADCC against human cytomegalovirus *J. Clin. Invest.* **131** e139296

[44] Pelegrin M, Naranjo-Gomez M and Piechaczyk M 2015 Antiviral monoclonal antibodies: can they be more than simple neutralizing agents? *Trends Microbiol.* **23** 653–65

[45] Fukasawa M, Nagase S, Shirasago Y, Iida M, Yamashita M, Endo K *et al* 2015 Monoclonal antibodies against extracellular domains of claudin-1 block hepatitis C virus infection in a mouse model *J. Virol.* **89** 4866–79

[46] Harris H J, Davis C, Mullins J G L, Hu K, Goodall M, Farquhar M J *et al* 2010 Claudin association with CD81 defines hepatitis C virus entry *J. Biol. Chem.* **285** 21092–102

[47] Patel S, Saxena B and Mehta P 2021 Recent updates in the clinical trials of therapeutic monoclonal antibodies targeting cytokine storm for the management of COVID-19 *Heliyon* **7** e06158

[48] Westendorf K, Žentelis S, Wang L, Foster D, Vaillancourt P, Wiggin M *et al* 2022 LY-CoV1404 (bebtelovimab) potently neutralizes SARS-CoV-2 variants *Cell Rep.* **39** 110812

[49] Ilan Y, Shailubhai K and Sanyal A 2018 Immunotherapy with oral administration of humanized anti-CD3 monoclonal antibody: a novel gut-immune system-based therapy for metaflammation and NASH *Clin. Exp. Immunol.* **193** 275–83

[50] Vercauteren K, Van Den Eede N, Mesalam A A, Belouzard S, Catanese M T, Bankwitz D *et al* 2014 Successful anti-scavenger receptor class B type I (SR-BI) monoclonal antibody therapy in humanized mice after challenge with HCV variants with *in vitro* resistance to SR-BI-targeting agents *Hepatology* **60** 1508–18

[51] Horvath P and Barrangou R 2010 CRISPR/Cas, the immune system of bacteria and archaea *Science* **327** 167–70

[52] Guo Z, Li Y and Ding S W 2019 Small RNA-based antimicrobial immunity *Nat. Rev. Immunol.* **19** 31–44

[53] Gao G F 2021 ERASE: a novel nucleic-acid based antiviral mechanism *Cell Res* **31** 1142–3

[54] Paris T K, Khan C, Robson K S, Ng F and Rocchi W L 2021 Nucleic acid-based technologies targeting coronaviruses *Trends Biochem. Sci.* **46** 351–65

[55] Asha K, Kumar P, Sanicas M, Meseko C A, Khanna M and Kumar B 2018 Advancements in nucleic acid based therapeutics against respiratory viral infections *J. Clin. Med.* **8** 6

[56] Roberts T C, Langer R and Wood M J A 2020 Advances in oligonucleotide drug delivery *Nat. Rev. Drug Discov.* **19** 673–94

[57] Qureshi A, Tantray V G, Kirmani A R and Ahangar A G 2018 A review on current status of antiviral siRNA *Rev. Med. Virol.* **28** e1976

[58] Li K, Li H, Bi Z, Song D, Zhang F, Lei D *et al* 2019 Significant inhibition of re-emerged and emerging swine enteric coronavirus *in vitro* using the multiple shRNA expression vector *Antiviral Res.* **166** 11–8

[59] Hadj Hassine I 2022 Covid-19 vaccines and variants of concern: a review *Rev. Med. Virol.* **32** e2313

[60] Faghfuri E, Pourfarzi F, Faghfouri A H, Abdoli Shadbad M, Hajiasgharzadeh K and Baradaran B 2021 Recent developments of RNA-based vaccines in cancer immunotherapy *Expert Opin. Biol. Ther.* **21** 201–18

[61] Yi C, Yi Y and Li J 2020 mRNA vaccines: possible tools to combat SARS-CoV-2 *Virol. Sin.* **35** 259–62

[62] Zhang C, Maruggi G, Shan H and Li J 2019 Advances in mRNA vaccines for infectious diseases *Front. Immunol.* **10** 594

[63] Vogel A B, Lambert L, Kinnear E, Busse D, Erbar S, Reuter K C *et al* 2018 Self-amplifying RNA vaccines give equivalent protection against influenza to mRNA vaccines but at much lower doses *Mol. Ther.* **26** 446–55

[64] Freyn A W, Ramos da Silva J, Rosado V C, Bliss C M, Pine M, Mui B L *et al* 2020 A multi-targeting, nucleoside-modified mrna influenza virus vaccine provides broad protection in mice *Mol. Ther.* **28** 1569–84

[65] Pantaleo G, Correia B, Fenwick C, Joo V S and Perez L 2022 Antibodies to combat viral infections: development strategies and progress *Nat. Rev. Drug Discov.* **21** 676–96

[66] Murin C D, Wilson I A and Ward A B 2019 Antibody responses to viral infections: a structural perspective across three different enveloped viruses *Nat. Microbiol.* **4** 734–47

[67] Bournazos S, Corti D, Virgin H W and Ravetch J V 2020 Fc-optimized antibodies elicit CD8 immunity to viral respiratory infection *Nature* **588** 485–90

[68] Kabanova A, Perez L, Lilleri D, Marcandalli J, Agatic G, Becattini S *et al* 2014 Antibody-driven design of a human cytomegalovirus gHgLpUL128L subunit vaccine that selectively elicits potent neutralizing antibodies *Proc. Natl Acad. Sci. USA* **111** 17965–70

[69] Zheng Q, Jiang J, He M, Zheng Z, Yu H, Li T *et al* 2019 Viral neutralization by antibody-imposed physical disruption *Proc. Natl Acad. Sci. USA* **116** 26933–40

[70] Lu L L, Suscovich T J, Fortune S M and Alter G 2018 Beyond binding: antibody effector functions in infectious diseases *Nat. Rev. Immunol.* **18** 46–61

Chapter 15

Pathophysiology of coronavirus disease 2019 (COVID-19)

Rajkishor Pandey, Arvind K Singh Chandel and Simran Sharma

This chapter provides an in-depth exploration of the pathophysiology of coronavirus disease 2019 (COVID-19), focusing on the intricate biological mechanisms of infection induced by severe acute respiratory syndrome coronavirus-2 (SARS-CoV-2). The discussion begins with an analysis of the virus's structural characteristics, its genetic adaptability, and the critical role of the spike protein in facilitating host cell entry through ACE2 receptors. It extends to the virus's ability to affect multiple organ systems, including the respiratory, cardiovascular, endocrine, and gastrointestinal systems, leading to a wide array of clinical manifestations. The chapter emphasizes the disruption of the renin–angiotensin system and the consequent metabolic and functional abnormalities in affected organs. Additionally, it examines the long-term repercussions of the virus, particularly post-acute sequelae of COVID-19 (long COVID), which involves persistent neurological, cardiovascular, and respiratory complications. The chapter also considers the evolution of SARS-CoV-2, highlighting the emergence of variants of concern and their public health implications. Through a comprehensive review of both acute and chronic effects, this chapter underscores the complexity of COVID-19 pathogenesis, offering valuable insights for developing effective diagnostic, therapeutic, and preventive strategies to combat the ongoing global health crisis.

15.1 Introduction

The coronavirus disease 2019 (COVID-19) pandemic started in Wuhan, China, in 2020 and spread worldwide. It was declared a pandemic by the WHO. COVID-19 is the most disastrous disease of the 21st century. It is a highly infectious viral disease caused by severe acute respiratory syndrome coronavirus-2 (SARS-CoV2). The recent report by WHO stated that there were more than 765 million confirmed cases in May 2023 and over 6.9 million globally recorded deaths [1, 2]. The literature noted that viruses are acellular pathogenic particles made up of nucleic acid (DNA or RNA)

doi:10.1088/978-0-7503-4987-1ch15

covered by a protective capsid and outermost lipid or carbohydrate sheath layer. Genetic structure and genome size give pathogenic versatility in the host environment. Similarly, coronaviruses (CoVs) are enveloped positive-single-stranded RNA (+ssRNA) viruses having unusually large (~30 kb) positive-sense RNA genomes with a 5′-cap structure and 3′-poly-A tail. The virus's outer envelope is covered with multiple spikes proteins (glycoproteins) that give a crown-like appearance. Therefore, Coronaviruses are given their name, where 'corona' means 'crown' [3].

It was reported that viruses are non-living acellular virion particles without cellular repair mechanisms to correct their wrong genomic sequences after each generation. Like other viruses, SARS-CoV-2 is also prone to changes in its nucleotide sequences (mutation) after each multiplication in new host cells. The resulting mutation forms different variants which might have different characteristics than the ancestral strain [4]. Several variants of SARS-CoV-2 have been observed during the pandemic courses, but only a few impact public health. According to the recent WHO report, the five most potent variants of concern are shown in table 15.1 [5]:

SARS-CoV2 primarily targets the epithelial cells of the human lungs. However, it can spread to other organs such as the lung, heart, digestive system, oral cavity, endocrine system, and brain (figures 15.1(A) and (B)) through blood circulation and

Table 15.1. Variants of concern of SARS-CoV-2. Data was taken from [5].

S. No.	WHO label	Pango lineage	Name of country origin and year
1	Alpha	B. 1. 1. 7	United Kingdom, Sep. 2020
2	Beta	B. 1. 351	South Africa, May. 2020
3	Gamma	P.1	Brazil, Nov. 2020
4	Delta	B. 1. 617. 2	India, Oct. 2020
5	Omicron	B. 1. 1. 529	Multiple countries, Nov. 2021

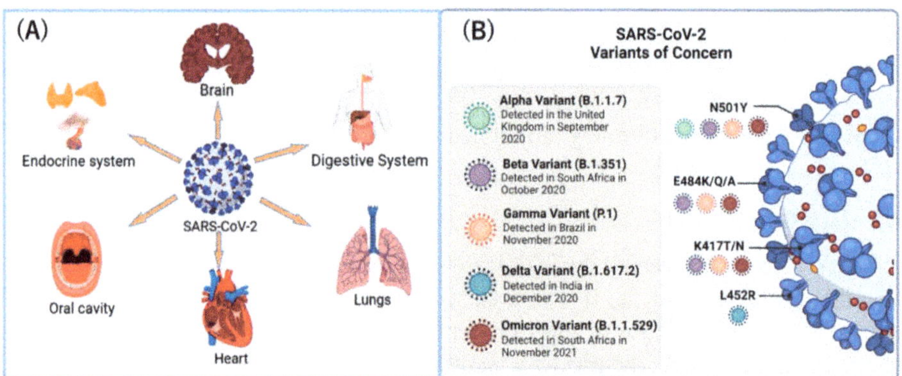

Figure 15.1. (A) SARS-Cov2 infection affecting different human body organs. (B) Currently circulating SARS-CoV-2 variants of concern and their receptor binding domain (RBD) amino acid substitutions of interest to virulence and immune evasion, adopted from Frontiers 2012 [6], CC BY 4.0.

affect their functions. At the expression level of ACE and other virus-compatible receptors, each organ affected by the virus showed multiple metabolic changes and abnormalities.

15.1.1 Biology of SARS-CoV-2

As per the literature, coronavirus is a group of viruses, and SARS-CoV-2 is the most infectious virus in this group. The virus transfer occurs from an infected person to a healthy person by coughing, sneezing, speaking, and breathing in respiratory droplets. The virus particles adhere on the surface of respiratory epithelial tissue, and like other viruses, coronavirus also depends on host cells for their proliferation and release of progeny. Stages of coronavirus multiplication and growth include attachment and entry to the host cells, the release of genetic material, replication, gene synthesis of viral genomic materials, translation of genes, arrangement, and release of new virus particles [7].

As noted, the SARS-CoV-2 strain is the leading cause of the COVID-19 pandemic. It is an RNA virus belonging to the Coronaviridae family. The SARS-CoV-2 genome contains 14 open reading frames (ORFs), including 27 proteins that reside at both the genome's 5′ and 3′ ends. The 5′ end of the SARS-CoV-2 genome ORF contains polyproteins, including replicase and transcriptase complex (RTC), which are involved in the virus's replication machinery. On the other side, the 3′ end of the viral genome contains ORFs encoding the four core structural proteins, namely spike (S), envelope (E), membrane (M), and nucleocapsid (N), as well as other putative additional protein factors [7, 8].

It is well established that SARS-CoV-2 enters the host cell by binding spike protein to host cell receptors. Spike glycoprotein (S) is the virus's outermost protein, which binds with host cells' angiotensin-converting enzyme 2 (ACE2) receptors. The S protein targets host immune cells, immunoglobulins, and many antiviral drugs and vaccines for viral entry inhibition. The host cell protease cleaves the S protein into S1 and S2 subunits where S1 is involved in attachment and S2 shows a fusion of protein with ACE2 receptor [8, 9]. After the triumphant entry of the virus into the host cells, The E and M proteins regulate the release of the viral genome into the host cell cytoplasm and localization to other organelles such as the endoplasmic reticulum (ER) and Golgi body of cell for their gene transcription and translation [10].

15.1.2 Pathophysiology of COVID-19

15.1.2.1 The renin-angiotensin system

The renin-angiotensin system (RAS) is a hormone system that regulates blood pressure and fluid balance in the body. It comprises a series of steps that lead to the production of the hormone angiotensin II, which constricts blood vessels and increases blood pressure [11]. The process begins when the kidneys detect low blood pressure or low blood volume, releasing the enzyme renin into the bloodstream. Renin cleaves a protein called angiotensinogen, produced by the liver, to produce angiotensin I. Angiotensin I is then converted into angiotensin II by the action of an enzyme called angiotensin-converting enzyme (ACE), primarily found in the lungs. Angiotensin II acts on various target tissues in the body, including the blood vessels, adrenal glands, and brain, to increase blood pressure and fluid retention. It constricts blood vessels, increasing blood flow resistance and raising blood pressure. It also stimulates the adrenal glands to produce the hormone aldosterone, which promotes sodium and water retention in the body, further increasing blood volume and blood pressure [11, 12]. The RAS plays a vital role in regulating blood pressure and fluid balance, and dysfunction in the system can contribute to conditions such as hypertension, heart failure, and kidney disease. Drugs that target the RAS, such as ACE inhibitors and angiotensin receptor blockers, are commonly used to treat hypertension and other related conditions. It has been proved that ACE2 receptors are crucial for virus binding to host cells and entering into the cells. SARS-CoV2 spikes protein decrease the expression of ACE2 receptors and increase the expression of ABR-I. The reduced expression of ACE2 causes severe acute respiratory failure [12].

15.1.2.2 Impact of SARS-Cov-2 on the respiratory system

Severe acute respiratory syndrome coronavirus-2 (SARS-CoV-2) viruses are the primary causative agent of the COVID-19 pandemic, a respiratory illness affecting the respiratory system. The virus primarily spreads through respiratory droplets of the infected person to healthy person when they talk, cough, or sneeze. The primary symptoms of COVID-19 are fever, dry cough, and shortness of breath. However, the virus can affect different individuals in different ways, ranging from no symptoms to mild-to-severe respiratory distress and ultimately death [13]. Here are some of the effects of COVID-19 on the respiratory system:

A. **Inflammation of the airways:** COVID-19 can cause inflammation, leading to difficulty in breathing, coughing, and wheezing. This inflammation can damage the lining of the airways, making it more difficult for oxygen to enter the body and carbon dioxide to leave [13, 14].
B. **Pneumonia:** COVID-19 can cause pneumonia, an infection of the lungs that can cause fever, cough, chest pain, and difficulty breathing. In severe cases, pneumonia can cause lung damage and respiratory failure. Acute respiratory distress syndrome (ARDS) is a severe lung condition that can occur in some people with COVID-19. Rapid breathing, low oxygen levels, and lung fluid buildup characterize ARDS. It can lead to respiratory failure and the need for mechanical ventilation [15].
C. **Blood clots:** Microclots and resistance to fibrinolysis (compared to plasma from controls) were found in the plasma samples of acute COVID-19 and long COVID (post-acute sequelae of COVID-19) patients. These microclots might block the blood vessels in the lungs and cause a condition called pulmonary embolism, which can cause shortness of breath and chest pain [16].
D. **Long-term effects:** Long COVID is a condition often encompassing severe symptoms that follow a SARS-CoV-2 infection. It occurs in approximately 10% of SARS-CoV-2 infections. More than 200 long COVID symptoms have been recognized, with effects on multiple organs, including the lungs, heart, pancreas, liver, immune system, kidney, spleen, gastrointestinal tract, nervous system, reproductive system, and blood vessels. At least 65 million individuals worldwide are estimated to have COVID, with cases increasing daily [17].

Overall, COVID-19 can significantly impact the respiratory system, causing inflammation, pneumonia, ARDS, blood clots, and long-term respiratory symptoms. It is important to take steps to prevent the spread of COVID-19, such as wearing a mask, washing your hands regularly, and practicing physical distancing. If you develop respiratory symptoms, it is important to seek medical attention.

15.1.2.3 SARS-Cov-2 impact on the cardiovascular system

SARS-CoV-2 primarily affects the respiratory organ tissue and damages the lungs' alveoli, but it can also significantly affect the cardiovascular system. SARS-CoV-2 in the cardiac tissue has been reported to be directly associated with cardiac pathology. The higher expression of cardiac markers such as troponins, myoglobin, C-reactive protein, interleukins, and natriuretic peptides potentiate cardiac complications, including myocardial injury, ventricular dysfunction, and heart failure observed after COVID-19 infection [18]. Acute myocarditis (inflammation of the heart muscle) and Thromboembolic events (blood clots) also contribute to heart complications and heart failure after COVID-19 infection [19]. Additionally, SARS-CoV-2 invaded heart cells through different putative mechanisms such as changes in transcriptional factors in heart tissue, complement-mediated cascade activation and generation of coagulopathy, suppression of ACE2 receptors, dysregulation of the renin-angiotensin-aldosterone system, the release of a higher amount of pro-inflammatory cytokines, and activation of TGF-β signaling pathway [20].

It is important to note that not all COVID-19 patients will experience cardiovascular complications. However, those with underlying cardiovascular disease or risk factors are more likely to develop these complications. Healthcare providers should be aware of the potential cardiovascular effects of COVID-19 and monitor patients for these complications.

15.1.2.4 Impact of SARS-Cov-2 infection on the endocrine system

SARS-CoV-2 interacts with many organ tissues of the human body, including the endocrine system, which modulates the secretion of hormones and plays a crucial role in many biological functions. It has been reported that SARS-CoV-2 regulates endocrine glands such as the pituitary, adrenal, and thyroid glands, affecting glucose and mineral metabolism. The coronavirus targets the central nervous system (CNS) through the entry receptors ACE2 and cellular serine protease-TMPRSS2 receptors, which are also expressed in the hypothalamic-pituitary axis. Determination of the SARS-CoV-2 virus in the cerebrospinal fluid and autopsy studies of virus-infected patients revealed the presence of the virus in the hypothalamus of the brain [21].

The thyroid gland secretes another metabolic regulatory hormone, the thyroid (T3 and T4). The ACE2 receptors are expressed in the thyroid's follicular cells. SARS-Cov-2 has been found to affect thyroid function directly and indirectly. In some cases, T3 and T4 levels were reported to be lowered in SARS-CoV-2 infected patients [22, 23].

The research studies established that adults with diabetes mellitus, obesity, and hypertension are more prone to the infection of SARS-CoV-2 and associated complications and death [24]. SARS-CoV-2 affects male gonads more than female gonads. The literature reported that ACE2 and TMPRSS2 are expressed in spermatogonia and somatic cells of the testis (Leydig and Sertoli). Germ cell destruction, reduced sperm count, and lymphocytic infiltration in Sertoli and Leydig cells were reported in corona-infected patient autopsies. A semen sample of COVID-19 infected patients showed virus presence, but its role in male infertility is still under evaluation [25]. The ACE2 receptors are found in the ovary of female gonads, but TMPRSS2 is absent [26].

15.1.2.5 SARS-CoV-2 impact on the digestive system

The digestive system is a complex network of organs responsible for breaking down food, absorbing nutrients, and eliminating waste. COVID-19 primarily affects the respiratory system but can also impact the digestive system. Respiratory symptoms such as acute respiratory distress, lung cell injury, and organ failure are the leading cause of COVID-19 death. The literature reported that 20%–50% of patients with COVID-19 experienced the most common gastrointestinal (GI) symptoms, such as loss of appetite, abdominal pain, vomiting, and diarrhea [27]. The SARS-Cov-2 was isolated from the stool sample of COVID-19 infected patients, raising questions about other transmission modes [28]. It has been observed that SARS-Cov-2 enters into host cells mediated by the binding of angiotensin-converting enzyme 2 (ACE2) and transmembrane serine protease (TMPRSS2) receptors, which are expressed in pulmonary alveolar epithelial lung cells. However, both receptors are abundantly expressed in the intestinal epithelial cells [29].

An increasing number of COVID-19 studies showed that SARS-Cov-2 facilitates liver dysfunction. A higher impact of COVID-19 on the liver has been reported in severe and critically ill patients than in mildly affected patients. It has been found that the measurement of elevated levels of aspartate amino transaminase (AST), glutamate moderately amino transaminase (ALT), and total bilirubin (TBil) helps in determining the harmful impact of COVID-19 on the liver [30]. Additionally, it has been observed that patients with mild and moderate malnutrition conditions are more prone to COVID-19 [31]. Gastrointestinal dysfunction affects the observation of nutrition, leading to malnutrition. In COVID-19 patients, it has been observed that albumin levels decrease, which is positively correlated with COVID-19 infection [32].

15.1.2.6 Effects of SARS-Cov-2 on the central nervous system

COVID-19 is primarily a respiratory illness caused by the SARS-CoV-2 virus, but it can also affect other parts of the body, including the CNS. The CNS comprises the brain and spinal cord, and its involvement in COVID-19 can lead to various neurological symptoms and complications. Studies have shown that COVID-19 can cause inflammation and damage to the brain and other parts of the CNS. The virus can enter the brain through the olfactory nerve or by crossing the blood–brain barrier, a protective barrier that usually prevents harmful substances from entering the brain. SARS-Cov-2 infected patient's data revealed that the virus interacts with brain tissues and generates mild-to-moderate neurological symptoms, including headache, confusion, loss of memory, loss of smell and taste, depression, brain inflammation, encephalopathy, and stroke [33].

The cerebrospinal fluid (CSF) of acute COVID-19-infected living patients showed neuroinflammation and neuroimmune response. The CSF showed upregulation of interferon-regulated genes and activated T cells and NK cells [34, 35]. Additionally, infiltration of macrophages, CD8+ T lymphocytes, and activation of microglial cells in the entire section of the brain has been reported in autopsy studies of patients with acute COVID-19 [36].

Overall, COVID-19 can have significant effects on the CNS, leading to a range of neurological symptoms and complications. It is essential to continue studying the long-term impact of COVID-19 on the CNS and develop appropriate treatment strategies. While the effects of COVID-19 on the CNS are still being investigated, it is clear that the virus can cause neurological symptoms in some patients, and this should be taken into consideration when evaluating and treating patients with COVID-19.

15.1.2.7 SARS-Cov-2 effects on the oral cavity and dental complication
The COVID-19 virus primarily affects the respiratory system, but it can also have implications for oral health. However, maintaining good oral hygiene and seeking prompt treatment for any dental issues can help prevent complications. COVID-19 patients can experience dry mouth due to dehydration or side effects of medications used to treat the virus. This can increase the risk of cavities, gum disease, and other oral health issues. Some COVID-19 patients may develop oral lesions, such as ulcers, blisters, or white patches on the tongue or inside the cheeks. These lesions may be related to the virus or the body's immune response to the infection [37]. COVID-19 can weaken the immune system, making it easier for bacteria to thrive in the mouth. This can lead to inflammation of the gums (gingivitis) or more severe gum disease (periodontitis). Loss of taste and smell is a common symptom of COVID-19 infection. This can affect the patient's ability to taste and smell food, leading to poor nutrition and dehydration [38].

Abbreviations

ARDS	Acute respiratory distress syndrome
ACE2	Angiotensin-converting enzyme 2
COVID-19	Coronavirus disease 2019
CSF	Cerebrospinal fluid
DNA	Deoxyribonucleic acid
E	Envelope
ER	Endoplasmic reticulum
M	Membrane
N	Nucleocapsid
ORF	Open reading frames
RAS	Renin-angiotensin system
RTC	Replicase and transcriptase complex
RNA	Ribonucleic acid

S	Spike
SARS-CoV-2	Severe acute respiratory syndrome coronavirus-2
ssRNA	single-stranded RNA
TMPRSS2	Transmembrane serine protease
WHO	World Health Organization

References

[1] WHO 2023 *Weekly Epidemiological Update on COVID-19* https://who.int/publications/m/item/weekly-epidemiological-update-on-covid-19---13-april-2023

[2] Wong M C-S, Huang J, Wong Y-Y, Wong G L-H, Yip T C-F, Chan R N-Y, Chau S W-H, Ng S-C, Wing Y-K and Chan F K-L 2023 Epidemiology, symptomatology, and risk factors for long COVID symptoms: population-based, multicenter study *JMIR Public Health Surveill.* **9** e42315

[3] Yang Y, Xiao Z, Ye K, He X, Sun B, Qin Z, Yu J *et al* 2020 SARS-CoV-2: characteristics and current advances in research *Virol. J.* **17** 1–17

[4] Cascella M, Rajnik M, Aleem A, Dulebohn S and Di Napoli R 2023 Features, evaluation, and treatment of coronavirus (COVID-19) *StatPearls*

[5] WHO *Tracking SARS-CoV-2 Variants* https://who.int/activities/tracking-SARS-CoV-2-variants

[6] Mistry P, Barmania F, Mellet J, Peta K, Strydom A, Viljoen I M, James W, Gordon S and Pepper M S SARS-CoV-2 variants, vaccines, and host immunity *Front. Immunol.* **12** 809244

[7] Wang M-Y, Zhao R, Gao L-J, Gao X-F, Wang D-P and Cao J-M 2020 SARS-CoV-2: structure, biology, and structure-based therapeutics development *Front. Cell. Infect. Microbiol.* **10** 587269

[8] Satarker S and Nampoothiri M 2020 Structural proteins in severe acute respiratory syndrome coronavirus-2 *Arch. Med. Res.* **51** 482–91

[9] Yan W, Zheng Y, Zeng X, He B and Cheng W 2022 Structural biology of SARS-CoV-2: open the door for novel therapies *Signal Transduct. Targeted Therapy* **7** 26

[10] Mariano G, Farthing R J, Lale-Farjat S L M and Bergeron J R C 2020 Structural characterization of SARS-CoV-2: where we are, and where we need to be *Front. Mol. Biosci.* **7** 605236

[11] Fountain J H, Kaur J and Lappin S L 2023 Physiology, renin angiotensin system *StatPearls* (StatPearls Publishing)

[12] El-Arif G, Farhat A, Khazaal S, Annweiler C, Kovacic H, Wu Y, Cao Z, Fajloun Z, Khattar Z A and Sabatier J M 2021 The renin-angiotensin system: a key role in SARS-CoV-2-induced COVID-19 *Molecules* **26** 6945

[13] Lamers M M and Haagmans B L 2022 SARS-CoV-2 pathogenesis *Nat. Rev. Microbiol.* **20** 270–84

[14] Zhao F, Ma Q, Yue Q and Chen H 2022 SARS-CoV-2 infection and lung regeneration *Clin. Microbiol. Rev.* **35** e00188–21

[15] Menezes M C S, Pestana D V S, Gameiro G R, da Silva L F F, Baron Ė, Rouby J-J and Auler Jr J O C 2021 SARS-CoV-2 pneumonia—receptor binding and lung immunopathology: a narrative review *Critical Care* **25** 1–13

[16] Pretorius E, Vlok M, Venter C, Bezuidenhout J A, Laubscher G J, Steenkamp J and Kell D B 2021 Persistent clotting protein pathology in Long COVID/post-acute sequelae of

COVID-19 (PASC) is accompanied by increased levels of antiplasmin *Cardiovasc. Diabetol.* **20** 1–18
[17] Davis H E, McCorkell L, Vogel J M and Topol E J 2023 Long COVID: major findings, mechanisms and recommendations *Nat. Rev. Microbiol.* **21** 133–46
[18] Zhu J-Y, Wang G, Huang X, Lee H, Lee J-G, Yang P, van de Leemput J *et al* 2022 SARS-CoV-2 Nsp6 damages Drosophila heart and mouse cardiomyocytes through MGA/MAX complex-mediated increased glycolysis *Commun. Biol.* **5** 1039
[19] Jone P-N, John A, Oster M E, Allen K, Tremoulet A H, Saarel E V, Lambert L M, Miyamoto S D and De Ferranti S DAmerican Heart Association Leadership Committee and Congenital Cardiac Defects Committee of the Council on Lifelong Congenital Heart Disease and Heart Health in the Young; Council on Hypertension, and Council on Peripheral Vascular Disease 2022 SARS-CoV-2 infection and associated cardiovascular manifestations and complications in children and young adults: a scientific statement from the American Heart Association *Circulation* **145** e1037–52
[20] Xie Y, Xu E, Bowe B and Al-Aly Z 2022 Long-term cardiovascular outcomes of COVID-19 *Nat. Med.* **28** 583–90
[21] Zhou L, Zhang M, Wang J and Gao J 2020 Sars-Cov-2: underestimated damage to nervous system *Travel Med. Infect. Dis.* **36** 101642
[22] Scappaticcio L, Pitoia F, Esposito K, Piccardo A and Trimboli P 2020 Impact of COVID-19 on the thyroid gland: an update *Rev. Endocr. Metab. Disorders* **22** 803–15
[23] Çabuk S A, Cevher A Z and Küçükardalı Y 2022 Thyroid function during and after COVID-19 infection: a review *Touch Rev. Endocrinol.* **18** 58
[24] Miller R, Ashraf A P, Gourgari E, Gupta A, Kamboj M K, Kohn B, Lahoti A *et al* 2021 SARS-CoV-2 infection and paediatric endocrine disorders: risks and management considerations *Endocrinol., Diab. Metab.* **4** e00262
[25] Yang M, Chen S, Huang B O, Zhong J-M, Su H, Chen Y-J, Cao Q *et al* 2020 Pathological findings in the testes of COVID-19 patients: clinical implications *Eur. Urol. Focus* **6** 1124–9
[26] Soldevila B, Puig-Domingo M and Marazuela M 2021 Basic mechanisms of SARS-CoV-2 infection. What endocrine systems could be implicated? *Rev. Endocrine Metab. Disord.* **23** 137–50
[27] Lin L, Jiang X, Zhang Z, Huang S, Zhang Z, Fang Z, Gu Z *et al* 2020 Gastrointestinal symptoms of 95 cases with SARS-CoV-2 infection *Gut* **69** 997–1001
[28] Zhou J, Li C, Liu X, Chiu M C, Zhao X, Wang D, Wei Y *et al* 2020 Infection of bat and human intestinal organoids by SARS-CoV-2 *Nat. Med.* **26** 1077–83
[29] Jiao L, Li H, Xu J, Yang M, Ma C, Li J, Zhao S *et al* 2021 The gastrointestinal tract is an alternative route for SARS-CoV-2 infection in a nonhuman primate model *Gastroenterology* **160** 1647–61
[30] Zhang C, Shi L and Wang F-S 2020 Liver injury in COVID-19: management and challenges *Lancet Gastroenterol. Hepatol.* **5** 428–30
[31] Huang J, Cheng A, Kumar R, Fang Y, Chen G, Zhu Y and Lin S 2020 Hypoalbuminemia predicts the outcome of COVID-19 independent of age and co-morbidity *J. Med. Virol.* **92** 2152–8
[32] Viana-Llamas M C, Arroyo-Espliguero R, Silva-Obregón J A, Uribe-Heredia G, Núñez-Gil I, García-Magallón B, Torán-Martínez C G *et al* 2021 Hypoalbuminemia on admission in COVID-19 infection: an early predictor of mortality and adverse events. A retrospective observational study *Med. Clin.* **156** 428–36

[33] Natale N R, Lukens J R and Petri Jr W A 2022 The nervous system during COVID-19: caught in the crossfire *Immunol. Rev.* **311** 90–111

[34] Song E, Bartley C M, Chow R D, Ngo T T, Jiang R, Zamecnik C R, Dandekar R *et al* 2021 Divergent and self-reactive immune responses in the CNS of COVID-19 patients with neurological symptoms *Cell Rep. Med.* **2** 100288

[35] Matschke J, Lütgehetmann M, Hagel C, Sperhake J P, Schröder A S, Edler C, Mushumba H *et al* 2020 Neuropathology of patients with COVID-19 in Germany: a post-mortem case series *Lancet Neurol.* **19** 919–29

[36] Ciardo A, Simon M M, Sonnenschein S K, Büsch C and Kim T-S 2022 Impact of the COVID-19 pandemic on oral health and psychosocial factors *Sci. Rep.* **12** 4477

[37] Qi X, Northridge M E, Hu M and Wu B 2022 Oral health conditions and COVID-19: a systematic review and meta-analysis of the current evidence *Aging Health Res.* **2** 100064

[38] Dickson-Swift V, Kangutkar T, Knevel R and Down S 2022 The impact of COVID-19 on individual oral health: a scoping review *BMC Oral Health* **22** 422

IOP Publishing

Viral Diseases

History and new developments in diagnostics and therapeutics

Arvind K Singh Chandel, Bhakti Tanna, Amisha Parmar, Gopal Patel and Neeraj S Thakur

Chapter 16

Advances in COVID-19 diagnosis and treatment interventions

Meha Bhatt, Yesha Upadhyaya, Bhakti Tanna, Neeraj S Thakur and Sonal Sharma

The first case of the SARS-CoV-2 virus was recorded in Wuhan (China) in December 2019, and it spread throughout the world very quickly, resulting in rapid 14 million active cases with 582 000 deaths as of July 2020. The rising number of COVID-19 cases provoked the need of technologies for complete and reliable identification of SARS-CoV-2 for efficient COVID-19 prevention and management. During the initial outbreak of COVID-19, various imaging techniques such as CT scans and x-ray scans were developed. C-reactive protein (CRP), lactate dehydrogenase (LDH), creatine phosphokinase (CPK), D-dimer, and Erythrocyte sedimentation rate (ESR) are all tested in the lab, along with SpO_2 monitoring. By that time several immunological and serological tests like enzyme-linked immunosorbent assay (ELISA), lateral flow, and chemiluminescence immunoassays had also been developed. RT-qPCR using particular primers, which is the gold standard for early and late COVID-19 detections, is one of the most common molecular diagnostic procedures. In addition, novel and advanced diagnostic approaches based on next-generation sequencing (NGS), CRISPR-based detection, loop-mediated isothermal amplification (LAMP), and droplet digital polymerase chain reaction (DDPCR) are being developed in the present day. In this chapter, we have given an overview of these conventional and advanced diagnostic techniques. Finally, we'll go over the benefits and drawbacks of each approach and methodology, as well as their approximate cost, accuracy, and turnaround time. The second section of the chapter will cover effective treatment interventions for COVID-19. Drug lead molecules from synthetic as well as natural resources are reported for treating the virus. In addition, many monoclonal antibodies have been developed and tested for their efficacy against SARS-CoV-2. We have also given an overview of some emerging treatment interventions.

doi:10.1088/978-0-7503-4987-1ch16

16.1 Introduction

Coronaviruses include a varied group of viruses that can infect equally animals as well as humans, and cause acute and chronic respiratory, gastrointestinal, and central nervous system (CNS) illnesses [1, 2]. They are enveloped, spherical-shaped viruses approximately 125 nm in diameter with spike proteins originating from their surface giving them the appearance of a 'corona' or a crown, thus the name 'coronavirus' was given [3]. They are positive-sense, single-stranded RNA-containing viruses with their genome about 26–32 kb in length [4]. The nucleocapsid (N) protein, the transmembrane (M) protein, the envelope (E) protein, and the spike (S) protein are the four key structural proteins found in the virus. They are divided into four genera: Alphacoronavirus, Betacoronavirus, Gammacoronavirus, and Deltacoronavirus [5].

Historically, severe acute respiratory syndrome (SARS) initially emerged in November 2002, in Foshan, Guangdong Province, China, and from there, it spread rapidly worldwide with more than 8000 infected persons and 776 fatalities [6, 7]. A man in Saudi Arabia succumbed to severe pneumonia and renal failure in June 2012, ten years after SARS-CoV first appeared. Middle East Respiratory Syndrome coronavirus (MERS-CoV), a new coronavirus, was isolated from his sputum [8]. According to the World Health Organization, the MERS coronavirus infected around 2428 people, resulting in 838 fatalities [9]. Both SARS-CoV and MERS-CoV belong to the Betacoronavirus group of Coronaviruses and have been the causes of an epidemic during their respective outbreaks [10].

The first case of the novel Coronavirus disease of 2019 (COVID-19) was reported in December 2019 from a seafood market in Wuhan, Hubei province, China [11]. Severe Acute Respiratory Syndrome Coronavirus 2 (SARS-CoV-2) is the causative pathogen for COVID-19. SARS-CoV-2 falls under the Betacoronavirus group of Coronaviruses. Given its somewhat distant link to the prototype SARS-CoV in a species tree and the distance space, the name SARS-CoV-2 was chosen following the custom of naming viruses in this species [3].

COVID-19 patients presented with symptoms similar to SARS and MERS, such as fever, coughing, breathing difficulty, and chest pain [1]. Patients who had been infected had pneumonia and widespread alveolar injury, resulting in acute respiratory distress syndrome. The earliest COVID-19 symptoms emerge around 5 days after incubation [12]. The average time from COVID-19 incubation to symptom presentation is 5.1 days, and those infected had symptoms for 11.5 days [13]. SARS-CoV-2 infections can cause a variety of clinical symptoms, such as breathing problems, fever, shortness of breath, cough, dyspnea, pneumonia, severe acute respiratory syndrome, heart failure, kidney failure, and even death in severe cases [14]. It is of utmost importance that the detection of SARS-CoV2 is done accurately at the early stages of infection. During the initial outbreak of COVID-19, various imaging techniques were developed for the detection of the virus. Over time, more efficient and precise methods including molecular, immunological, and serological tests for diagnosis have been developed (figure 16.1) [15]. This review includes a comprehensive overview of most of the techniques employed for viral detection.

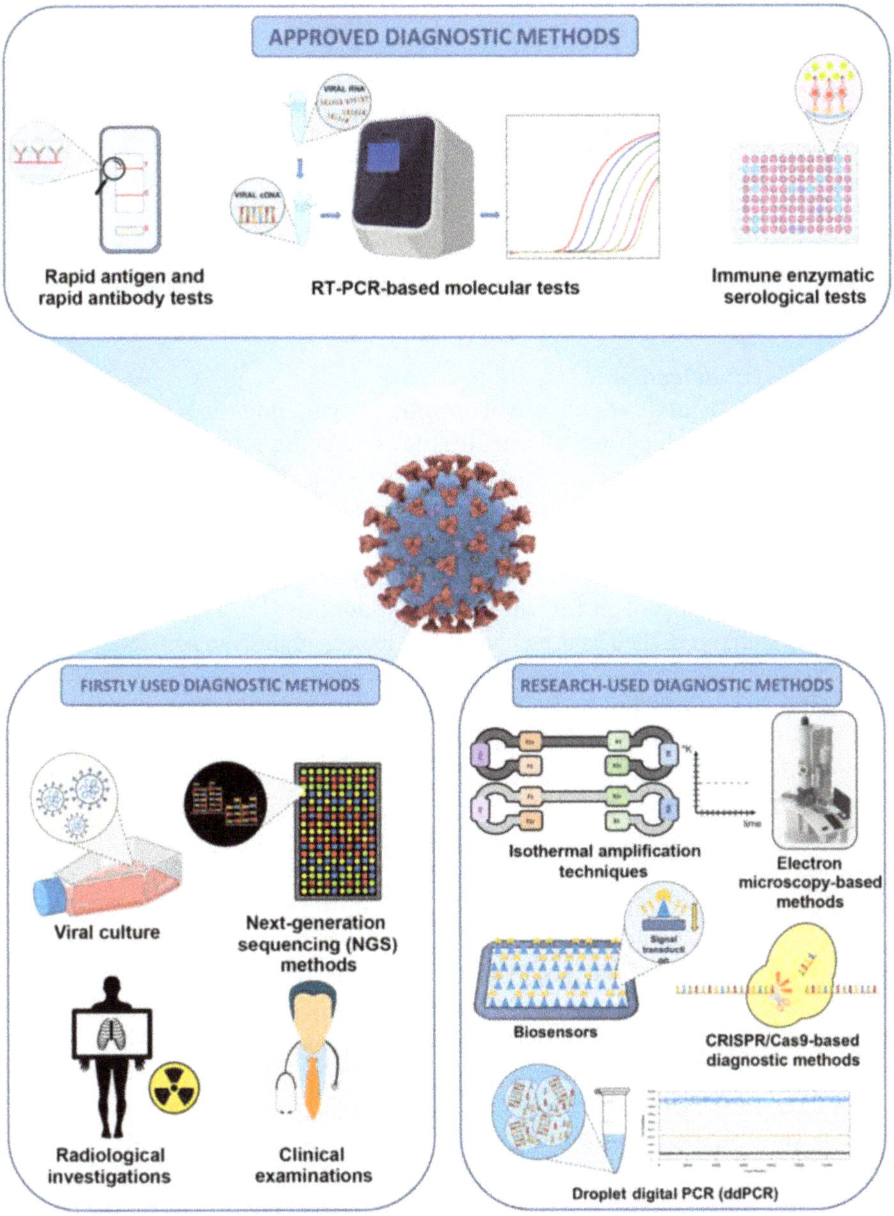

Figure 16.1. Available clinical, diagnostic, and research strategies for effectively diagnosing COVID-19 infection. Adapted with permission from [15], copyright Falzone *et al.*

COVID-19 has also been associated with hypercoagulable disease, which raises the risk of venous thrombosis. There is also information on neurological symptoms (such as weariness, dizziness, and altered awareness), ischemic and hemorrhagic strokes, and muscular injury [6].

16.2 Diagnostics

16.2.1 Conventional methods of virus testing

Viruses are ubiquitous entities that depend on the host cell for their propagation. Structurally, virus consists of two core components: either RNA or DNA as genome and a capsid made up of protein. The host range of most viruses is not well defined, and this plays an important role in the emergence of viruses [16].

Viruses may evolve and migrate between hosts so quickly, so dynamic approaches for detecting existing and emerging viral strains are required. Viral diagnostics is broadly divided into two categories: direct and indirect detections.

16.2.1.1 Indirect detection

One of the methods involves virus isolation by propagating virus particles via their introduction to a suitable host cell line. It is considered an important method since it provides a means to propagate viruses for further analysis and characterization. Despite the development of various modernized methods that have allowed the improvement in the turnaround time, virus detection through infection of cell lines is considered as slow with the requirement of technical expertise, but meanwhile, it is the 'gold standard' approach for viral disease diagnosis [16, 17].

Centrifuge-enhanced shell vial techniques or cluster plates use low-level centrifugation to expedite adsorption of the virus into the host cell line. This allows shorter turnaround time for detection and easy microscopic analysis [17]. The application of co-cultured cell lines is another advance in cell culture techniques for virus isolation [16]. After growth in cell culture, viruses are diagnosed with methods that employ observation of cytopathic effects (CPE) or molecular methods which are known as pre-CPE. Cells that are infected with cytopathic viruses have evident damage and subsequent morphological changes. These CPE can be inspected under light microscopy but the appearance of CPE can take between 48 h to several weeks. Therefore, this method cannot necessarily provide rapid results [16]. Moreover, this method has limitations in being applied universally as it can only be used for CPE-inducing viruses.

Molecular methods in conjunction with virus cell culture can provide a more accurate and rapid diagnosis. This approach is called a 'pre-CPE' diagnosis. This method can detect the virus before the cells present CPE after the entry of the virus in cell lines. It enables them to provide faster results [16]. Detection can be done directly by using coverslips obtained from shell vial cultures. Detection is facilitated by staining the coverslip with an antibody [17]. Antibodies can be labeled with any reporter enzyme or any fluorescent dye and applied to the monolayer of cells on the coverslip. This can be used to detect viruses. Comparatively, pre-CPE methods provide faster diagnosis with results as reliable as traditional cell culture methods [16, 17].

16.2.2 Immunological and serological methods of virus testing

Immunological assays employ antibodies as a primary means to detect the presence of viruses within a sample. Antibodies can be monoclonal, polyclonal, and recombinant forms. They are used according to the specificity needed in diagnosis and the desired outcome. Polyclonal antibodies can bind to different epitopes on target organisms and thus are polyspecific and can be used where the end goal is the simultaneous detection of all viral strains from a sample, whereas monoclonal antibodies and some recombinant antibodies possess single-epitope specificity, i.e. they are monospecific. They offer targeted detection of distinct regions on the target molecule [16].

There are multiple applications of using virus-targeting antibodies in virology, but two major applications include: (1) detection; and (2) determining seroprevalence essentially that are being used to identify patients who have been exposed to a virus.

One of the most widely applied immunoassays is ELISA, which can be performed in several different formats like direct, indirect, competitive, and sandwich ELISA. In both, direct and indirect formats the antigen is initially, coated to the surface of the ELISA well through passive adsorption, or it can also be chemically linked. For direct ELISA, a labeled, anti-target primary antibody is applied to the well, whereas in indirect ELISA, the primary antibody is unlabelled, and a secondary antibody is required for detection. These methods are being implicated in measuring antibody response against a given antigen after the development of an immune response post-viral infection. In these formats of ELISA when the goal is the detection of viruses from crude biological samples like blood, stool, or other tissues, inaccurate quantitation can be possible. Presence of a combination of target proteins and other proteins can cause false results due to competition for the absorption on the assay wells' surface. These limitations can be overcome by competitive and sandwich formats of ELISA.

In competitive ELISA after the first immobilization of the target antigen to an ELISA the antibody and the sample are added simultaneously to the same well. There is competition between antigens to bind with antibodies, leaving fewer antibodies available for binding to the immobilized antigen. A secondary antibody is added to detect the remaining bound antibody after washing the sample. Thus, in this assay format, the final detection signal is negatively correlated to the amount of analyte in the sample [18]. This assay format is useful when considering the rapid-development of viral detection assays as it only requires one target-specific antibody but the sensitivity and the specificity of the assay would be compromised.

This issue of cross-reactivity can be tackled by using sandwich ELISA since it uses two antibodies, and both antibodies are specific for different epitopes on the target. The plate is coated with immobilized antibody followed by application of the antigen-containing sample. This immobilized antibody binds with the antigen. After washing unbound entities, the second antibody is applied which can be labeled directly or detected with a labeled secondary antibody. It increases the specificity as it requires the binding of two antibodies to produce a signal.

Despite high potency, virus detection by ELISA may be prone to the risk of cross-reactivity of antibodies to other co-infecting viruses, resulting in false positives or inaccurate quantification. At the very early stage when the quantities of viral antigen present would be very low false-negative results can occur. Moreover, ELISA procedures take several hours to perform, limiting the possibility of rapid testing.

Lateral flow immunoassays (LFIAs) can also be used in the detection of virus antigens. LFIAs are also based on the principle of labeled antibodies binding to their cognate antigens. The assays are formatted in either sandwich or competitive immunoassay formats [19]. Colour change at the test line is considered as the signal. In sandwich format, positive results are when the colour changes, whereas in competitive format colour should not be changed which is indicative of the presence of virus antigen. Control lines are incorporated to ensure test validity. For the detection of viruses, LFIAs offer an appealing alternative to ELISA or blotting methods. The primary advantage is a rapid turnaround time, in minutes rather than hours. Furthermore, LFIA can detect viral antigens from crude samples like blood and viral transport media, efficiently. Also, LFIAs are cost-effective, easy to use, require minimal sample preparation and results are visible to the naked eye. The only drawback of LFIAs is that they offer only qualitative results.

Overall, viral detection using immunoassays is an effective approach. However, sensitivity similar to nucleic acid detection methods are not offered by these immunoassays, particularly at the early stages of infection. However, they come with the advantage of a reduced cost, reduced complexity, and higher utility for use by untrained personnel [16].

16.2.3 Molecular diagnosis

Molecular diagnostic approaches target the genomic sequence or proteome of the organism, which makes them precise and dependable as compared to other diagnostic techniques [20]. For the diagnosis of a novel pathogen, sequencing is vital in the recognition of the genomic sequence. Deep sequencing and random amplification helped sequence SARS-CoV-2 and opened doors to a lot of possibilities in its diagnostics [21]. There are various approaches for molecular diagnosis as discussed below.

16.2.3.1 PCR-based tests

Real-time reverse transcription polymerase chain reaction (real-time RT-PCR), the nucleic acid-based technique was recommended by WHO after the identification of virus. This technique proved to be a frontline diagnostic approach in the detection of SARS-CoV-2 infection as it is really sensitive and detects even a little viral load as well (figure 16.2) [22]. The technique amplifies the target gene/nucleotide sequence in a sample, which helps in the detection of the targeted pathogen and differentiates it from other correlated pathogens. There are two possible strategies for RT-PCR: two-step or one-step assay. In a two-step assay, reverse transcription and PCR amplification steps are performed in two separate tubes sequentially, which makes it time-consuming but sensitive. In a one-step assay, both sequential steps are performed in one tube, which makes it a faster and reproducible detection method but leads to lower target amplicon generation [23].

The commonly used COVID-19 testing procedure involves: (a) Collecting patient samples and placing potential SARS-CoV-2 viral particles in a transport medium; (b) inactivating the virus using detergent/chaotropic reagents or heat treatment; (c) extracting RNA from the sample; (d, e) transferring the extracted RNA to PCR

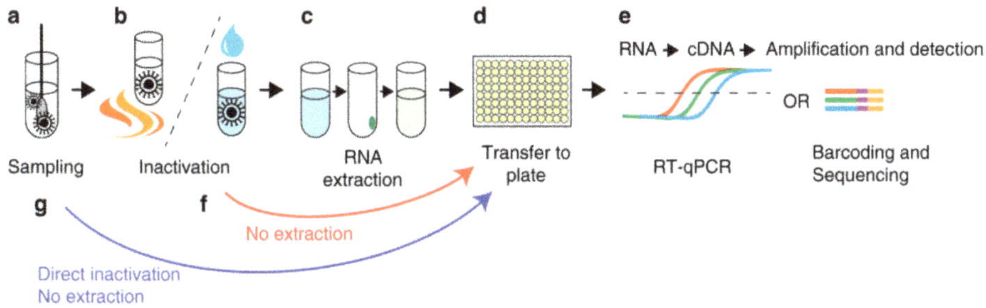

Figure 16.2. Schematic overview of SARS-CoV-2 RT-PCR testing procedure. Reproduced from [22] CC BY 4.0.

plates (96/384-well format) for cDNA synthesis by reverse transcription (RT) and detection by quantitative PCR (qPCR). Alternatively, detection can be done through sample barcoding and high-throughput DNA sequencing; (f, g) In contrast to the widely used approach that includes an RNA extraction step (c) using industrial RNA extraction kits, direct sample testing bypasses this process. After depositing clinical samples in transport medium, viral particles are inactivated either by heating or direct lysis in a detergent-containing buffer. These inactivated samples are then used directly in the downstream RT-PCR diagnostic reaction.

National Medical Product Administration (NMPA) in China has approved 11 nucleic acid-based assays and eight antibody detection kits, but still PCR was the preferred diagnostic technique among all. The Centres for Disease Control and Prevention (CDC) in the US uses a one-step PCR format for the diagnosis of COVID-19 [22]. The methodology of the assay is the isolation of RNA from the sample, followed by the addition of a master mix that contains forward and reverse primers, a reaction mixture containing the required enzymes (polymerase, nucleotides, reverse transcriptase, magnesium, and other additives). PCR thermocycler is loaded with reaction mixture and the PCR reaction is run. The fluorophore quencher gets cleaved in the reaction that generates a fluorescence signal which is detected by the thermocycler as the amplification progresses [24]. To make the interpretation stringent and easy, positive and negative controls have to be added in the RT-PCR reaction setup. Untreated sewage water can contain SARS-CoV-2 viruses to survive up to hours or even days. Thus, analysis of sewage water or fecal samples using RT-PCR and some biosensor-based diagnostic kits have been used to estimate warnings of infectious disease outbreaks in certain areas [25].

RT-PCR is a rapid and sensitive detection technique in molecular diagnostics. It can also amplify and detect a small amount of genomic sequence in a sample, however, it relies on various aspects such as proper collection, storage, transport, and processing of the sample [26]. It can be used for various viruses such as Rotavirus, Adenovirus, and numerous enteric viruses obtained from fecal samples [27]. However, there is one disadvantage of this technique: that it requires a high-equipped laboratory and technical personnel to perform the experiment, which cannot be easy when the demand for rapid testing is increased in pandemic-like conditions [28]. The kits are also expensive and it takes time to deliver the results, which makes it essential to look for alternate faster, and dependable diagnostic techniques [29, 30].

16.2.3.2 Isothermal amplification-based tests

PCR and its different variations as Rt-PCR, digital PCR is the gold standard technique in the field of molecular biology-based diagnosis. Isothermal amplification techniques have the benefit that they can be implicated without the need for a specific instrument such as a thermal cycler. Various methods are available which are based on the principle of amplification on the constant temperature. These methods include: strand displacement amplification (SDA), LAMP, rolling circle amplification (RCA), helicase-dependent amplification (HAD), and multiple displacement amplification (MDA). In all of these methods, the common part is the application of DNA polymerase enzyme which can extend the new strand at a constant temperature and have the activity of strand displacement which can displace the older DNA strand. Several good reviews have been written in which these methods have been detailed nicely. These techniques have also been implemented successfully as the detection methods of SARS-CoV2.

16.2.3.3 CRISPR-Cas-based methods

The advent of CRISPR-Cas systems has offered various opportunities to be applied for various bio-medical and bioengineering purposes. The implication of CRISPR-Cas systems is in the development of point-of-care diagnostics [31].

CRISPR-Cas-based nucleic acid detection methods contain three steps: (1) amplification of target region; (2) interrogation of target with guide RNA and activation of the Cas enzyme; and (3) due to collateral cleavage activity, Cas enzymes cleaved the reporter ssRNA/ssDNA/dsDNA. These reporter probes can be detected through sensing fluorescence, colorimetric, or electrochemical signals (figure 16.3) [32, 33]. CRISPR-Cas-based methods are mostly combined with isothermal amplification

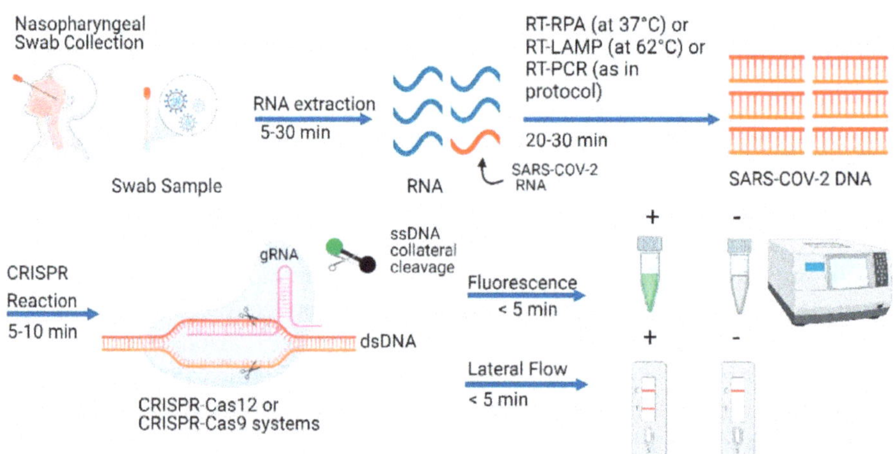

Figure 16.3. Diagram depicting the CRISPR-based amplification assay procedure for SARS-CoV-2 detection. Adapted from reference [33], copyright (2022) with permission from Elsevier.

technologies for the amplification of the target region. This will eliminate the need for sophisticated lab instruments as well as increase the specificity and sensitivity of the methods which are solely based on isothermal amplification. In most of the CRISP-Cas detection methods CRISPR-Cas 9, Cas12, Cas13, and Cas14 have been used as the enzymes. These enzymes have different activities as Cas12 can recognize dsDNA molecule as a reporter, Cas14 is more efficient for the ssDNA reporter and lastly, Cas13 has been used for recognizing ssRNA reporter molecules.

DETECTR, SHEROLOCK, STOPCovid, and AIOD-CRISPR, CARMEN, SHINE, FELUDA are examples of CRISPR/Cas-based nucleic acid detection systems for SARS-CoV-2 [34]. SARS-CoV-2 DNA Endonuclease-Targeted CRISPR Trans Reporter (DETECTR) was reported by [35]. Amplification in the assay was based on the RT-LAMP mediated amplification of N (N2 region) and E gene and then implicated Cas12 to cleave the reporter probes. The system was found more efficient than the CDC SARS-CoV-2 real-time RT-PCR assay, it can be completed in less than 40 min rather than 24 h as in the case of RT-PCR-based testing. They did not consider the N1 and N3 regions due to the lack of essential PAM sequences in these regions. However, Liang *et al* have developed a CRISPR-Cas12a-based detection method to differentiate the wild type of virus with the variants of concern as alpha, beta, and delta. The method has been combined with the reverse transcription PCR (Rt-PCR). They have introduced the PAM site near the mutation sites through the PCR primers in order to enable the detection of those mutations that are not near the PAM site for recognition and then cleavage by Cas enzyme [36]. Exclusion of PAM sequence essentiality for specific interrogation of target by CRISPR-Cas system has successfully been demonstrated by [37]. They have developed a single-pot assay which was named All-In-One Dual CRISPR-Cas12a (AIOD-CRISPR). In this method, they introduced two different Cas12a-crRNA complexes to bind to two different but close to the recognition sites of primers used in RPA-mediated amplification of the target. The second advantage of these methods is that it was a single-pot assay which eliminated the chances of contamination while transferring the reaction mixture from the pre-amplification step to the CRISPR-Cas step. All the components were mixed in a single tube and incubated at 37 °C. Further, the detection was made possible through naked eyes under a blue LED or UV light illuminator. Cas enzymes obtained from different sources are not similarly efficient. Nguyen *et al* (2020) have found that LbCas12a has higher trans-cleavage activity than the AsCas12a or FnCas12a [38]. Moreover, they also demonstrated that additional ssDNA extensions of crRNA at the 3′ end enhanced the trans-cleavage activity of LbCas12a. The method they named was CRISPR-ENHANCE (ENHanced Analysis of Nucleic acids with CrRNA Extensions). This will improve the sensitivity of the assay up to 23-fold in comparison to the wild-type systems. Ramachandran *et al* (2020) used the isotachophoresis (ITP) technique combined with microfluidic chips for enhancement of CRISPR assay [39]. It is an separation technique in which ionic analytes can be separated using electric gradient. ITP was also introduced in nucleic acid extraction step to develop method of automated. It will reduce the manual handling of samples as well as minimal reagent consumption.

Patchsung *et al* (2020) used Cas13 from *Leptotrichia wadei* to develop a specific high-sensitivity enzymatic reporter unlocking (SHERLOCK) assay [40]. They were able to obtain 100% specificity and 96%–97% sensitivity with different signal read-out methods. They also used Rnase inhibitors to stop the nuclease-mediated degradation of crRNA or the reporter RNA. Joung *et al* (2020) have improvised the SHERLOCK system and turned it into a single-pot assay [41]. They utilized the Cas12b from *Alicyclobacillus acidiphilus.* This enzyme was found more thermostable in a higher temperature range of 55 °C–60 °C which allows being added with the LAMP components to make it the single-pot assay. However, in this method, they have used the sgRNA from other bacteria such as *Alicyclobacillus acidoterrestris* which helped in the enhancement of the activity of the Cas enzyme. The assay is referred to as the STOPCovid.

Arizti-Sanz *et al* (2020) have also improvised the SHERLOCK system by combining it with the HUDSON (Heating Unextracted Diagnostic Samples to Obliterate Nucleases). In this combinatorial method (SHINE-SHERLOCK and HUDSON Integration to Navigate Epidemics) RNA extraction step was not needed as the swab samples can be directly used as the source for template after heat inactivation of nucleases and lysis of the virus [42].

Other than the CRISPR-Cas-based nucleic acid-mediated detection of SARS-CoV2, CRISPR-Cas systems have been reported to be used to detect viral proteins. Liu *et al* (2022) have developed antibody-assisted proximity ligation assay integrated with CRISPR technologies [43]. They have introduced the aptamer which can detect the viral nucleocapsid. This assay is based on the competitive binding of antigen or the Cas12a-crRNA complex to the aptamer. In the presence of antigen, aptamer binds to the antigen which makes the aptamer less available to the Cas enzyme. This causes the low activity of the enzyme. Meanwhile, they have developed an electronic system to detect the active/inactive Cas12a. Their electronic system is fabricated with the DNA architecture through rolling circle amplification on the gold electrode. Active Cas enzyme cleaved the DNA on the electrode due to its collateral cleavage activity, resulting in lowering the resistance which will be detected as a signal by electrochemical impedance spectroscopy. The input of the trigger DNA for Cas enzyme activation can affect the sensitivity of the detection. Zhao *et al* (2022) designed a hybrid DNA which is the tandem array of dsDNA and ssDNA which is linked to the aptamer [44]. Upon binding with the antigen (nucleocapsid protein) the aptamer released the HyDNA which further worked as the trigger for Cas12 activation. This strategy helped to increase the sensitivity of the assay (one copy/μl of viral RNA). They named their biosensing platform CaT-Smelor-Covid.v1 (CRISPR/Cas12a and aptamer-mediated detector of diverse analytes for COVID-19). This is based on the detection of fluorescent signals. CRISPR/Cas12a-derived electrochemical aptasensor has also been developed by Han *et al* (2022) [45]. In this method, an electrochemical sensing interface was fabricated by immobilizing methylene blue labeled poly adenine DNA sequence (polyA-MB electrochemical reporter) on a gold electrode surface and aptamer was linked with an activator strand to activate the Cas enzyme. The limit of detection of the technique was to 16.5 pg ml^{-1}.

16.2.3.4 RPA-based methods

Recombinase polymerase amplification, or RPA, is a more simplified technique than LAMP as it requires only two primers as in PCR. However, a bunch of enzymes are needed for the completion of the process. Recombinase enzyme is required to bind with the primers and help them to bind with the dsDNA at their complementary site. Strand displacement polymerase does the extension of new strands with the help of single-strand binding proteins which helps in inhibiting the reannealing of the parent strand. Amplification reaction is followed by signal readouts by fluorescence detection or colorimetric detection.

A point of need for reverse transcription recombinase polymerase amplification (RT-RPA) has been developed by El Wahed *et al* (2020) [46]. All the components or the instrument for detection can be packed in the solar-powered suitcase and can be ported to the place of need. The primers were developed for the RNA-dependent RNA polymerase (RdRP), envelope protein (E), and nucleocapsid protein (N) genes of SARS-CoV-2. The assay was found to be specific as no amplification has been observed in other closely related respiratory pathogens. For detection fluorescent exo-probe has been used. The assay took only 15 min to complete and results were found to be comparable with the Rt-PCR test.

Penn-RAMP, a two-step isothermal amplification COVID-19 detection assay has been developed by El-Tholoth *et al* (2020) [47]. In the first step, RPA assay occurred on the tube cap which was further subjected to LAMP-based detection on the higher temperature inside the tube. This combination has made the assay more specific and with minimum noise.

Lau *et al* (2021) have developed a lateral flow assay test for COVID-19 test which was based on the RPA. The specificity and sensitivity in the clinical samples were found as 98% and 100%, respectively [48].

An RT-RPA-based point-of-care multiplex assay has been demonstrated by Cherkaoui *et al* (2021) [49]. They use primers and probes for the E gene and RdRp gene. Signal readouts were made possible by a portable real-time fluorescent reader as well as a dipstick-based system. Another multiplex RPA-based lateral flow assay has been developed by Sun *et al* (2021) which can detect the SARS-CoV-2 and Flu viruses (Flu A and Flu B) simultaneously in a single assay [50]. In the clinical setup the assay has shown 100% accuracy. Further, advancement in the detection system of RPA products has been demonstrated by Liu *et al* (2021) [51]. In this method, a single-chambered microfluidic chip has been developed which encompasses a place for both the RPA assay and detection of analytes using lateral flow assay. It can detect the single copy of RNA present in one microliter of the solution and has high sensitivity in the clinical samples also [52].

The specificity and sensitivity also depend upon the probe or the system we are using for signal readouts. Choi *et al* (2021) used the rkDNA-Graphene oxide probe based system to detect the products of RPA assay [53]. rkDNA is the stretch of DNA having the modified nucleotide morpholine naphthalimide deoxyuridine (dUrkTP) which can be incorporated into DNA through primer extension. Exonuclease can be used to separate rkDNA from its complementary sequence which gives the fluorescence. When combined with graphene oxide (GO) the fluorescence of the free rkDNA was quenched [54]. RPA amplified products then replaced the rkDNA on GO and then again started to give fluorescence. The authors claimed the high selectivity of the whole system.

16.3 Treatment of COVID-19

Allopathic treatment or Western-style treatment involves the usage of synthetic drugs. The drugs that are still under investigation require stringent and lengthy laboratory and clinical studies, which is not possible in the crisis of a pandemic. The treatment of COVID-19 was done using various antiviral drugs and in emergency conditions, oxygen also needed to be given to the patients. Previously used antiviral and antimalarial drugs were utilized for the treatment. The current approaches to COVID-19 treatment comprised virus targeting and host targeting (figure 16.4) [55, 56].

The drugs such as remdesivir, favipiravir, tenofovir, and sofosbuvir are nucleoside and nucleotide analogs. Other drugs like lopinavir, atazanavir and ritonavir, and peptideomimetic drugs. Umifenovir is an indole derivative [57]. Remdesivir (RDV), a promising antiviral drug had been shown to slow down SARS-CoV-2 infections. There has been a study involving SARS-CoV-2 infecting Vero E6 cells with MOI (multiplicity of infection) of 0.05 for 48 h. The EC50 (half-maximal effective concentration) values and cytotoxicity activities by qRT-PCR and CCK-8 assay, respectively, were evaluated which showed the effectiveness of remdesivir, favipiravir, chloroquine, nitazoxanide, and ribavirin. It was observed that a low-micromolar concentration of remdesivir was effective against fatal corona disease as too much dosage caused organ damage [56, 58]. Chloroquine has also been used for the treatment of COVID-19 as it has shown antiviral activity. It is a well-known antimalarial drug. It inhibits the viral infection by increasing endosomal pH which is necessary for viral growth and glycosylation of cellular receptors of coronavirus

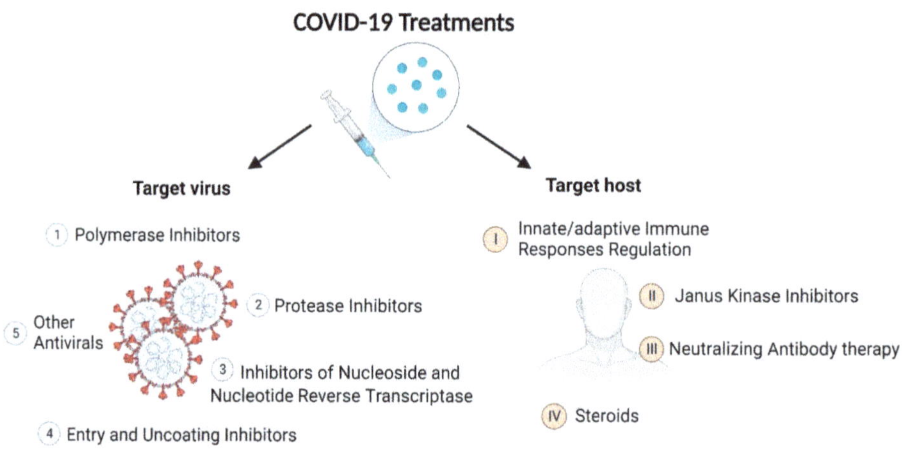

Figure 16.4. Classification of COVID-19 treatment approaches. COVID-19 treatments can be categorized into two main groups based on their targets: (1) antiviral agents: these directly target the SARS-CoV-2 virus; (2) host-directed therapies: these focus on modulating the host's response to the viral infection. Adapted from reference [55]. Copyright (2023) Authors published at Frontiers CC BY 4.0.

[56, 58]. A derivative of chloroquine, hydroxychloroquine (HCQ) has also been approved to be used for corona disease treatment. The main difference between the two drugs is that hydroxychloroquine is less orally toxic, more soluble, comparatively safer than chloroquine, and easily available. Synergistic effects were observed when given azithromycin drug; both are cheap and commercially available drugs. In the study, it was observed that a >400 mg dose given twice a day for at least 5 days was very effective against viral infection. However, there have been various side effects such as damage to retina tissue, and the central nervous system, the genotoxicity of DNA, and liver cells, thus WHO has recommended banning the drug for COVID-19 treatment [56].

Favipiravir or favilavir is a very good antiviral drug. It has also been tested on corona patients and shown to inhibit viral clearance with high chest CT scans and showed improvements in patients with medium severity of COVID-19 in comparison to patients with Ritonavir [56, 59]. Another drug ivermectin has been approved by FDA (Food and Drug Administration) as an antiparasitic drug and also has evident antiviral activity. It has shown broad-spectrum antiviral activity against coronaviruses *in vitro*. It has shown a powerful effect against SARS-CoV-2 infections in the vero-hSLAM cell model by suppressing pathogenic viruses. It has also been shown to have higher effectiveness against infected cells in comparison to dimethyl sulfoxide vehicles. The drug exposure was kept for 48 h, which showed decreased cell-associated viral RNA as compared to control. The sample preparation was done using viral load via real-time PCR; IC50 values were attained for cell-associated virus by using GraphPad prism and the supernatant was treated against different concentrations of the drug against E: and RdRp gene and showed to be very effective against COVID-19 [56, 60].

There have been plenty of treatments repurposed or developed to fight against COVID-19. Monoclonal antibodies (mAbs) are also one of the therapeutic approaches that have been used for the treatment which mainly acts by neutralizing the virus in the infected patients' B cells. The neutralizing mAbs can be acquired from recovering COVID-19 patients or humanized mice. These mAbs decrease virulence and are a type of passive immunotherapy. Identification of specific antibodies towards the virus is done through high throughput screening of B cells, its ability to bind the virus with high affinity to block the entry of the virus, thus negating the productive infection pathology [61].

There has been emergency use authorization (EUA) for bamlanivimab mAb for the treatment of SARS-CoV-2 infected patients with mild-to-moderate symptoms in the United States; it can also be given as monotherapy or in combination with estevimab or casirivimab with imdevimab [61]. There have been other antibodies such as P2C-1F11, CB6-LALA, C105, C002, nAB cc12.1, B38, 311mAb-31B5, and CV30 isolated from COVID-19 patients have been tested for the use [62]. There are different binding sites for different mAbs. Some mAbs bind to RBM (receptor-binding motif) only when RBD (receptor-binding domain) is in the open state (mAbs e.g., REGN10933, ADG2, AZD8895, LY-CoV016, Brii-196, CT-P59 and ABBV-2B04). However, some mAbs recognize RBD in open and closed states (mAbs e.g., BGB-DXP593, LY-CoV555, and AZD1061) [63].

It has been shown in studies that patients with comorbidities who received monoclonal antibodies had declined rates of hospitalization as compared to patients without treatment [64, 65]. Thus, it is recommended to use mAb treatments despite the lack of social, and racial support [65]. Anti Ig (Immunoglobulin)-E antibody omalizumab has been shown to lower COVID-19 duration and severity. IgE can play an important role in respiratory infection susceptibility as it activates mast cells during hypersensitivity reactions. Hence IgE blockage by mAb has been shown to provide immunotherapy in the treatment of corona in clinical studies [66]. During the coronavirus infection, cytokine surge occurs with disease development. Thus, clinical trials have been conducted to evaluate if inhibiting this type of surge may help COVID-19 infection. Compilations of these types of studies showed that IL-6 (Interleukin-6) inhibitor Tocilizumab has been shown to be effective in controlling the cytokine surge correlated with COVID-19 [67]. Due to the COVID-19 crisis and the urgency of the situation in the pandemic condition, researchers have gathered more knowledge of mAbs use for anti-infective purposes in one year than in the last 20 years. However, there are a few challenges in the approval of mAbs for COVID-19 treatment, such as large-scale manufacturing, route of administration requirements to be shifted from a hospital setting, etc. Thus, filling these gaps could eventually lead to the use of mAbs on a global scale for the reduction of morbidity and mortality caused by COVID-19 [63].

Abbreviations

AIOD-CRISPR	All-in-one dual CRISPR-Cas12a
CDC	Centers for Disease Control and Prevention
COVID-19	Coronavirus disease of 2019
CPE	Cytopathic effects
CPK	Creatine phosphokinase
CRISPR	Clustered regularly interspaced short palindromic repeats
CRP	C-reactive protein
CT	Computed tomography
CT	Computed tomography
DDPCR	Droplet digital polymerase chain reaction
DETECTR	DNA endonuclease-targeted CRISPR trans reporter
EC50	Half-maximal effective concentration
ELISA	Enzyme-linked immunosorbent assay
ESR	Erythrocyte sedimentation rate
EUA	Emergency use authorization
FDA	Food and Drug Administration
HAD	Helicase-dependent amplification
HCQ	Hydroxychloroquine
HUDSON	Heating unextracted diagnostic samples to obliterate nucleases
LAMP	Loop-mediated isothermal amplification
LDH	Lactate dehydrogenase
LFIA	Lateral flow immunoassay
mAbs	Monoclonal antibodies
MDA	Multiple displacement amplification

MERS-CoV	Middle East respiratory syndrome coronavirus
NGS	Next-generation sequencing
NMPA	National Medical Product Administration
Penn-RAMP	Pennsylvania-recombinase amplification
RBD	Receptor-binding domain
RBM	Receptor-binding motif
RCA	Rolling circle amplification
RdRP	RNA-dependent RNA polymerase
RPA	Recombinase polymerase amplification
RT-PCR	Real-time reverse transcription polymerase chain reaction
SARS	Severe acute respiratory syndrome
SARS-CoV-2	Severe acute respiratory syndrome Coronavirus 2
SDA	Strand displacement amplification
SHERLOCK	Specific high-sensitivity enzymatic reporter unlocking
SHINE	SHERLOCK and HUDSON integration to navigate epidemics
SpO2	Peripheral oxygen saturation

References

[1] Hu B, Guo H, Zhou P and Shi Z L 2021 Characteristics of SARS-CoV-2 and COVID-19 *Nat. Rev. Microbiol.* **19** 141–54

[2] Weiss S R and Navas-Martin S 2005 Coronavirus pathogenesis and the emerging pathogen severe acute respiratory syndrome Coronavirus *Microbiol. Mol. Biol. Rev.* **69** 635–64

[3] Malik Y A 2020 Properties of Coronavirus and SARS-CoV-2 *Malays. J. Pathol.* **42** 3–11

[4] Yang H and Rao Z 2021 Structural biology of SARS-CoV-2 and implications for therapeutic development *Nat. Rev. Microbiol.* **19** 685–700

[5] Hasöksüz M, Kiliç S and Saraç F 2020 Coronaviruses and SARS-CoV-2 *Turkish J. Med. Sci.* **50** 549–56

[6] Mohamadian M, Chiti H, Shoghli A, Biglari S, Parsamanesh N and Esmaeilzadeh A 2021 COVID-19: virology, biology and novel laboratory diagnosis *J. Gene Med.* **23** e3303

[7] Zhong N S *et al* 2003 Epidemiology and cause of severe acute respiratory syndrome (SARS) in Guangdong, People's Republic of China, in February, 2003 *Lancet* **362** 1353–8

[8] Zaki A M, van Boheemen S, Bestebroer T M, Osterhaus A D M E and Fouchier R A M 2012 Isolation of a novel Coronavirus from a man with pneumonia in Saudi Arabia *N. Engl. J. Med.* **367** 1814–20

[9] Rahman A and Sarkar A 2019 Risk factors for fatal Middle East respiratory syndrome coronavirus infections in Saudi Arabia: analysis of the WHO line list, 2013–2018 *Am. J. Public Health* **109** 1288–93

[10] Rabaan A A, Al-Ahmed S H, Haque S, Sah R, Tiwari R, Malik Y S, Dhama K, Yatoo M I, Bonilla-Aldana D K and Rodriguez-Morales A J 2020 SARS-CoV-2, SARS-CoV, and MERS-COV: a comparative overview *Le Infez. Med.* **2** 174–84

[11] Gralinski L E and Menachery V D 2020 Return of the coronavirus: 2019-nCoV *Viruses* **12** 135

[12] Shereen M A, Khan S, Kazmi A, Bashir N and Siddique R 2020 COVID-19 infection: origin, transmission, and characteristics of human coronaviruses *J. Adv. Res.* **24** 91–8

[13] Lauer S A, Grantz K H, Bi Q, Jones F K, Zheng Q, Meredith H R, Azman A S, Reich N G and Lessler J 2020 The incubation period of coronavirus disease 2019 (CoVID-19) from publicly reported confirmed cases: estimation and application *Ann. Intern. Med.* **172** 577–82

[14] Rai P, Kumar B K, Deekshit V K, Karunasagar I and Karunasagar I 2021 Detection technologies and recent developments in the diagnosis of COVID-19 infection *Appl. Microbiol. Biotechnol.* **105** 441–55

[15] Falzone L, Gattuso G, Tsatsakis A, Spandidos D A and Libra M 2021 Current and innovative methods for the diagnosis of COVID-19 infection (review) *Int. J. Mol. Med.* **47** 100

[16] Cassedy A, Parle-McDermott A and O'Kennedy R 2021 Virus detection: a review of the current and emerging molecular and immunological methods *Front. Mol. Biosci.* **8** 637559

[17] Leland D S and Ginocchio C C 2007 Role of cell culture for virus detection in the age of technology *Clin. Microbiol. Rev.* **20** 49–78

[18] He J 2013 Practical guide to ELISA development *Immunoassay Handbook: Theory and Applications of Ligand Binding, ELISA and Related Techniques* (Elsevier) pp 381–93

[19] Sajid M, Kawde A N and Daud M 2015 Designs, formats and applications of lateral flow assay: a literature review *J. Saudi Chem. Soc.* **19** 689–705

[20] Zhou P *et al* 2020 A pneumonia outbreak associated with a new coronavirus of probable bat origin *Nature* **579** 270–3

[21] Briese T, Mishra N, Jain K, Zalmout I S, Jabado O J, Karesh W B, Daszak P, Mohammed O B, Alagaili A N and Ian Lipkin W 2014 Middle East Respiratory Syndrome coronavirus quasispecies that include homologues of human isolates revealed through whole- genome analysis and virus cultured from dromedary camels in Saudi Arabia *MBio* **5** e01146-14

[22] Smyrlaki I *et al* 2020 Massive and rapid COVID-19 testing is feasible by extraction-free SARS-CoV-2 RT-PCR *Nat. Commun.* **11** 1–12

[23] Wong M L and Medrano J F 2005 Real-time PCR for mRNA quantitation *Biotechniques* **39** 75–85

[24] Centers for Disease Control and Prevention (U.S.), 2020 CDC - 2019-nCoV real-time RT-PCR diagnostic panel: acceptable alternative primer and probe sets

[25] Orive G, Lertxundi U and Barcelo D 2020 Early SARS-CoV-2 outbreak detection by sewage-based epidemiology *Sci. Total Environ.* **732** 139298

[26] Afzal A 2020 Molecular diagnostic technologies for COVID-19: limitations and challenges *J. Adv. Res.* **26** 149–59

[27] Kowada K, Takeuchi K, Hirano E, Toho M and Sada K 2018 Development of a multiplex real-time PCR assay for detection of human enteric viruses other than norovirus using samples collected from gastroenteritis patients in Fukui Prefecture, Japan *J. Med. Virol.* **90** 67–75

[28] Bustin S A and Nolan T 2004 Pitfalls of quantitative real- time reverse-transcription polymerase chain reaction *J. Biomol. Tech.* **15** 155–66

[29] Hofman P, Puchois P, Brest P, Lahlou H and Simeon-Dubach D 2020 Possible consequences of the COVID-19 pandemic on the use of biospecimens from cancer biobanks for research in academia and bioindustry *Nat. Med.* **26** 809–10

[30] Sheridan C 2020 Fast, portable tests come online to curb coronavirus pandemic *Nat. Biotechnol.* **38** 515–8

[31] Kaminski M M, Abudayyeh O O, Gootenberg J S, Zhang F and Collins J J 2021 CRISPR-based diagnostics *Nat. Biomed. Eng.* **5** 643–56

[32] Ganbaatar U and Liu C 2021 CRISPR-based COVID-19 testing: toward next-generation point-of-care diagnostics *Front. Cell. Infect. Microbiol.* **11** 663949

[33] Filchakova O, Dossym D, Ilyas A, Kuanysheva T, Abdizhamil A and Bukasov R 2022 Review of COVID-19 testing and diagnostic methods *Talanta* **244** 123409

[34] Palaz F, Kalkan A K, Tozluyurt A and Ozsoz M 2021 CRISPR-based tools: Alternative methods for the diagnosis of COVID-19 *Clin. Biochem.* **89** 1–13

[35] Broughton J P *et al* 2020 CRISPR–Cas12-based detection of SARS-CoV-2 *Nat. Biotechnol.* **38** 870–4

[36] Liang Y *et al* 2021 CRISPR-Cas12a-based detection for the major SARS-CoV-2 variants of concern *Microbiol. Spectr.* **9** e01017-21

[37] Ding X, Yin K, Li Z, Lalla R V, Ballesteros E, Sfeir M M and Liu C 2020 Ultrasensitive and visual detection of SARS-CoV-2 using all-in-one dual CRISPR-Cas12a assay *Nat. Commun.* **11** 1–10

[38] Nguyen L T, Smith B M and Jain P K 2020 Enhancement of trans-cleavage activity of Cas12a with engineered crRNA enables amplified nucleic acid detection *Nat. Commun.* **11** 1–13

[39] Ramachandran A, Huyke D A, Sharma E, Sahoo M K, Huang C, Banaei N, Pinsky B A and Santiago J G 2020 Electric field-driven microfluidics for rapid CRISPR-based diagnostics and its application to detection of SARS-CoV-2 *Proc. Natl. Acad. Sci. USA* **117** 29518–25

[40] Patchsung M *et al* 2020 Clinical validation of a Cas13-based assay for the detection of SARS-CoV-2 RNA *Nat. Biomed. Eng.* **4** 1140–9

[41] Joung J *et al* 2020 Point-of-care testing for COVID-19 using SHERLOCK diagnostics *medRxiv Prepr. Serv. Heal. Sci.* https://www.medrxiv.org/content/10.1101/2020.05.04.20091231v1

[42] Arizti-Sanz J *et al* 2020 Integrated sample inactivation, amplification, and Cas13-based detection of SARS-CoV-2 *bioRxiv Prepr. Serv. Biol.* https://www.biorxiv.org/content/10.1101/2020.05.28.119131v1

[43] Liu N, Liu R and Zhang J 2022 CRISPR-Cas12a-mediated label-free electrochemical aptamer-based sensor for SARS-CoV-2 antigen detection *Bioelectrochemistry* **146** 108105

[44] Zhao X *et al* 2021 Integrating PCR-free amplification and synergistic sensing for ultrasensitive and rapid CRISPR/Cas12a-based SARS-CoV-2 antigen detection *Synth. Syst. Biotechnol.* **6** 283–91

[45] Han C, Li W, Li Q, Xing W, Luo H, Ji H, Fang X, Luo Z and Zhang L 2022 CRISPR/Cas12a-derived electrochemical aptasensor for ultrasensitive detection of COVID-19 nucleocapsid protein *Biosens. Bioelectron.* **200** 113922

[46] El Wahed A A *et al* 2021 Suitcase lab for rapid detection of SARS-CoV-2 based on recombinase polymerase amplification assay *Anal. Chem.* **93** 2627–34

[47] El-Tholoth M, Bau H H and Song J 2020 A single and two-stage, closed-tube, molecular test for the 2019 Novel Coronavirus (COVID-19) at home, clinic, and points of entry *ChemRxiv Prepr. Serv. Chem.* https://doi.org/10.26434/chemrxiv.11860137.v1

[48] Lau Y L *et al* 2021 Development of a reverse transcription recombinase polymerase amplification assay for rapid and direct visual detection of Severe Acute Respiratory Syndrome Coronavirus 2 (SARS-CoV-2) *PLoS One* **16** e0245164

[49] Cherkaoui D, Huang D, Miller B S, Turbé V and McKendry R A 2021 Harnessing recombinase polymerase amplification for rapid multi-gene detection of SARS-CoV-2 in resource-limited settings *Biosens. Bioelectron.* **189** 113328

[50] Sun Y *et al* 2022 Rapid and simultaneous visual screening of SARS-CoV-2 and influenza virufses with customized isothermal amplification integrated lateral flow strip *Biosens. Bioelectron.* **197** 113771

[51] Liu D, Shen H, Zhang Y, Shen D, Zhu M, Song Y, Zhu Z and Yang C 2021 A microfluidic-integrated lateral flow recombinase polymerase amplification (MI-IF-RPA) assay for rapid COVID-19 detection *Lab Chip* **21** 2019–26

[52] Shelite T R, Uscanga-Palomeque A C, Castellanos-Gonzalez A, Melby P C and Travi B L 2021 Isothermal recombinase polymerase amplification-lateral flow detection of SARS-CoV-2, the etiological agent of COVID-19 *J. Virol. Methods* **296** 114227

[53] Choi M H, Lee J and Seo Y J 2021 Combined recombinase polymerase amplification/rkDNA–graphene oxide probing system for detection of SARS-CoV-2 *Anal. Chim. Acta* **1158** 338390

[54] Choi M H, Ravi Kumara G S and Seo Y J 2020 rkDNA–graphene oxide as a simple probe for the rapid detection of miRNA21 *Bioorgan. Med. Chem. Lett.* **30** 127398

[55] Yuan Y, Jiao B, Qu L, Yang D and Liu R 2023 The development of COVID-19 treatment *Front. Immunol.* **14** 1125246

[56] Farooq S and Ngaini Z 2021 Natural and synthetic drugs as potential treatment for Coronavirus disease 2019 (COVID-2019) *Chem. Africa* **4** 1

[57] Batalha P N, Forezi L S M, Lima C G S, Pauli F P, Boechat F C S, de Souza M C B V, Cunha A C, Ferreira V F and da Silva F C 2021 Drug repurposing for the treatment of COVID-19: pharmacological aspects and synthetic approaches *Bioorg. Chem.* **106** 104488

[58] Wang M, Cao R, Zhang L, Yang X, Liu J, Xu M, Shi Z, Hu Z, Zhong W and Xiao G 2020 Remdesivir and chloroquine effectively inhibit the recently emerged novel coronavirus (2019-nCoV) *in vitro Cell Res. 2020 303* **30** 269–71

[59] Arab-Zozani M, Hassanipour S and Ghoddoosi-Nejad D 2020 Favipiravir for treating patients with novel coronavirus (COVID-19): protocol for a systematic review and meta-analysis of randomised clinical trials *BMJ Open* **10** e039730

[60] Caly L, Druce J D, Catton M G, Jans D A and Wagstaff K M 2020 The FDA-approved drug ivermectin inhibits the replication of SARS-CoV-2 *in vitro Antiviral Res* **178** 104787

[61] Taylor P C, Adams A C, Hufford M M, de la Torre I, Winthrop K and Gottlieb R L 2021 Neutralizing monoclonal antibodies for treatment of COVID-19 *Nat. Rev. Immunol.* **21** 382–93

[62] Jaworski J P 2021 Neutralizing monoclonal antibodies for COVID-19 treatment and prevention *Biomed. J.* **44** 7–17

[63] Corti D, Purcell L A, Snell G and Veesler D 2021 Tackling COVID-19 with neutralizing monoclonal antibodies *Cell* **184** 3086–108

[64] Verderese J P *et al* 2022 Neutralizing monoclonal antibody treatment reduces hospitalization for mild and moderate coronavirus disease 2019 (COVID-19): a real-world experience *Clin. Infect. Dis.* **74** 1063–9

[65] Bierle D M, Ganesh R, Wilker C G, Hanson S N, Moehnke D E, Jackson T A, Ramar P, Rosedahl J K, Philpot L M and Razonable R R 2021 Influence of social and cultural factors on the decision to consent for monoclonal antibody treatment among high-risk patients with mild-moderate COVID-19 *J. Prim. Care Commun. Heal.* **12** 21501327211019282

[66] Farmani A R, Mahdavinezhad F, Moslemi R, Mehrabi Z, Noori A, Kouhestani M, Noroozi Z, Ai J and Rezaei N 2021 Anti-IgE monoclonal antibodies as potential treatment in COVID-19 *Immunopharmacol. Immunotoxicol.* **43** 259–64

[67] Patel S, Saxena B and Mehta P 2021 Recent updates in the clinical trials of therapeutic monoclonal antibodies targeting cytokine storm for the management of COVID-19 *Heliyon* **7** e06158

Chapter 17

Theranostics: a hope for viral diseases

Pradeep Singh Thakur and Muniappan Sankar

The continuous worldwide difficulties presented by viral diseases emphasise the crucial need for novel and multifaceted approaches to treatment and diagnosis. This chapter discusses the transformational potential of theranostics, an integrated approach integrating medicines and diagnostics for enhanced management of viral diseases. Theranostics, which focuses on cutting-edge technologies, including molecular diagnostics, precision medicine, and nanotechnology, presents a potential solution to the problems caused by viral infections. The chapter emphasizes how important theranostics is for accurate early diagnosis and customized treatment plans. Through the application of nanotechnology, biomarker identification, and tailored therapies, theranostics assesses and eliminates adverse effects while optimizing medicine delivery and real-time therapy responses. Newly developed CRISPR/Cas technology and ongoing clinical trials highlight theranostics' practical applications and demonstrate how it could revolutionize current medical practices.

17.1 Introduction

Recurrent outbreaks of viral infections have significantly influenced the trajectory of human history. These include the deadly Spanish Flu in 1918 [1, 2] and the more recent challenges encountered with human immunodeficiency virus (HIV), Zika virus, hepatitis virus, Ebola virus, and the ongoing SARS-CoV-2 caused COVID-19 pandemic. These rapidly mutating infectious pathogens constantly challenge our understanding of disease mechanisms and force us to develop novel, cutting-edge solutions for diagnosing and treating them. More sophisticated and adaptable approaches must be developed as we confront the complexities of managing viral illnesses in the twenty-first century. Viral diseases have had a significant impact on people's lives all over the world, with pandemics having a particularly lasting effect on healthcare systems worldwide. The path has been one of ongoing discovery and adaption, starting with the early attempts to comprehend the nature of these pathogenic threats and continuing through the invention of

doi:10.1088/978-0-7503-4987-1ch17

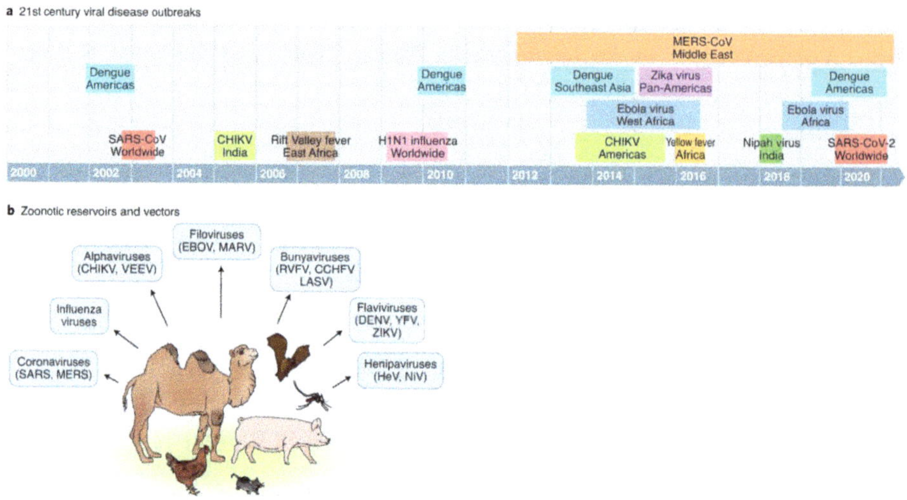

Figure 17.1. Historic overview of the 21st-century viral outbreaks. (a) Timeline of twenty-first-century viral outbreaks, from 2000 to the present day. Viral strains and the area of outbreak are indicated along with the timeline. (b) Animals such as the ones shown are zoonotic reservoirs or vectors for many virus families with pandemic potential. Adapted from reference [3] with permission from Springer Nature.

vaccinations and antiviral medications. Due to the persistent danger of viral mutations and the perpetual appearance of novel infectious infections, disease treatment requires dynamic and comprehensive strategies (figure 17.1) [3, 4].

In this regard, theranostics emerges as a beacon of hope since it marks a paradigm change in our approaches to fighting viral illnesses. The term 'theranostics' refers to a comprehensive approach that integrates both therapeutic and diagnostic modalities into a single framework [3]. Fundamentally, theranostics aims to obfuscate the distinction between diagnosis and treatment by offering an adjunctive technique that has the potential to transform the management of viral infections completely. Theranostics is centered on the integration of cutting-edge technologies like nanotechnology, which is highly versatile and precise and plays a significant role in drug delivery systems and molecular recognition. This strategy makes use of specially designed medications to lessen collateral damage to healthy tissues while treating and imaging the damaged tissue only.

Molecular diagnostics, a crucial part of theranostics, provides the ability to accurately and early detect viral infections. This enables prompt intervention and forms the basis for individualized treatment plans that consider the unique genetic composition of each patient. With precision medicine-based theranostics, treatment regimens are tailored to the specific characteristics of individual viral infections and the patient's response. This specified strategy reduces the likelihood of drug resistance, a recurring issue with antiviral treatments, while also boosting efficacy. In light of theranostics' progress, doctors can now monitor therapy responses in real time, improving patient outcomes and allowing for intervention modifications [5].

Theranostics's integration with artificial intelligence (AI) signals a paradigm shift in the treatment of viral infections. By leveraging the capabilities of machine learning, predictive analytics, and data-driven insights, AI-driven theranostics holds the potential to revolutionize the precision medicine space. While research and technology advance, the synergy between AI and theranostics will undoubtedly result in more efficient, tailored, and timely interventions in the battle against viral infections [6].

This chapter aims to illustrate theranostics' significant contribution to changing the narrative surrounding the treatment of viral illness through an extensive analysis of the field. Through an examination of historical analogies, contemporary issues, and the opportunities of theranostics, we chart the progression from previous pandemics to the forefront of medical breakthroughs. This expedition offers a diverse and flexible approach to combat the forthcoming viral adversaries, encapsulating the optimism and promise that theranostics brings to the worldwide battle against viral diseases.

17.2 Theranostics a hope

Theranostics shines as a ray of hope against evolving viral threats, offering a complete and efficient strategy to combat infections. Theranostic approach improves patient outcomes by addressing challenges like treatment resistance and viral mutation. As we navigate the intricacies of viral diseases, theranostics emerges as a potential paradigm shift that could bring about a new era in medicine where precision medicine and targeted treatment converge to minimize the global burden of viral infections. Some developments related to theranostic moieties have been furnished in table 17.1.

Table 17.1. Summary table for theranostics for viral diseases.

Theranostic system	Viral disease	Therapeutic mechanism	Diagnostic mechanism	References
Protease-responsive peptide-conjugated mitochondrial-targeting AIEgens	COVID-19 (SARS-CoV-2-infected cells)	Enzyme-instructed self-assembly (EISA) process	Aggregation-induced emission (AIE) effect	[7]
Covalent aptamer	COVID-19 (SARS-CoV-2 Proteins)	Blocking SARS-CoV-2 RBD-ACE2 interaction (functional blocking neutralizers of SARS-CoV-2 proteins)	Aptamers-based sandwich ELISA	[8]
SELEX based aptamers	COVID-19	Inhibited the entry of a SARS-CoV-2 virus	SELEX screening	[9]
Fe(III)-doped mesoporous silica nanoparticles	COVID-19	Remdesivir delivery	MRI	[10]

(*Continued*)

Table 17.1. (*Continued*)

Theranostic system	Viral disease	Therapeutic mechanism	Diagnostic mechanism	References
Anti-spike antibody attached Gold nanoparticle	COVID-19	Inhibiting the virus from binding to cell receptors	SERS	[11]
Nanoformulations of ritonavir, atazanavir, and curcumin	HIV	Antiretroviral therapy	Fluorescence signal	[12]
Multimodal imaging theranostic nanoprobes	HIV	Long-acting, slow-release antiretroviral therapy	MRI	[13]
Rilpivirine (RPV) ^{177}lutetium labeled bismuth sulfide nanorods (^{177}LuBSNRs)	HIV	Long-acting, slow-release antiretroviral therapy	SPECT, LA-ICP-MS imaging	[14]
Nano MOF	HIV/AIDS	Antiretroviral therapy	MRI	[15]
Curcumin/Gd loaded apoferritin	Hepatitis	Hepatoprotective action of Curcumin	MRI	[16]
Deoxyribozyme-loaded nano-graphene oxide	Hepatitis C	Cleaving the HCV gene and ultimately blocking viral replication	Fluorescence recovery	[17]

17.3 Application of biosensors for infectious disease diagnosis

17.3.1 COVID-19

The coronavirus disease 2019 (COVID-19) pandemic has severely and catastrophically impacted human health over the last three years. Since the pandemic started, scientists have focused a great deal of work on stopping the spread of COVID-19 and developing effective COVID-19 therapies and vaccination strategies. The pathogen responsible for COVID-19 is designated as Severe Acute Respiratory Syndrome Coronavirus 2 (SARS-CoV-2). This virus is the seventh identified member of the human coronavirus family. According to the World Health Organisation's coronavirus (COVID-19) dashboard, it caused over 774 million human infections and over 7.0 million deaths as of January 2024 [18]. The development of fast and accurate diagnostic techniques is a crucial first step in combating the threats posed by novel and deadly viruses. The current infrastructure of accessible point-of-care (POC) testing is incompatible with the two primary diagnostic procedures employed today, RT-qPCR and ELISA. In order to facilitate efficient diagnosis, more time, money, and resources are now required to ensure that laboratories are compatible with clinics, hospitals, and other healthcare facilities [19].

To reduce and eventually stop viral transmission, it is imperative to precisely treat SARS-CoV-2-infected cells and watch their movements in real time. But it is still difficult to precisely start and monitor the healing process in infected cells. So, to overcome this issue, Cheng *et al* [7] reported that a modular peptide-conjugated AIEgen probe (PSGMR) that targets mitochondria is responsive to main protease (M^{pro}, also known as $3CL^{pro}$), and may be used to selectively inhibit and image SARS-CoV-2-infected TMPRSS2-Vero cells by the aggregation-induced emission (AIE) effect and enzyme-instructed self-assembly (EISA) process. They confirmed that the cleavage of PSGMR led to progressive aggregation accompanied by bright yellow fluorescence and increased cytotoxicity, resulting in mitochondrial interference in the infected cells. This was achieved by logically constructing an AIE luminogen (AIEgen) with modular peptides and M^{pro}. Overall, the use of modular peptide-conjugated probes with protease-responsive organelle targeting may result in the development of potential theranostic agents for the treatment of SARS-CoV-2 and other developing viral diseases [7].

Metalloporphyrins have been reported to be employed for both diagnostic and therapeutic purposes owing to their intrinsic therapeutic properties and the capability to fine-tune their electrochemical properties [20]. Inspired by this approach, Wang *et al* developed a novel detection technique with excellent sensitivity for identifying viral nucleic acids. This technique utilizes nanoscale porphyrinic metal–organic frameworks (NPMOFs) as a photodynamic probe and magnetite nanoparticles as a trapping agent [21]. NPMOFs demonstrate an impressive photodynamic effect by utilizing the high concentration of porphyrin molecules as superior organic linkers. This effect efficiently transfers energy to molecular oxygen (O_2), generating highly reactive singlet oxygen ($^1O_2$) upon light irradiation. Through gene complementary hybridization, target nucleic acids help magnetite nanoparticles capture NPMOF probes, which in turn causes photodynamic action to produce significant amounts of singlet oxygen quickly. In order to enable signal readout, the indicator is then broken down using the singlet oxygen that is produced. As per the findings, SARS-CoV-2-associated RNA can be identified with this technique in simulated swabs using less than 30 min with a detection limit of 4.94 fM. This has enormous promise for quick, easy, and sensitive detection of viral nucleic acids without the need for RNA amplification treatment. This approach opens up new possibilities for signal transduction using nanomaterials in biosensing applications for COVID-19 [21].

The evolution of aptamer-based detection and therapy for SARS-CoV-2 has overcome hurdles relating to cost and adaptability. However, the inherent conformational instability of aptamers usually limits their performance under severe conditions, limiting sensitivity and therapeutic efficacy. Addressing this, Wang *et al* [8] developed a new covalent aptamer approach, providing increased detection and neutralization of essential SARS-CoV-2 proteins. They engineered covalent aptamers to transform dynamic aptamer-protein complexes into stable, irreversible covalent complexes that are resistant to environmental stressors. This is achieved by utilizing particular cross-link electrophilic groups. Even in severe washing conditions, the covalent aptamer-based ELISA for nucleocapsid protein performs better than antibody-based techniques, with an eight-fold increase in sensitivity.

Leveraging nucleic acid-based amplification further boosts detection sensitivity by two orders of magnitude [8].

Furthermore, under shear stress conditions, the covalent aptamer method outperforms conventional aptamers and antibodies in functional inhibition of the spike protein receptor binding domain (RBD). Although covalent aptamers are now effective against the wild-type SARS-CoV-2, further structural knowledge may enable them to be adapted for variant strains [8].

It is anticipated that the strong covalent aptamer-based approach would stimulate further applications in precise molecular modification, the identification of disease biomarkers, and other theranostic domains.

17.3.2 HIV/AIDS

Human Immunodeficiency Virus (HIV)/Acquired Immune Deficiency Syndrome (AIDS), caused by (HIV), remains a global health challenge defined by a progressive weakening of the immune system. As of present, according to the WHO report [22], around 39 million individuals are living with HIV worldwide, with over 40.4 million having lost their lives to AIDS-related illnesses. The burden of HIV/AIDS extends beyond health, impacting social, economic, and developmental elements of affected areas. Despite breakthroughs in antiretroviral therapy (ART) that can effectively control the infection and prolong life, problems continue. Access to treatment, potential drug resistance, and the necessity for lifelong medication adherence pose continuous barriers. The intricacy of the disease needs novel techniques, leading to the rise of theranostic systems as a crucial answer.

Singh *et al* [12] report the development of a theranostic nanoformulation encapsulating multiple drugs for HIV-1 antiretroviral therapy, utilizing laser ablation techniques. Ultrasmall nanoformulations comprising atazanavir, ritonavir, and Curcumin were synthesized through femtosecond laser ablation in an aqueous medium containing Pluronic® F127. These formulations, measuring 20–25 nm, demonstrated better water dispersibility and higher cellular absorption, notably in microglia. In an *in vitro* blood–brain barrier (BBB) model, F127-containing formulations displayed improved BBB crossing. The curcumin-loaded nanoparticles displayed cytoplasmic localization, demonstrating cellular absorption. Moreover, formulations with F127 dramatically reduced viral p24 levels by 36-fold compared to those without F127, showing potential efficacy in brain therapy and highlighting their usefulness as a solvent-free strategy for brain theranostics [12].

Iron(III) based porous metal–organic frameworks (nanoMOFs) emerge as remarkable non-toxic nanocarriers for efficient drug delivery, particularly addressing issues in retroviral medicines for AIDS treatment [15]. These nanoMOFs give high drug loadings and regulated release, surpassing traditional carriers. Engineered with adjustable architectures, they display superior medication interactions. Notably, these porous nanoMOFs exhibit dual functionality by possibly combining diagnostics and therapeutic qualities, opening the door for theranostics in customized AIDS care. These nanoMOFs contain various medications, such as potent antiviral agents, and release them gradually in physiological conditions. NanoMOFs demonstrated established anti-HIV efficacy when loaded with azidothymidine triphosphate (AZT-TP). These nanoMOFs could be used as potential contrast agents in magnetic resource imaging because of the iron-based core's beneficial relaxivities. Taking into account all the factors, porous nanoMOFs' diverse qualities make them a potential theranostics platform for improved HIV treatment, fusing individualized medication delivery with diagnostic imaging abilities [15].

In the ongoing worldwide effort to combat this persistent pandemic, addressing the multiple challenges of HIV/AIDS through theranostics may dramatically improve patient outcomes, limit adverse effects, and optimize the utilization of healthcare resources.

17.3.3 Hepatitis virus (HBV and HCV)

In many cases, viral infections cause liver damage and, consequently, viral hepatitis, a common illness with inflammatory liver damage that can be extremely dangerous for a patient's health. Hepatitis B (HBV) and C viruses primarily target hepatocytes. (HCV), as well as recurring infections with HBV and HCV, can result in a number of issues, including liver cancer and chronic cirrhosis [23].

Hepatitis C virus (HCV), a positive-sense single-stranded RNA virus, infects over 180 million individuals globally. It constitutes a primary etiological factor in hepatocellular carcinoma and chronic liver pathology [24]. Despite its seriousness, there is still no permanent treatment or vaccine for hepatitis C. The prevailing therapeutic regimen for HCV infection involves a combination of two medications: ribavirin, serving as a broad-spectrum inhibitor of viral replication, and interferon-α, functioning as an immunomodulatory agent. These medications are acknowledged to exhibit restricted efficacy and to be associated with notable adverse effects, including depression, cough, anemia, and myalgia. DNAzyme (deoxyribozyme, Dz) stands as a promising candidate therapeutic agent poised to cleave the HCV gene, thereby impeding viral replication within human host cells. This represents one of the endeavors aimed at developing a direct-acting anti-HCV drug, pivotal for the efficacious treatment of hepatitis C. Taking inspiration from this, Kim *et al* [17] developed a graphene oxide (nGO)-based nano-sized theranostic system for the monitoring of HCV non-structural gene 3 (NS3) mRNA and intracellular delivery of Dz. The findings demonstrated the efficacy of the FAM-Dz/nGO complex for monitoring the presence of NS3 mRNA within living cells. This was achieved through the fluorescence recovery of FAM-Dz, facilitated by detachment from nGO and subsequent hybridization with target mRNA.

Additionally, the complex exhibited the potential to suppress HCV replication in human cells by downregulating HCV NS3 gene expression. The current method offers numerous benefits as a promising theranostic nanomedicine for the management of viral infections. First off, the entire nanocomplex is reasonably priced; Dz is more affordable than ribozyme and siRNA, while nGO is easily synthesized from graphite at a lower cost than other nanomaterials such as carbon nanotubes and noble metal nanomaterials. Secondly, Dz has an effective catalytic action that is sequence-specific and does not depend on RNAi, which needs RISC. Furthermore, compared to RNA, Dz has a higher chemical stability. Third, Dz can be delivered intracellularly or loaded without undergoing any chemical changes. Ultimately, one of the most promising theranostic tools for HCV infection in the future is predicted to be the Dz/nGO complex, as it is potentially helpful in treating other viral illnesses [17].

Similarly, Cutrin *et al* [16] invented the first 'theranostic' agent, Apo-CUR-Gd, utilizing apoferritin as a carrier to deliver therapeutic and imaging agents to hepatocytes at the same time. This strategy aims to mitigate hepatocellular damage in toxic-induced acute hepatitis. The process involved encasing the polyphenolic compound curcumin with apoferritin, which has anti-inflammatory, antioxidant, and antineoplastic properties in conjunction with GdHPDO3A, an MRI contrast agent. Apoferritin's encapsulation of Curcumin significantly increased both the drug's stability and bioavailability without sacrificing its therapeutic anti-inflammatory properties. The study evaluated the effectiveness of Apo-CUR-Gd in reducing thioacetamide-induced hepatitis and used magnetic resonance imaging to assess drug delivery efficiency [16].

Reduced alanine aminotransferase (ALT) activity in plasma and histological analysis demonstrated that Apo-CUR-Gd effectively shielded hepatocytes from acute damage caused by thioacetamide. Additionally, the study also emphasized the potential application of Apo-CUR-Gd for real-time assessment of drug concentration in the liver, providing guidance for personalized treatment plans based on efficacious monitoring and biodistribution. The findings highlight the potential utility of apoferritin-based theranostic agents for liver-targeted drug delivery [16].

17.3.4 Influenza

The public often underestimates the severe health risks associated with influenza. It affects a wide range of people, including infants, expectant mothers, obese individuals, and those with weakened immune systems. Complications such as otitis and pneumonia can lead to artificial ventilation. During pandemics and annually, influenza causes excess mortality. Secondary bacterial pneumonia from enhanced viral replication is a substantial contributor to death. Severe influenza leads to severe lung injury, viral pneumonia, systemic inflammation, cytokine storms, and immune-mediated abnormalities, often culminating in mortality. Effective therapy choices are limited, making it challenging to improve outcomes for severe hypoxemic patients. A multitude of influenza virus (IV) subtypes have been observed to infect and circulate within the human population, thereby contributing significantly to the occurrence of seasonal influenza outbreaks, which represent a significant source of morbidity and mortality worldwide. It is still challenging to come up with practical solutions for quickly monitoring and blocking IVs. A novel theranostic strategy is required to prevent influenza from becoming severe [25].

As an alternative to conventional fluorescence probes, which depend on a fluorimetric shift for influenza virus (IV) detection, Wang *et al* [26] introduced a simple method involving the assembly of 'Supra-dots.' These are formed by combining a blue-emitting polymer dot with red-emitting sialyl glycan probes in an aqueous medium, enabling ratiometric IV detection. Through the precise modulation of Förster resonance energy transfer from polymer dots to glycan probes via selective sialyl glycan-virus recognition, the Supra-dots facilitate fluorescence ratiometric evaluation of influenza viruses (IVs). Furthermore, the Supra-dots have been validated to effectively inhibit the infiltration of human-infecting influenza viruses (IVs) into a human cell line, thus positioning them as a distinctive bifunctional supramolecular probe for influenza theranostics [26].

Influenza A virus (IAV) is a prevalent respiratory pathogen capable of infecting a diverse array of animal hosts, encompassing avian species (avian influenza virus, AIV), pigs (swine influenza virus, SIV), as well as humans. Monitoring swine and avian influenza viruses in agricultural settings, natural habitats, and live poultry markets is imperative for safeguarding public health, both for humans and animals. The demand for portable, sensitive, and quantitative immunoassay equipment is expected to be significant, particularly in rural and resource-limited regions [27]. To address this need, Wu *et al* [27] developed the *Z*-Lab POC device, which requires minimal sample handling and laboratory expertise for the sensitive and specific detection of swine influenza viruses. In their investigation, IAV nucleoprotein (NP) and pure H3N2 viruses were detected using a portable, quantitative immunoassay platform based on giant magnetoresistive (GMR) technology. *Z*-Lab provides quantitative results in under 10 min, with pure H3N2v and IAV NP sensitivities as low as 125 TCID50/ml and 15 $ng\,ml^{-1}$, respectively. This platform expands the use of immunoassays in nonclinical contexts and permits outdoor lab testing [27].

17.4 CRISPR/Cas system-based theranostics

Jennifer Doudna and Emmanuelle Charpentier were awarded the 2020 Nobel Prize in Chemistry for their groundbreaking discovery of the CRISPR/Cas (Clustered Regularly Interspaced Short Palindromic Repeats/CRISPR-associated) system [28]. This discovery marked a major milestone in molecular biology, opening new opportunities for advanced theranostics, especially in the context of viral diseases. Initially discovered as a bacterial defense system against viral infections, CRISPR/Cas has been used by scientists to edit the genome precisely. In the realm of theranostics for viral diseases, the CRISPR/Cas system has exhibited exceptional potential [29].

In the CRISPR/Cas system, specific DNA sequences are directed by RNA molecules to the Cas enzyme, allowing for targeted modifications. Researchers have investigated its potential to disrupt viral genomes during infections, thereby increasing the challenge for viruses to spread and evade the immune system. CRISPR/Cas is an excellent tool for creating therapeutic interventions that are tailored to the genetic composition of various viruses due to its accuracy and adaptability [30].

CRISPR/Cas-based theranostics for viral diseases has advanced significantly in the past few years. Research efforts are targeting numerous viruses, including influenza, hepatitis, COVID-19, and HIV. To render host cells resistant to viral infections, one technique is to alter them using CRISPR/Cas. To mitigate the virus's ability to cause harm, a different strategy investigates directly modifying and targeting its DNA. Additionally, CRISPR/Cas makes it easier to develop diagnostic tools that use its precise gene-editing abilities to rapidly and accurately identify genetic material [31–33].

In February 2020, as the world started to realize how dangerous the new coronavirus was, a team of virologists from Temple University tested a CRISPR gene-editing technique developed by Excision BioTherapeutics. With this method, a portion of humanized mice that were HIV-positive were cured successfully. By integrating its genome into the host's DNA, HIV can survive even after antiretroviral medications have completely eradicated it. Excision BioTherapeutics guided the application of CRISPR-Cas9 to target and cleave HIV genetic sequences within host cells after the mice were given high-dose antiretroviral treatment. This method successfully cured the mice of HIV infection and eliminated viral reservoirs [34].

17.5 Conclusion and future prospectives

To sum up, the field of theranostics offers a comprehensive strategy that seamlessly integrates treatments and diagnostics, making it a game-changing paradigm in the ongoing battle against viral illnesses. Theranostics provides a versatile and dynamic method of understanding, diagnosing, and treating viral infections with uses ranging from previous pandemics to the challenges presented by recently emerging infectious diseases. The field of precision medicine, molecular diagnostics, and nanotechnology is expanding and shows significant potential for efficient and customized management of viral diseases. The future of the field of theranostics appears bright. New insights into viral pathogenesis are anticipated to emerge from ongoing research and clinical trials, and the application of AI may enhance predictive capabilities. Beyond customized treatment, theranostics can revolutionize public health strategies by providing early warning systems and enabling targeted responses to potential epidemics. In addition to providing cutting-edge hope in the face of growing viral threats, theranostics lays the foundation for a strong and flexible plan that will influence world health in the future as we continue to combat viral diseases.

Abbreviations

ACE2	Angiotensin-converting enzyme 2
AIDS	Acquired immune deficiency syndrome
HIV	Human immunodeficiency virus
LA-ICP-MS	Laser ablation inductively coupled plasma mass spectrometry
MOF	Metal–organic frameworks
MRI	Magnetic resonance imaging
NS3	Non-structural gene 3
RBD	Receptor binding domain
SELEX	Systematic evolution of ligands by exponential enrichment
SERS	Surface-enhanced Raman spectroscopy
SPECT	Single photon emission computed tomography

References

[1] Reid A H, Fanning T G, Hultin J V and Taubenberger J K 1999 Origin and evolution of the 1918 'Spanish' influenza virus hemagglutinin gene *Proc. Natl Acad. Sci. USA* **96** 1651–6

[2] Oxford J S, Sefton A, Jackson R, Innes W, Daniels R S and Johnson N P A S 2002 World war I may have allowed the emergence of 'Spanish' influenza *Lancet Infect. Dis.* **2** 111–4
[3] Meganck R M and Baric R S 2021 Developing therapeutic approaches for twenty-first-century emerging infectious viral diseases *Nat. Med.* **27** 401–10
[4] Zhou P *et al* 2020 A pneumonia outbreak associated with a new coronavirus of probable bat origin *Nature* **579** 270–3
[5] Valenzuela-Sánchez F, Valenzuela-Méndez B, Rodríguez-Gutiérrez J F and Rello J 2016 Personalized medicine in severe influenza *Eur. J. Clin. Microbiol. Infect. Dis.* **35** 893–7
[6] Taniguchi M *et al* 2021 Combining machine learning and nanopore construction creates an artificial intelligence nanopore for coronavirus detection *Nat. Commun.* **12** 1–8
[7] Cheng Y *et al* 2022 Protease-responsive peptide-conjugated mitochondrial-targeting AIEgens for selective imaging and inhibition of SARS-CoV-2-Infected Cells *ACS Nano* **16** 12305–17
[8] Wang D *et al* 2023 Robust covalent aptamer strategy enables sensitive detection and enhanced inhibition of SARS-CoV-2 proteins *ACS Cent. Sci.* **9** 72–83
[9] Halder S *et al* 2023 SELEX based aptamers with diagnostic and entry inhibitor therapeutic potential for SARS-CoV-2 *Sci. Rep.* **13** 1–18
[10] Arkaban H, Jaberi J, Bahramifar A, Zolfaghari Emameh R, Farnoosh G, Arkaban M and Taheri R A 2023 Fabrication of Fe(III)-doped mesoporous silica nanoparticles as biocompatible and biodegradable theranostic system for Remdesivir delivery and MRI contrast agent *Inorg. Chem. Commun.* **150** 110398
[11] Pramanik A, Gao Y, Patibandla S, Mitra D, McCandless M G, Fassero L A, Gates K, Tandon R and Chandra Ray P 2021 The rapid diagnosis and effective inhibition of coronavirus using spike antibody attached gold nanoparticles *Nanoscale Adv.* **3** 1588–96
[12] Singh A, Kutscher H L, Bulmahn J C, Mahajan S D, He G S and Prasad P N 2020 Laser ablation for pharmaceutical nanoformulations: multi-drug nanoencapsulation and theranostics for HIV *Nanomed. Nanotechnol., Biol. Med.* **25** 102172
[13] Kevadiya B D *et al* 2018 Multimodal theranostic nanoformulations permit magnetic resonance bioimaging of antiretroviral drug particle tissue-cell biodistribution *Theranostics* **8** 256–76
[14] Kevadiya B D *et al* 2020 Rod-shape theranostic nanoparticles facilitate antiretroviral drug biodistribution and activity in human immunodeficiency virus susceptible cells and tissues *Theranostics* **10** 630–56
[15] Horcajada P *et al* 2010 Porous metal-organic-framework nanoscale carriers as a potential platform for drug deliveryand imaging *Nat. Mater.* **9** 172–8
[16] Cutrin J C, Crich S G, Burghelea D, Dastrù W and Aime S 2013 Curcumin/Gd loaded apoferritin: a novel 'theranostic' agent to prevent hepatocellular damage in toxic induced acute hepatitis *Mol. Pharm.* **10** 2079–85
[17] Kim S, Ryoo S R, Na H K, Kim Y K, Choi B S, Lee Y, Kim D E and Min D H 2013 Deoxyribozyme-loaded nano-graphene oxide for simultaneous sensing and silencing of the hepatitis C virus gene in liver cells *Chem. Commun.* **49** 8241–3
[18] World Health Organization 2023 *COVID-19 Cases WHO COVID-19 Dashboard* https://data.who.int/dashboards/covid19/cases
[19] Tang Y N, Jiang D, Wang X, Liu Y and Wei D 2024 Recent progress on rapid diagnosis of COVID-19 by point-of-care testing platforms *Chin. Chem. Lett.* **35** 108688

[20] Thakur P S, Gautam L, Vyas S P and Sankar M 2023 Metalloporphyrin nanoparticles for diverse theranostic applications *Inorganic Nanosystems: Theranostic Nanosystems* **Vol. 2** (New York: Academic) pp 489–507

[21] Wang Y, Chen J, Wu C and Zhu Y 2024 Nanoscale porphyrinic metal-organic frameworks as a photodynamic probe for highly sensitive detection of SARS-CoV-2 related RNA *Sens. Actuators B Chem.* **406** 135413

[22] World Health Organization 2023 *HIV* https://www.who.int/data/gho/data/themes/hiv-aids (accessed 2024-02-22)

[23] Llovet J M, Kelley R K, Villanueva A, Singal A G, Pikarsky E, Roayaie S, Lencioni R, Koike K, Zucman-Rossi J and Finn R S 2021 Hepatocellular carcinoma *Nat. Rev. Dis. Prim.* **7** 6

[24] Brody H 2011 Hepatitis C *Nature* **474** S1–1

[25] Rello J 2017 Theranostics in severe influenza *Lancet Respir. Med.* **5** 91–2

[26] Wang C Z, Han H H, Tang X Y, Zhou D M, Wu C, Chen G R, He X P and Tian H 2017 Sialylglycan-assembled supra-dots for ratiometric probing and blocking of human-infecting influenza viruses *ACS Appl. Mater. Interfaces* **9** 25164–70

[27] Wu K, Klein T, Krishna V D, Su D, Perez A M and Wang J P 2017 Portable GMR handheld platform for the detection of influenza A virus *ACS Sens.* **2** 1594–601

[28] Davies K 2020 CRISPR pioneers Doudna and Charpentier Win 2020 Nobel Prize for chemistry *Genet. Eng. Biotechnol. News* **40** 8–10

[29] Kong H, Ju E, Yi K, Xu W, Lao Y H, Cheng D, Zhang Q, Tao Y, Li M and Ding J 2021 Advanced nanotheranostics of CRISPR/Cas for viral hepatitis and hepatocellular carcinoma *Adv. Sci.* **8** 2102051

[30] Pickar-Oliver A and Gersbach C A 2019 The next generation of CRISPR–Cas technologies and applications *Nat. Rev. Mol. Cell Biol.* **20** 490–507

[31] Sridhara S, Goswami H N, Whyms C, Dennis J H and Li H 2021 Virus detection via programmable type III-A CRISPR-Cas systems *Nat. Commun.* **12** 1–10

[32] Kabay G, DeCastro J, Altay A, Smith K, Lu H, Capossela A M, Moarefian M, Aran K and Dincer C 2022 Emerging biosensing technologies for the diagnostics of viral infectious diseases *Adv. Mater.* **34** 2201085

[33] Liu Y *et al* 2019 CRISPR-Cas13a nanomachine based simple technology for avian influenza A (H7N9) virus on-site detection *J. Biomed. Nanotechnol.* **15** 790–8

[34] Burdo T H *et al* 2023 Preclinical safety and biodistribution of CRISPR targeting SIV in non-human primates *Gene Ther.* **2023** 1–10

www.ingramcontent.com/pod-product-compliance
Ingram Content Group UK Ltd.
Pitfield, Milton Keynes, MK11 3LW, UK
UKHW051900100926
8556IPUK00005B/709

9 780750 349857